Atlas of Spinal Imaging

Atlas of Spinal Imaging

Phenotypes, Measurements, and Classification Systems

EDITED BY

PHILIP K. LOUIE
Spine Surgeon, Neuroscience Institute, Virginia Mason Medical Center, Seattle, WA, United States

HOWARD S. AN
Professor and Morton International Endowed Chair, Director of Spine Fellowship Program Department of Orthopaedic Surgery, Rush University Medical Center, Chicago, IL, USA

DINO SAMARTZIS
Director, International Spine Research and Innovation Initiative (ISRII) and an Associate Professor, Department of Orthopedic Surgery, Rush Medical College, Chicago, IL, USA

ELSEVIER

Elsevier
Radarweg 29, PO Box 211, 1000 AE Amsterdam, Netherlands
The Boulevard, Langford Lane, Kidlington, Oxford OX5 1GB, United Kingdom
50 Hampshire Street, 5th Floor, Cambridge, MA 02139, United States

Notices

Knowledge and best practice in this field are constantly changing. As new research and experience broaden our understanding, changes in research methods, professional practices, or medical treatment may become necessary.

Practitioners and researchers must always rely on their own experience and knowledge in evaluating and using any information, methods, compounds, or experiments described herein. In using such information or methods they should be mindful of their own safety and the safety of others, including parties for whom they have a professional responsibility.

To the fullest extent of the law, neither the Publisher nor the authors, contributors, or editors, assume any liability for any injury and/or damage to persons or property as a matter of products liability, negligence or otherwise, or from any use or operation of any methods, products, instructions, or ideas contained in the material herein.

Library of Congress Cataloging-in-Publication Data
A catalog record for this book is available from the Library of Congress

British Library Cataloguing-in-Publication Data
A catalogue record for this book is available from the British Library

ISBN: 978-0-323-76111-6

For information on all Elsevier publications
visit our website at https://www.elsevier.com/books-and-journals

Publisher: Cathleen Sether
Acquisitions Editor: Humayra Khan
Editorial Project Manager: Mona Zahir
Production Project Manager: Niranjan Bhaskaran
Cover Designer: Alan Studholme

Typeset by SPi Global, India

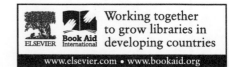
Working together
to grow libraries in
developing countries
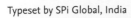
www.elsevier.com • www.bookaid.org

Contents

SECTION III
FULL-LENGTH SPINE

Contributors

Tae-Keun Ahn
Department of Orthopedic Surgery, CHA Bundang Medical Center, CHA University, Pocheon-si, South Korea

Howard S. An
Department of Orthopedic Surgery, Rush University Medical Center, Chicago, IL, United States
International Spine Research and Innovation Initiative (ISRII), Rush University Medical Center, Chicago, IL, United States

Carrie E. Andrews
Department of Neurological Surgery, Thomas Jefferson University, Philadelphia, PA, United States

Ronald Bartels
Department of Neurosurgery, Radboud University Medical Center, Nijmegen, The Netherlands

Martine van Bilsen
Department of Neurosurgery, Radboud University Medical Center, Nijmegen, The Netherlands

Scott Blumenthal
Center for Disc Replacement at Texas Back Institute, Plano, TX, United States

Stephane Bourret
Polyclinique Bordeaux Nord Aquitaine, Vertebra Spine Unit, Bordeaux, France

Zorica Buser
Department of Orthopaedic Surgery, Keck School of Medicine of the University of Southern California, Los Angeles, CA, United States

Meghan Cerpa
Department of Orthopaedic Surgery, Columbia University Irving Medical Center, New York, NY, United States

Thomas D. Cha
Department of Orthopedic Surgery, Massachusetts General Hospital, Harvard Medical School, Boston, MA, United States

Andrew Chung
Department of Orthopaedic Surgery, Keck School of Medicine of the University of Southern California, Los Angeles, CA, United States

Thibafvult Cloché
Polyclinique Bordeaux Nord Aquitaine, Vertebra Spine Unit, Bordeaux, France

Ashlyn A. Fitch
Department of Orthopaedic Surgery, Rush University Medical Center, Chicago, IL, United States

Evan M. Fitchett
Department of Neurological Surgery, Thomas Jefferson University, Philadelphia, PA, United States

Erik B. Gerlach
Northwestern Memorial Hospital, Department of Orthopaedic Surgery, Chicago, IL, United States

Morgan B. Giers
School of Chemical, Biological and Environmental Engineering, Oregon State University, Corvallis, OR, United States

Atul Goel
Department of Neurosurgery, K.E.M. Hospital and Seth G.S. Medical College, Mumbai, India

Glenn A. Gonzalez
Department of Neurological Surgery, Thomas Jefferson University, Philadelphia, PA, United States

Vadim Goz
Department of Orthopaedic Surgery, Rothman
    Institute, Thomas Jefferson University,
    Philadelphia, PA, United States

Garrett K. Harada
Department of Orthopaedic Surgery, Rush University
    Medical Center, Chicago, IL, United States

James S. Harrop
Department of Neurological Surgery, Thomas Jefferson
    University, Philadelphia, PA, United States

Fayyazul Hassan
Department of Orthopaedic Surgery, Rush University
    Medical Center, Chicago, IL, United States

Alexander L. Hornung
Department of Orthopaedic Surgery, Rush University
    Medical Center, Chicago, IL, United States

Nassim Lashkari
Department of Orthopaedic Surgery, Keck School of
    Medicine of the University of Southern California,
    Los Angeles, CA, United States

Jean-Charles Le Huec
Polyclinique Bordeaux Nord Aquitaine, Vertebra Spine
    Unit, Bordeaux, France

Lawrence G. Lenke
Department of Orthopaedic Surgery, Columbia
    University Irving Medical Center, New York, NY,
    United States

Kayla L. Leverich
Department of Orthopaedic Surgery, Rush University
    Medical Center, Chicago, IL, United States

Wylie Y. Lopez
Department of Orthopedic Surgery, Massachusetts
    General Hospital, Harvard Medical School, Boston,
    MA, United States

Philip K. Louie
Department of Neurosurgery, Virginia Mason Medical
    Center, Seattle, WA, United states
Department of Orthopaedic Surgery, Rush University
    Medical Center, Chicago, IL, United States

Michael L. Martini
Icahn School of Medicine at Mount Sinai,
    New York, NY, United States

Michael H. McCarthy
Indiana Spine Group, Carmel, IN, United States

Domingo Molina, IV
Texas Back Institute, Plano, TX, United States

Thiago S. Montenegro
Department of Neurological Surgery, Thomas
    Jefferson University, Philadelphia, PA,
    United States

Thomas E. Mroz
Cleveland Clinic, Cleveland, OH, United States

Sean N. Neifert
Icahn School of Medicine at Mount Sinai,
    New York, NY, United States

Richard W. Nicolay
Northwestern Memorial Hospital, Department of
    Orthopaedic Surgery, Chicago, IL, United
    States

Stefan Parent
Department of surgery, Université de Montréal,
    Montréal, QC, Canada
Centre Hospitalier Universitaire Sainte-Justine,
    Montréal, QC, Canada

Mark A. Pastore
Department of Orthopaedic Surgery, Philadelphia
    College of Osteopathic Medicine, Philadelphia, PA,
    United States

Omair A. Qureshi
Department of Orthopaedic Surgery, Keck School of
    Medicine of the University of Southern California,
    Los Angeles, CA, United States

Jonathan J. Rasouli
Cleveland Clinic, Cleveland, OH, United States

Cecile Roscop
Polyclinique Bordeaux Nord Aquitaine, Vertebra Spine
    Unit, Bordeaux, France

Samuel S. Rudisill
Department of Orthopaedic Surgery, Rush University
Medical Center, Chicago, IL, United States

Dino Samartzis
Department of Orthopedic Surgery, Rush University
Medical Center, Chicago, IL, United States
International Spine Research and Innovation Initiative
(ISRII), Rush University Medical Center, Chicago,
IL, United States

Eric J. Sanders
Northwestern Memorial Hospital, Department
of Orthopaedic Surgery, Chicago, IL,
United States

Andrew N. Sawires
Department of Orthopaedic Surgery, Lenox Hill
Hospital, New York, NY, United States

Zakariah K. Siyaji
Department of Orthopaedic Surgery, Rush University
Medical Center, Chicago, IL, United States
Department of Neurological Surgery, Rush University
Medical Center, Chicago, IL, United States

Eloise Stanton
Department of Orthopaedic Surgery, Keck School of
Medicine of the University of Southern California,
Los Angeles, CA, United States

Peter R. Swiatek
Northwestern Memorial Hospital, Department of
Orthopaedic Surgery, Chicago, IL, United States

Noor Tamimi
Department of Orthopaedic Surgery, Rothman
Institute, Thomas Jefferson University,
Philadelphia, PA, United States

Wendy Thompson
Polyclinique Bordeaux Nord Aquitaine, Vertebra Spine
Unit, Bordeaux, France

Alexander Vaccaro
Department of Orthopaedic Surgery, Rothman
Institute, Thomas Jefferson University,
Philadelphia, PA, United States

Anthony Viola
Department of Orthopaedic Surgery, Philadelphia
College of Osteopathic Medicine, Philadelphia, PA,
United States

Jeffrey C. Wang
Department of Orthopaedic Surgery, Keck School of
Medicine of the University of Southern California,
Los Angeles, CA, United States

I dedicate this book to my wife Alice Louie, for her continued support throughout my training and career; to my parents, Douglas and Belinda, for their ongoing inspiration and belief; and to all my mentors, colleagues, and patients who provide me with the constant motivation to learn and educate.

Louie

Dedicated to my wife, Sue Kao An, M.D., for her love and support throughout my entire career.

An

I dedicate this textbook to my father, Steve (my hero), mother, Joanna, my wife, Imelda, and my two beautiful daughters, Yianna and Isabella. I thank them for their undying support, belief, inspiration, and love throughout my life and career. I also thank all the students, residents, fellows, colleagues, and friends in the spine community for being exceptional in every capacity and for all their support.

Samartzis

Foreword

A surgical trainee's earliest exposure to musculoskeletal disorders of the spine begins with a dedicated understanding of spinal anatomy. Once an understanding of basic anatomy is mastered through reading and clinical dissections, students may now evolve into correlating spinal morphology with two- and three-dimensional imaging representation of spinal anatomy via plain radiography and advanced imaging modalities. Surgeons can use this opportunity to understand the differences between normal and abnormal anatomy and their disease correlates. Students can use this educational process to understand the differences radiographically between races, gender, and ages in spinal morphology. Part of the study of spinal care is understanding these differences in morphology and image-related motion parameters, as it can mean the difference between understanding which patients have normal anatomic variants versus someone with an impending neurologic abnormality. In my experience, I have seen halo rings mistakenly placed on patients with normal cervical spines because of instability patterns that may be abnormal in an adult but are normal variants in a developing child.

For the first time, experts in the field of spinal care have come together to create a textbook illustrating imaging features of normal and abnormal spinal morphology in all age-groups, genders, and racial backgrounds. No longer will one have to reference multiple sources to find out if a spinal anomaly is normal or abnormal or if the distance measured at the atlanto-dens interval is normal or abnormal in a patient with rheumatoid arthritis.

Various spine study groups over the last ten years have provided rich data on normal and pathologic spinal alignment in all age-groups using various imaging modalities such as plain radiography and advanced imaging such as CT and MRI. This information is presented to the reader in an understandable and easily referenced manner. Furthermore, this book provides an in-depth analysis of imaging characteristics focusing on the complicated junctions of the spine such as the occipital cervical junction, cervicothoracic junction, and especially the lumbosacral junction. This information is brought together and assimilated in classification systems that allow surgeons to correlate a patient's neurological examination and spinal imaging into a language of communication facilitating disease categorization and appropriate treatment guidelines. The book concludes with where we are heading in terms of the future of spinal imaging. We are all eager to see an imaging modality developed that can prognosticate recovery in the setting of a spinal cord injury or determine the potential for progressive deformity if nonoperative treatment is chosen in the setting of a spinal fracture.

This book is the brainchild of two great institutions, the Hospital for Special Surgery and Midwestern Orthopaedics at Rush. I have met and worked with Howard An at Rush who introduced me to the love of spinal care and have recently begun to work with one of the top clinical researchers in this country, Dino Samartzis, who is the director of the International Spine Research and Innovation Institute at Rush. Only could such acclaimed clinical scientists put together such a useful, clinically applicable book that is a must-read and reference source for medical students, residents, fellows, and attending surgeons. This book is a one-stop shop for spine-related imaging and clinical correlation. Nowhere can one experience the variety, depth, and perspective provided by an international experienced group of spinal care physicians.

I am proud to be chosen as one of the authors of this textbook and I hope you enjoy this masterpiece as much as I enjoyed participating in its development.

Sincerely yours,
Alexander R. Vaccaro

In this first edition of the *Atlas of Spinal Imaging: Phenotypes, Measurements, and Classification Systems*, Drs. Louie, An, and Samartzis have brought together world experts in the field of spine care and research to contribute to this comprehensive imaging offering. As spine surgeons, researchers, and academic leaders, these three individuals have provided yet another excellent contribution to the education of residents, fellows, and early career and senior specialists who seek refresher and updates on these topics. In this comprehensive text, Dr. Louie and his colleagues provide a "one-stop shop" of common imaging findings associated with the spine and their clinical implications.

The textbook is all-inclusive and consists of 17 chapters describing the phenotypes, measurements, and critical evaluation of plain radiographs, MRI, and CT imaging as provided by experts throughout the world. However, Drs. Louie, An, and Samartzis understand the value of correlating these imaging findings to the clinical picture and have provided incredible correlations with classification systems and clinical outcomes based on the role of diverse image presentations. They have presented a well-organized way of facilitating learning the critical evaluation of spine imaging and how to correlate these findings with patient care.

Although spine care has gone through several waves of advancement over the past few decades, the principles of evaluation and workup based on clinical findings as well as multiparametric imaging remain incredibly important. However, the diagnostic value of such imaging has exponentially increased over the years as studies have described new measurements, phenotypes, and clinical correlations based on these common imaging modalities. In fact, recent studies over the past decade alone and attributed to big data approaches and focused attention on imaging nuances have further illustrated some of the predictive utility of imaging with respect to outcomes. This aspect in part is critical as it will feed into a component of precision-based spine care aimed to incorporate several dimensions of a patient's profile to determine the best treatment, for the right patient at the right time to obtain the most optimal outcome. From that perspective, understanding of imaging, as the editors and their esteemed authors have comprehensively illustrated, is key in the aforementioned movement. However, this Atlas also definitely underlines the spine specialists' claim to competently assess by himself/herself the imaging of spinal pathology *in the light of the clinical findings* of the affected patient. In spinal disorders in particular, it is of utmost importance to consider all the imaging modalities only as a tool to better understand and define the individual spinal problem in order not to treat X-rays, MRIs, and CT scans—but to treat the suffering patient.

In order to maximize the value of imaging studies, provide evidence-based care for patients, and grow the field of spine care, it is imperative that trainees and clinicians have a reliable resource as a unique compilation of objective assessment and measurements of image modalities that form the base of reproducible, evidence-based treatment plans for specific spinal disorders.

In this sense, this textbook will not only serve clinicians as a daily companion in patient management, but will also be an invaluable resource to the scientific and research community.

I am confident that this textbook will become the "go-to" resource on the subject and will stand the test of time. I congratulate Drs. Louie, An, and Samartzis in this endeavor, which without question will be an immensely invaluable resource for current and future generations of students, clinicians, and researchers alike throughout the world.

Max Aebi
McGill University, Montreal, QC, Canada
University of Bern, Bern, Switzerland
European Academy of Sciences, Biel, Switzerland

Preface

Spine-related pain is the world's leading disabling condition, affecting every population and a main reason necessitating medical consultation. The healthcare and socioeconomic consequences of these conditions are substantial and unfortunately continue to rise. As we have experienced rapid advances in the workup, identification, prevention, and treatment of such spine conditions, comprehensive resources are lacking as to how to best evaluate the various imaging studies often obtained on these patients.

Numerous spinal phenotypes (i.e., observations/ traits) and their respective measurements performed on various spine imaging have been shown to directly correlate and predict clinical outcomes as well as assist in the management algorithm of the clinician. Furthermore, research into spinal phenotypes on imaging has also increased, in particular in this era of big data and a drive for more precision-based approaches toward spine care whereby genomics and other omics platforms have taken center stage. Understanding these spinal phenotypes will facilitate new targeted drug discovery, novel diagnostics and biomarker discovery, and outcome predictions. More importantly, in the age of artificial intelligence and machine learning, there is a need for understanding the various spinal phenotypes to assist in standardization to facilitate multicenter studies and global impact. However, there is currently no comprehensive resource that acts as an easy-to-comprehend "visual atlas" to highlight various spinal phenotypes on imaging and describe their clinical and pathophysiological relevance along with extensive discussion and illustration of their respective measurement techniques and classifications. Such a resource will be an invaluable resource to clinicians and researchers worldwide.

We hope that this book will provide a comprehensive resource for common radiographic measurements and their direct clinical correlations often described in spine pathology. Exhaustive internet and literature searches are often required to identify descriptions of common imaging findingseven more scarce instructions on performing the numerous radiographic measurements that are utilized in both the clinical and academic setting. Trainees and clinicians have often lamented on the lack of a single resource that can serve as a comprehensive visual atlas for these descriptions and instructions. This textbook will be a "one-stop shop" that will highlight traditional and unique imaging findings/measurements that will serve as "the" key reference for clinicians and researchers alike.

Philip K. Louie
Howard S. An
Dino Samartzis

CHAPTER 1

Introduction

PHILIP K. LOUIE[a] • DINO SAMARTZIS[b,c] • HOWARD S. AN[b,c]
[a]Department of Neurosurgery, Virginia Mason Medical Center, Seattle, WA, United States
[b]Department of Orthopedic Surgery, Rush University Medical Center, Chicago, IL, United States
[c]International Spine Research and Innovation Initiative (ISRII), Rush University Medical Center, Chicago, IL, United States

HISTORY OF SPINE IMAGING

The idea of imaging to provide information on osseous anatomy dates back to 1895, when Wilhelm Conrad Roentgen demonstrated the existence and application of X-rays. Although introduced as a form of novel photography, physicians soon realized the medical utility of Roentgen's discovery. X-rays rapidly developed into an invaluable diagnostic tool to image the spine by the early 1900s.[1] By the 1920s, practitioners discovered that they could manipulate adjacent tissue densities, resulting in differentiation between adjacent structures. In one scenario, Sicard and Forestier may have accidentally introduced an iodine-based solution into the epidural space when attempting to target a patient's lumbar muscles (a technique considered as effective management for sciatica).[2] This experiment led to take radiographs after injections to evaluate for additional pathology, which subsequently led to the discovery that iodine enhances the anatomy of the spinal cord and subarachnoid space. Over the next few years, several improvements and innovations were described that improve the safety of these iodine-based contrast agents. Practitioners soon began to regularly inject these solutions into the dural sac and intervertebral discs.[3]

Due to limitations revolving around computing power, it would not be until 1973, when modern CT would emerge. Historians hypothesize that Dr. Godfrey Hounsfield conceived of CT in a thought experiment, where he reasoned it would be possible to identify the contents of a box by taking X-rays at every possible angle around it.[4] He further extrapolated that there may be medical utility with this technique, specifically to identify human skull contents. Over the next few months, Dr. Hounsfield successfully produced the initial CT images of a patient's brain and the original CT scanner was quickly adapted for full-body use, including the spine.[5] Concurrently, around the same time, a chemist by the name of Paul Lauterbur was working heavily with nuclear magnetic resonance (NMR) spectroscopy. During his experiments, he conceived that the application of a magnetic field on a large object could produce images based on its chemical structure.[6] This incredible theory laid the foundation for modern magnetic resonance imaging (MRI). MRI continued to evolve during the1970s, producing images with a low spatial resolution that advanced the discrimination of soft tissue proving superiority to CT, allowing earlier diagnoses. Furthermore, unlike CT, MRI had the advantage of not requiring ionizing radiation to produce high-resolution images. This accomplishment was eventually rewarded as a Nobel Prize in physiology and medicine.[7] The technology quickly improved during the late 1980–1990s that resulted in high-resolution descriptions of spinal anatomy and pathology that were soon cleared for human use.[8, 9]

COMMON IMAGING MODALITIES

In today's era, the imaging techniques continue to evolve, especially in the evaluation of spine anatomy. With the improved resolution of modern CT scanners, techniques such as myelography are not nearly as popular as they once were. Similarly, discography recommendations and indications have significantly narrowed due to increased rates of pain postoperatively induced associated with a discogram.[10] With the discovery of additional MRI pulse sequences and technological advances with electromagnetic fields to provide greater accuracy, the resolution of present-day T1- and T2-weighted images has dramatically improved, making possible diagnoses of spinal pathology that was invisible at the turn of the century.

The workhorse imaging modalities that continue to persist for the evaluation of spine pathology are plain radiographs, MRI, and CT. Plain radiographs remain the first-line imaging study for the evaluation of pain,

Atlas of Spinal Imaging. https://doi.org/10.1016/B978-0-323-76111-6.00005-5

1

numbness, weakness, or any other symptoms localizing to the spine. This form of imaging also serves as the initial diagnostic study in the setting of trauma, malignancy, infection, deformity, and degenerative spine pathology, due largely to the ease in acquisition and relatively low cost. Another strength of plain radiographs is the ability to implement specialized views to evaluate stability and flexibility. In parallel with standard anteroposterior and lateral views of the spine, flexion-extension, sitting, and bending views allow providers the ability to appreciate anatomical changes that occur with movement. Due to the high-resolution multiplanar images of vertebral and soft tissue anatomy, MRI remains a first-line advanced imaging study to evaluate spine pathology, avoiding risks associated with radiation exposure. As such, MRI is routinely ordered in the clinic setting and offers relatively high sensitivity and specificity for infections, tumors, disc degeneration, pathologic fractures, and herniations. However, MR imaging does carry a relatively expensive cost and has varying degrees of utility in obese, claustrophobic, and pacemaker-dependent individuals. CT imaging provides for a greater detailed evaluation of the bony anatomy, largely due to its ability to reconstruct three-dimensional and multiplanar images. However, this study comes with the risk of elevated radiation exposure compared to other imaging modalities.

GOALS OF THIS TEXTBOOK

Over the years, the evaluation of spine anatomy and pathology with plain radiographs, MRIs, and CTs has rapidly developed with a multitude of studies describing various phenotypes and measurements. From these descriptions, various classification systems have been developed to bridge the radiographic findings and measurements with clinical practice. It is important that trainees and providers understand the basics of the radiographic parameters and clinical associations.

However, no comprehensive manual exists that describes important phenotypes and measurements based on plain radiographs, MRI, and CT imaging of the cervical, thoracic, and lumbosacral spine. The goal of this textbook was to provide a single source that outlines common radiographic parameters based on these three common spine imaging modalities. There will also be a focus on the clinical application of these imaging phenotypes through the description of classification systems that are often utilized to guide the evaluation, diagnosis, and treatment of spine pathology.

REFERENCES

1. Dewing SB. *Modern Radiology in Historical Perspective.* Thomas; 1962.
2. Hoeffner EG, Mukherji SK, Srinivasan A, Quint DJ. Neuroradiology back to the future: spine imaging. *Am J Neuroradiol.* 2012;33:999–1006. https://doi.org/10.3174/ajnr.a3129.
3. Hesselink JR. Spine imaging: history, achievements, remaining frontiers. *AJR Am J Roentgenol.* 1988;150:1223–1229.
4. Isherwood I. Sir Godfrey Hounsfield. *Radiology.* 2005;234:975–976.
5. Hounsfield GN. Computerized transverse axial scanning (tomography): part 1. Description of system. *BJR Suppl.* 1973;46:1016–1022.
6. Lauterbur PC. Image formation by induced local interactions: examples employing nuclear magnetic resonance. *Nature.* 1973;242:190–191. https://doi.org/10.1038/242190a0.
7. Bradley WG. History of medical imaging. *Proc Am Philos Soc.* 2008;152:349–361.
8. Edelman RR, Shoukimas GM, Stark DD, et al. High-resolution surface-coil imaging of lumbar disk disease. *AJR Am J Roentgenol.* 1985;144:1123–1129.
9. Modic MT, Steinberg PM, Ross JS, Masaryk TJ, Carter JR. Degenerative disk disease: assessment of changes in vertebral body marrow with MR imaging. *Radiology.* 1988;166:193–199.
10. Carragee EJ, Alamin TF. Discography: a review. *Spine J.* 2001;1:364–372.

CHAPTER 2

Radiographic Evaluation of the Upper Cervical Spine

MARK A. PASTORE[a] • ANTHONY VIOLA III[a] • VADIM GOZ[b] •
NOOR TAMIMI[b] • ALEXANDER VACCARO[b]
[a]Department of Orthopaedic Surgery, Philadelphia College of Osteopathic Medicine, Philadelphia,
PA, United States, [b]Department of Orthopaedic Surgery, Rothman Institute, Thomas Jefferson
University, Philadelphia, PA, United States

INTRODUCTION

The upper cervical spine contains the craniocervical junction (CCJ), the atlas or C1, and the axis or C2. A large proportion of overall cervical motion comes from the upper cervical spine between the CCJ and C2. The CCJ accommodates approximately 45 degrees of flexion extension.[1] This is more than any other single cervical level. The C1–2 joint is responsible for approximately 40 degrees of axial rotation in each direction,[2] that is, 40% of total axial rotation of the cervical spine. Due to the significant amount of motion in the upper cervical spine, the ligamentous support of this region is pivotal to maintaining adequate stability.

Ligaments of the CCJ and atlantoaxial (AA) articulations are separated into two groups: intrinsic and extrinsic ligaments. Intrinsic ligaments include the tectorial membrane (rostral continuation of the posterior longitudinal ligament), the cruciate ligament complex, and the alar and apical ligaments (Fig. 1). The cruciate ligament complex contains the transverse atlantoaxial ligament (TAL), the most structurally important part of the complex, as well as longitudinal fibers that extend from the foramen magnum to the axis. The TAL is an essential stabilizer of the AA articulation. Extrinsic ligaments include the ligamentum nuchae, cranial continuation of the anterior longitudinal ligaments, as well as the ligamentum flavum.[3] Three ligaments traverse from the odontoid to the occipital condyles; these include the paired alar ligaments that extend from the cranial tip of the odontoid process to the occipital condyles and a central apical ligament that extends from the tip of the odontoid to the basion.

Plain radiographs were historically the primary tool for the evaluation of cervical trauma. While modalities such as CT and MRI scans have largely taken over the role of initial imaging in the setting of high-energy blunt trauma, radiographs remain as a useful adjunct in the evaluation of the upper cervical spine. Not only are plain radiographs inexpensive and reduce radiation exposure to the patient, they are easy to obtain in the emergency department and in the office postoperatively.[4] Flexion-extension plain radiographs can also be obtained providing information that is not obtained via CT and MRI. Radiographic evaluation of the upper cervical spine begins with obtaining an anteroposterior (AP) view, an open-mouth odontoid view, and a lateral view. When performed correctly, radiographs will include the base of the skull to the upper border of T1 on lateral radiographs and the C3-T1 vertebrae on AP radiographs.[4] The spinous processes and facet joints should be well aligned and symmetrical as any asymmetry would indicate rotation.[4] A number of specific injuries, classifications, and measurement techniques are discussed later.

OCCIPITAL CONDYLE FRACTURES

Occipital condyle fractures are most reliably identified with a thin-slice CT scan of the cervical spine. However, these injuries may be present on plain radiographs, and a general knowledge of their morphology is useful in order to maintain a high level of suspicion for their presence in the setting of blunt trauma. Currently, the most commonly used classification system is the Anderson and Montesano classification.[5] This system describes three types of occipital condyle fractures: Type 1, comminuted; Type 2, extension of a basilar skull fracture; and Type 3, avulsion. It is important to note that Type 3

Atlas of Spinal Imaging. https://doi.org/10.1016/B978-0-323-76111-6.00008-0

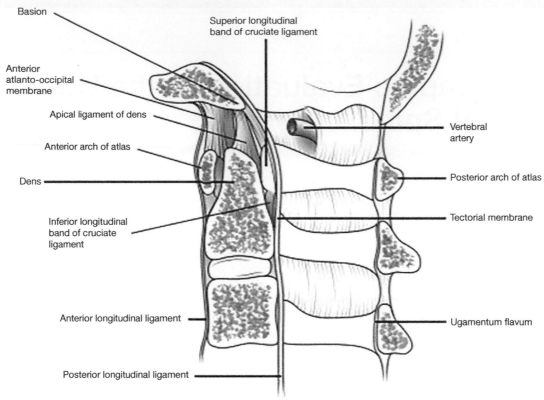

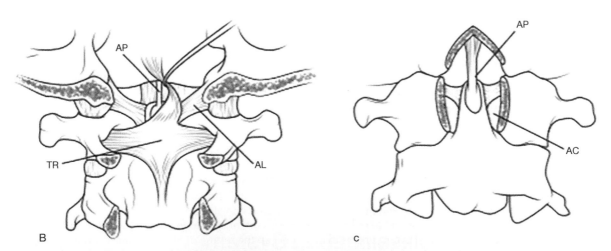

FIG. 1 (A) Illustration demonstrating sagittal view of the occipitocervical articulation. Posterior (B) and anterior (C) illustrations of the atlantoaxial articulation. AC = accessory ligament, AL = alar ligament, AP = apical ligament, TR = transverse atlantal ligament. (From Bransford RJ, Alton TB, Patel AR, Bellabarba C. Upper cervical spine trauma. *J Am Acad Orthopaed Surg* 2014;22(11): Figure 1, page 719.)

fractures are associated with craniocervical dissociation (CCD) injuries. Occipital condyle fractures are not obvious on plain radiographs, and thus, a CT scan should be used if there is suspicion for this injury.[5]

CRANIOCERVICAL DISSOCIATION

A craniocervical dissociation (CCD), otherwise known as "occipitocervical dissociation" (OCD), is a rare, but severe injury in which the stability between the cranium and the cervical spine has been compromised. This requires disruption of the stabilizing intrinsic and extrinsic craniocervical junction (CCJ) ligaments. Injuries to the CCJ typically require a high-energy mechanism, which usually involves a rapid deceleration with or without cranial impact.[6] These are most commonly seen in the setting of motor vehicle accidents or falls from significant height and are often fatal.[7] Accurate and early diagnosis and treatment of these patients is critical to optimize their outcomes.[8] The osseous anatomy of the craniocervical junction in the traumatized patient is rather difficult on plain radiographs due to the complex anatomy and overlying structures. Many methods have been described to evaluate the craniocervical junction on plain radiographs. These radiographic parameters help define normal anatomy and aid in the diagnosis of various pathologic conditions such as instability and superior migration of the dens. Radiographic parameters have inherent weaknesses as the variability exists in magnification, interobserver measurements, and normal anatomy.

Harris Lines (BAI and BDI)

Harris lines are a common measurement used to diagnose potential occipitocervical dissociations on a lateral cervical spine radiograph. This was first described by Harris et al.[9] They involve two measurements: the basion-dental interval (BDI) and the basion-axial interval (BAI). The BDI is measured from the basion to the tip of the dens and is considered abnormal above 12 mm. The BAI measures the distance from the tip of the basion to a line extending superiorly from the dorsal aspect of the dens, or the posterior axis line (PAL). The BAI should also be less than 12 mm. Together the two Harris line values are thought to be more diagnostically accurate than the Power's index/ratio in identifying CCD injuries[9] (Fig. 2).

Power's Ratio

The Power's ratio is another measurement used in the diagnosis of occipitocervical dissociation. It is

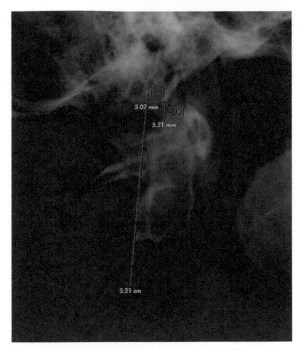

FIG. 2 The lateral cervical spine radiograph shown here demonstrates the Harris lines. The BAI is measured from the tip of the basion to a line extending from the posterior cortex of C2, measured here at 5.07 mm. The BDI is measured from the tip of the basion to the tip of the dens, or odontoid process, and is measured here at 5.21 mm.

calculated from the ratio of the distance from the basion to the ventral aspect of the posterior arch of C1, compared with the distance from the tip of the opisthion (posterior foramen magnum) to the center of the dorsal aspect of the anterior arch of C1. An accepted ratio is less than or equal to 1, with value greater than one considered abnormal and suggestive of ventral atlanto-occipital dissociation. Ratios approaching 0.7 or less are concerning for dorsal atlanto-occipital dislocation[10] (Fig. 3). A concern with the Power's ratio is that if both of the distances used in the ratio increase proportionally, such as in a primarily distraction injury; therefore, the ratio would remain normal in the presence of an OCD injury.

Wackenheim's Line

Wackenheim's line is drawn along the superior surface of the clivus and extending caudally. The odontoid process should not protrude posterior to the projection of this line on the lateral X-ray[11] (Fig. 4).

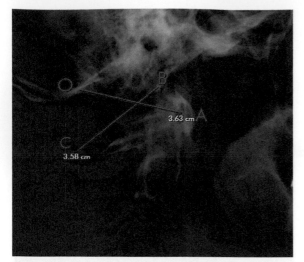

FIG. 3 Demonstrated on a neutral lateral cervical spine radiograph is an example of Power's ratio. The first measurement is drawn from the tip of the basion (B) to the midpoint of the posterior laminar line of C1 (C). The second measurement is drawn from the opisthion (O) to the dorsal aspect of the anterior arch of C1 (A). The ratio is then calculated by the distance from B to C over the distance from O to A, often represented as BC/OA. In this example, the Power's ratio is 3.58 cm/3.63 cm, or 0.986, and therefore < 1, which is considered normal.

Chamberlain's Line

Chamberlain's line is drawn from the posterior tip or pole of the hard palate to the opisthion, or dorsal margin of the foramen magnum. The tip of the odontoid should project less than 3 mm above Chamberlain's line. A projection of the odontoid above this point suggests a basilar invagination.[12] (Fig. 5).

McGregor's Line

McGregor later developed a modification of Chamberlain's line that can be applied when the opisthion cannot be accurately identified on X-ray. This line, termed McGregor's line, extends from the posterior tip or pole of the hard palate to the lowest point of the midline occipital curve. In a normal study, the tip of the odontoid should project less than 4.5 mm above this line. Typically, the odontoid will lie below or just tangent to Chamberlain's line and McGregor's line[13] (Fig. 6).

McRae's Line

Another tool to evaluate the craniocervical junction is McRae's line. This line is drawn across the foramen magnum from the basion to the opisthion. In a normal study, the tip of the odontoid process should not project above McRae's line; i.e., the odontoid process should not enter the foramen magnum[14] (Fig. 7).

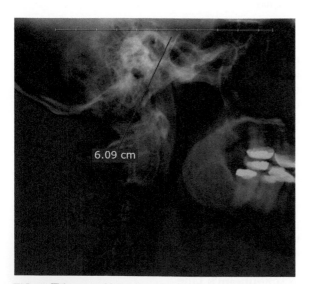

FIG. 4 This neutral lateral cervical spine radiograph demonstrates Wackenheim's line, as demonstrated by the *orange line* projecting along the superior surface of the clivus. In this patient, the odontoid process is anterior to this projection.

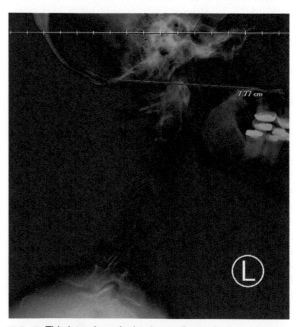

FIG. 5 This lateral cervical spine radiograph demonstrates Chamberlain's line, as demonstrated by the orange line projecting from the posterior pole of the hard palate to the opisthion.

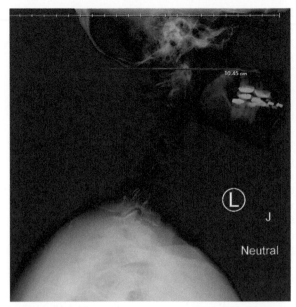

FIG. 6 The lateral cervical spine radiograph shown here demonstrates McGregor's line, drawn in *orange* from the posterior pole of the hard palate to the lowest point of the midline occipital curve.

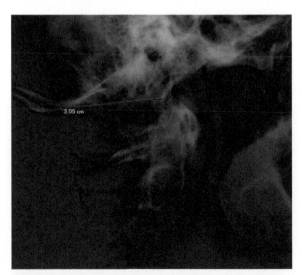

FIG. 7 Demonstrated in the neutral lateral cervical spine X-ray shown is McRae's line. This is drawn from the tip of the basion to the opisthion.

Clark's Station

Clark et al.[15] developed a system to categorize the relationship of the anterior ring of the C1 with the odontoid process. The odontoid process is divided into three equal thirds in the sagittal plane, with station I being

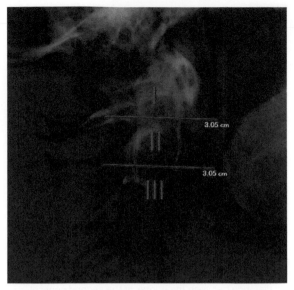

FIG. 8 The image on the left is a lateral cervical spine X-ray demonstrating Clark's station. The odontoid is divided into equal thirds. In this image, the anterior ring of C1 is level with Clark station I, which is considered normal.

most superior and station III most inferior. The anterior ring of C1 should lie within station I. Lying within station II or III is considered an abnormal finding and suspicious for basilar invagination[15] (Fig. 8).

Ranawat Criterion

The Ranawat criterion uses a measurement made using a line from the midpoint of the pedicle of C2 through the center of the odontoid process, and a line spanning the transverse axis of C1. The measurement of the midpoint of the C2 pedicle to where the lines intersect should be > 15 mm in men and > 13 mm in women. Any values less than 15 mm in men or 13 mm in women are considered abnormal and concerning for cranial settling[16] (Fig. 9).

Fischgold-Metzger Line

The Fischgold-Metzger line, also known as "the digastric line," spans between the tips of the mastoid processes on an open-mouth odontoid view. The apex of the odontoid process should be below the line and any extension above the line would indicate cranial settling.[17]

Redlund-Johnell Criterion

The Redlund-Johnell criterion utilizes a line drawn from the midpoint on the inferior endplate of the body of C2 to where it intersects with McGregor's line (spanning from the posterosuperior aspect of the hard palate to

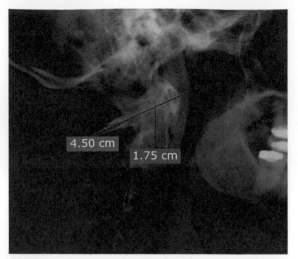

FIG. 9 The lateral cervical spine radiograph shown demonstrates the Ranawat criterion. This is a measure of the distance between the center of the second cervical pedicle and the transverse axis of the atlas drawn along the longitudinal axis of the odontoid process. This was measured at 1.75 cm in this particular patient.

the inferior most point on the midline of the occipital curve). Measurements > 34 mm in males and > 29 mm in females are within normal limits. Values < 34 mm in males and < 29 mm in females are considered positive for basilar invagination[18] (Fig. 10).

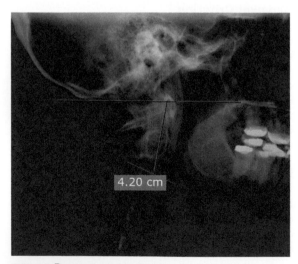

FIG. 10 Demonstrated in the lateral cervical spine radiograph shown here is the Redlund-Johnell criterion. This is a measurement from McGregor's line to the midpoint of the caudal margin of the second cervical vertebra. In this particular patient, the Redlund-Johnell criterion was 42 mm/4.20 cm. (69-year-old female).

INJURIES OF THE ATLAS (C1) AND AXIS (C2)

Injury to the atlanto-axial (AA) complex is very common in patients over 60 years old representing nearly 70% of cervical spine injuries in that population.[19] The atlanto-axial complex is clinically most significant for providing axial rotation to the cervical spine and has been found to provide 47 degrees of rotation, which accounts for up to 50% of overall cervical rotation.[4,19] Injury to the atlas and axis can be a result of hyperflexion, hyperextension, rotation, axial compression, traction, or a combination of multiple forces.[3,4] Injuries of C1 or C2 can involve associated injury of the transverse, apical, or alar ligaments.[3] Pathology of C1 and C2 can have multiple contributing factors, including degenerative, congenital, autoimmune, and traumatic processes.[19,20]

A lateral plain radiograph remains the initial screening tool essential to the diagnosis of any injury to the atlas and axis.[3] Additional views such as flexion and extension radiographs, upright films, and the open-mouth odontoid view can be utilized to further evaluate for any asymmetry or diastasis at the junction of C1 and C2.[3,19] There are several well-established measurements assessed on plain radiographs that aid in appropriate diagnosis and appropriate treatment.

Atlanto-Dens Interval (ADI)

A key measurement utilized in the assessment of AA injuries is the atlanto-dens interval (ADI). The ADI is initially assessed on a cross-table lateral plain radiograph; however, it is critical to obtain flexion-lateral and extension-lateral radiographs to assess for dynamic instability. These images are best obtained in the upright position as supine imaging can be misleading and result in false measurements secondary to gravitational forces and the pull of the cervical muscles.[3] Measurement of the atlanto-dens interval is critical to assessing atlanto-axial instability and determination of treatment. Keep in mind that dynamic films are not obtained in the acute setting and are best utilized when healing of a suspected structure is thought to be complete to avoid iatrogenic neurologic injury.

The ADI describes the distance from the posterior cortex of the C1 arch to the anterior cortex of the odontoid process[3] (Fig. 1) Normal values for this measurement are less than 3 mm in adults and less than 5 mm in children.[4] A measurement greater than 3 mm represents insufficiency of the transverse atlantal ligament (TAL).[19] In addition to the ADI, the posterior atlanto-dens interval is a particularly useful measurement to evaluate for AA pathology and injury to the TAL.[20]

Posterior Atlanto-Dens Interval (PADI)

As with the ADI, the posterior atlanto-dens interval (PADI) assesses subluxation of the atlanto-axial complex secondary to trauma, degenerative disease, or autoimmune processes such as rheumatoid arthritis. PADI describes a measurement from the posterior cortex of the odontoid process to the anterior surface of the posterior arch of C1 and thus effectively measures the space that is available for [spinal] cord (SAC), Fig. 11.[4,20] As with the ADI, this measurement is routinely assessed on neutral lateral plain radiographs with the valuable addition of flexion-lateral and extension-lateral plain radiographs. Advanced imaging such as CT may also be utilized for the assessment of additional injuries as well as the locations of the occipital condyles. MRI is a useful tool for the assessment of AA injuries, especially in assessing injury to the TAL and calculating the SAC.[4]

Clinically, the PADI has been shown to correlate more closely with the severity of neurological injury that occurs with atlanto-axial subluxation than the ADI as the diameter of the atlas varies from person to person.[20] In a study of rheumatoid arthritis patients with atlantoaxial subluxation, Boden et al. demonstrated that a PADI of less than 14 mm was associated with the development of paralysis and surgical stabilization or decompression was successful in improving the neurological outcomes compared with the nonoperative cohort.[20] The PADI can be effectively utilized in the trauma setting.

Combined Lateral Mass Overhang

Axial loads applied to the cervical spine can result in isolated fractures of the anterior or posterior arches of C1, the lateral masses of C1, or burst fractures. In any case of a C1 fracture, it is critical to obtain an open-mouth odontoid radiograph or coronal CT to measure the combined lateral mass overhang.

The combined lateral mass overhang is a measurement by which to evaluate for diastasis or asymmetry between the odontoid process and the lateral masses of C1 as is often seen in burst (Jefferson) fractures of C1.[3,4,21] This measurement effectively assesses the integrity of the TAL and determines if a fracture is potentially unstable.[3,4,21] This measure describes the combined horizontal distance from the lateral border of C1 to the lateral border of C2; hence, the measurement assesses the amount of displacement of the C1 lateral masses[3,4] (Fig. 12). The reported normal value for this measure varies but studies have consistently demonstrated that when measured greater than 6.9 mm, or 8.1 mm when accounting for X-ray magnification on the open-mouth odontoid view, there is rupture to the TAL indicating potential instability.[3,4]

Fractures of the Axis

Fractures of the second cervical vertebrae are common and are often missed secondary to the inherent difficulty of assessing imaging of the upper cervical spine.[19] These fractures can occur as a result of multiple mechanisms,

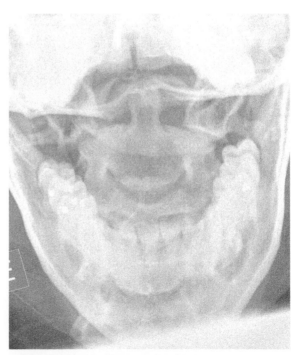

FIG. 12 Open-mouth odontoid radiograph demonstrating a widened lateral mass over hang in the setting of transverse alar ligament rupture. The sum of the lateral mass displacement should be less than 6.9 mm.

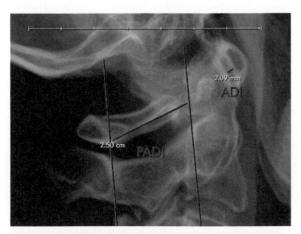

FIG. 11 Lateral cervical spine radiograph demonstrating values within normal limits for ADI (less than 3 mm) and PADI (greater than 14 mm).

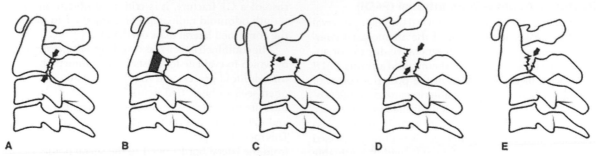

FIG. 13 Traumatic spondylolisthesis of the axis (i.e., hangman's fracture). (A) Type 1, (B) Type 1A, (C) Type 2, (D) Type 2A, and (E) Type 3. (From Bransford RJ, Alton TB, Patel AR, Bellabarba C. Upper cervical spine trauma. J Am Acad Orthopaed Surg 2014;22(11): Figure 6, page 727.)

although mostly fractures of the axis are secondary to hyperflexion or hyperextension injuries which can occur both from high-energy mechanisms in young patients or from low-energy mechanisms as in the case of the elderly with osteopenia. In addition to obtaining AP and lateral cervical plain radiographs, the open-mouth odontoid radiograph and dynamic radiographs are invaluable tool to both assess fractures of the axis and guide the spine surgeon towards appropriate management (Fig. 13).

Fractures of the odontoid process, or dens, constitute up to 20% of cervical spine fractures and are often missed secondary to a variety of factors especially in polytrauma or obtunded patients.[4,19] As with the combined lateral mass overhang, the addition of an open-mouth odontoid view along with AP and lateral plain films is essential to the diagnosis. Minimally displaced dens fractures can be missed on plain radiographs. A simple classification system that is commonly used to guide treatment is the Anderson and D'Alonzo classification.

Traumatic spondylolisthesis of the axis, also known as a "Hangman's fracture," is a common fracture that is a result of bilateral pars interarticularis fractures often sustained as a result of hyperextension and application of an axial load as seen in motor vehicle accidents.[3,4,19] The initial approach to diagnosis and selection of imaging is the same as stated above for other atlanto-axial injuries. This begins with plain AP and lateral radiographs as well as flexion and extension lateral films to assess for instability and subluxation. Often these fractures can be well visualized on plain films. However, computed tomography is the study of choice to further define the fracture pattern and thus establish a nonoperative or operative treatment plan.[22]

CONCLUSION

Throughout the course of this chapter, we discussed the evaluation of the upper cervical spine with the use of

radiographs. A thorough understanding of the relevant anatomy is critical when evaluating these cervical spine radiographs and interpreting the measurements and radiographic parameters discussed. These radiographic parameters may or may not adequately display the extent of injury and are routinely supplements by additional advanced imaging studies. Along with a history and physical including mechanism of injury and additional imaging modalities, the cervical spine plain radiographs should be a front-line assessment when caring for the injured patient. While cervical spine radiographs have their limitations, their ability to be obtained quickly at a relatively low cost and radiation exposure remain benefits for use in clinical practice. Therefore, understanding normal and abnormal findings on cervical spine radiographs will remain a pertinent skill.

REFERENCES

1. Panjabi M, Dvorak J, Oda T, Hilibrand A, Grob D. Flexion, extension, and lateral bending of the upper cervical spine in response to alar ligament transections. *J Spinal Disord.* 1991;4(2):157–167.
2. Maiman D, Yoganandan N. Biomechanics of cervical spine trauma. *Clin Neurosurg.* 1991;37:543.
3. Bransford RJ, Alton TB, Patel AR, Bellabarba C. Upper cervical spine trauma. *J Am Acad Orthop Surg.* 2014;22(11):718–729.
4. Benzel EC, Bransford RJ. *The Cervical Spine.* 5th ed. Philadelphia: Lippincott Williams & Wilkins; 2012:615–660.
5. Anderson PA, Montesano PX. Morphology and treatment of occipital condyle fractures. *Spine.* 1988;13(7):731–736.
6. Bellabarba C, Mirza SK, West GA, et al. Diagnosis and treatment of craniocervical dislocation in a series of 17 consecutive survivors during an 8-year period. *J Neurosurg Spine.* 2006;4(6):429–440.
7. Davis D, Bohlman H, Walker AE, Fisher R, Robinson R. The pathological findings in fatal craniospinal injuries. *J Neurosurg.* 1971;34(5):603–613.

8. Bellabarba C, Bransford RJ, Chapman JR. Timing to diagnosis and neurological outcomes in 48 consecutive craniocervical dissociation patients. *Spine J.* 2011;11(suppl 10):S57.

9. Harris Jr JH, Carson GC, Wagner LK. Radiologic diagnosis of traumatic occipitovertebral dissociation: normal occipitovertebral relationships on lateral radiographs of supine subjects. *Am J Roentgenol.* 1994;162(4):881–886.

10. Powers B, Miller MD, Kramer RS, et al. Traumatic anterior atlanto-occipital dislocation. *Neurosurgery.* 1979;4:12–17.

11. Wackenheim A. *Roentgen Diagnosis of the Craniovertebral Region.* New York, NY: Springer-Verlag; 1974.

12. Chamberlain WE. Basilar impression (Platybasia): a bizarre developmental anomaly of the occipital bone and upper cervical spine with striking and misleading neurologic manifestations. *Yale J Biol Med.* 1939;11:487–496.

13. McGreger M. The significance of certain measurements of the skull in the diagnosis of basilar impression. *Br J Radiol.* 1948;21:171–181.

14. McRae DL, Barnum AS. Occipitalization of the atlas. *Am J Roentgenol Radium Therapy, Nucl Med.* 1953;70:23–46.

15. Clark CR, Goetz DD, Menezes AH. Arthrodesis of the cervical spine in rheumatoid arthritis. *J Bone Joint Surg Am.* 1989;71(3):381–392.

16. Ranawat CS, O'Leary P, Pellicci P, Tsairis P, Marchisello P, Dorr L. Cervical spine fusion in rheumatoid arthritis. *J Bone Joint Surg Am.* 1979;61(7):1003–1010.

17. Fischgold H, Metzger J. Radio-tomography of the impression fractures of the cranial basis. *Rev Rhum Mal Osteoartic.* 1952;19:261–264.

18. Redlund-Johnell I, Pettersson H. Radiographic measurements of the cranio-vertebral region. Designed for evaluation of abnormalities in rheumatoid arthritis. *Acta Radiol Diagn (Stockh).* 1984;25(1):23–28.

19. Rothman RH, Simeone FA, Tay BKB, Eismont FJ. *Rothman-Simeone and Herkowitzs. Injuries of the Upper Cervical Spine. The Spine.* 7th ed. Philadelphia: Elsevier; 2018:1307–1329.

20. Boden SD, Dodge LD, Bohlman HH. Rheumatoid arthritis of the cervical spine: a long term analysis of predictors of paralysis and recovery. *J Bone Joint Surg.* 1993;75(9):1282–1295.

21. Spence Jr KF, Decker S, Sell KW. Bursting atlantal fracture associated with rupture of the transverse ligament. *J Bone Joint Surg Am.* 1970;52(3):543–549.

22. Schleicher P, Scholz M, Pingel A, Kandziora F. Traumatic spondylolisthesis of the axis vertebra in adults. *Global Spine J.* 2015;5:346–358.

CHAPTER 3

Upper Cervical Spine MRI

CARRIE E. ANDREWS • EVAN M. FITCHETT • THIAGO S. MONTENEGRO • GLENN A. GONZALEZ • JAMES S. HARROP
Department of Neurological Surgery, Thomas Jefferson University, Philadelphia, PA, United States

INTRODUCTION

Magnetic resonance imaging (MRI) is an essential modality in evaluating the ligamentous and soft tissue elements of the upper cervical spine. This region has horizontally oriented facets and no intervertebral discs; ligaments and membranes are thus crucial in stabilization at these levels.[1] This makes MRI an invaluable tool in assessing high cervical injury.[2] MRI also demonstrates prevertebral and posterior neck soft tissue edema in such injuries.[3] It is now considered the gold standard imaging study for the evaluation of patients with neurologic findings or when CT imaging findings are consistent with upper cervical spine trauma/injury. In one study, MRI demonstrated injury in 21% of the patients with normal radiographs or CT scans.[4] While several grading systems have been developed to classify and guide the management of these injuries, evaluation is based predominantly on the analysis of individual anatomic components.[3] Additionally, MRI can be utilized for the evaluation of congenital and degenerative conditions of the upper cervical spine. As in other areas of the spine, MRI also has utility in assessing the spinal cord and canal. In this chapter, we seek to describe utility and common applications of MRI of the upper cervical spine.

NORMATIVE CERVICAL SPINAL CORD DIMENSION

A fundamental understanding of normative values for cervical spine measurements is important when evaluating for pathology. Plain radiographs and CT scans have been utilized to obtain the measurements of spinal canal and spinal cord dimensions for decades. These imaging methods are inherently limited by effects of magnification and poor soft tissue resolution. MRI, specifically T2-weighted images, provides the detail necessary to accurately measure various components of the axial spine. As with most anatomical measurements in the body, there are significant variations based on age and sex.

Spinal Canal/Cord Diameter

The evaluation of the spinal canal diameter in the axial spine is best performed using midsagittal T2-weighted image, with a reference line drawn intersecting the most concave portions of both the anterior and posterior elements of C1. Measurements along this line can be used to define the spinal canal diameter of the axial spine that is the distance from the tectorial membrane to the anterior-most aspect of the posterior arch of C1. Similarly, the measurements of spinal cord diameter can be made along this same line (Fig. 1).

One prospective multicenter trial found both spinal canal and cord diameter in the axial spine are dependent on age, gender, and body height in normal volunteers with no known cervical pathology.[5] Therefore, there is no universal normal value that can be applied across all patients.

VERTEBRAL ARTERY ON MRI

The course of vascular structures is important in operative planning. In the axial spine, the vertebral artery is the largest and most significant vascular structure to be aware of, particularly with posterior surgical approaches to this region. In the typical course, the symmetric vertebral arteries course within the transverse foramen, exiting at C1 and coursing medially in a bony groove called the sulcus arteriosus before entering the foramen magnum. On MRI, vascular structures are best evaluated on MRA, though these may not routinely be included in studies of the cervical spine. Therefore, the course of the vertebral artery can be adequately assessed as a flow void on T2-weighted images (Fig. 2).

Both sagittal and axial views can be used to assess the course, with thin cut images allowing for a more comprehensive view of any vessel loops. Important considerations when evaluating the vertebral artery are tortuosity that may put the vessel at greater risk during surgical dissection. In addition, it is important to know of any anatomical variants such as dominance of one side or atypical courses of the vessel that may alter surgical planning or decision-making intra-operatively.[6]

Atlas of Spinal Imaging. https://doi.org/10.1016/B978-0-323-76111-6.00007-9

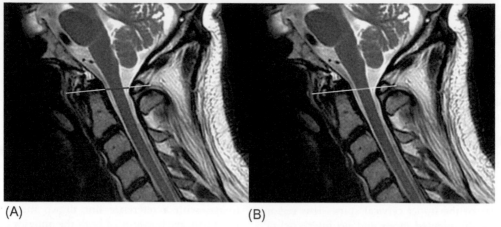

(A)   (B)

FIG. 1 Midsagittal T2 MRI demonstrating axial spine measurements. Reference line drawn intersecting the most concave portions of both the anterior and posterior elements of C1 (white line). (A) Spinal canal diameter measured from tectorial membrane to the anterior most aspect of the posterior arch of C1 (red line). (B) Spinal cord diameter measured from the anterior to posterior boundary of cord/cerebrospinal fluid (blue line).

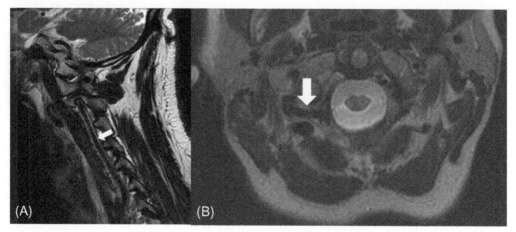

FIG. 2 (A) Sagittal T2 MRI with vertebral artery demonstrated as flow void traversing the transverse foramina (white arrow). (B) Axial T2 MRI showing medial path of the vertebral artery after exiting the transverse foramen of C1, before ascending through the foramen magnum.

TRAUMA

Fractures of the upper cervical spine account for an estimated half of all cervical fractures.[7] Injury in this region can be clinically fraught, as many of these patients have an associated cranial injury that can limit physical examination or may have only mild symptoms of neck pain and stiffness.[2,3] Instability of the upper cervical spine can have devastating neurologic consequences, making its prompt identification crucial to proper management. Several classification schemes have been devised to attempt to guide clinical decision making in these patients.[8-11]

In combination with radiographic and CT imaging, a holistic picture of a patient's injuries can be created. The indications to obtain a cervical spine MRI in the setting of trauma are diverse, including: to assess for ligamentous injury, to evaluate the spinal cord in patients with neurologic deficit (and prognosticate by differentiating hemorrhagic from nonhemorrhagic cord injury), to identify epidural hematoma, to rule out an occult bony injury with negative CT or radiographs, and to assess spinal stability to determine whether immobilization in a cervical collar is necessary.[12] The routine use of cervical spine MRI in trauma patients, however, is highly contested, particularly in the setting of an obtunded or comatose patient. Some authors argue that MRI is the gold standard for assessing cervical spine stability in patients unable to participate in neurologic exam, while others believe this study to be an unnecessary and costly endeavor that does not ultimately affect patient outcome.[4, 13]

Transverse Ligament Injury

The transverse ligament (TL) is crucial to atlantoaxial stability; its disruption is considered the most important pathologic contributor to instability at this level. When there is transverse ligament disruption associated with a dens fracture, there is a high rate of nonunion, as dens displacement or angulation is associated with injury to the transverse ligament.[8]

The transverse ligament can best be appreciated using axial sections of a gradient echo sequence, where it is visualized as a band of homogenous low-intensity signal between the synovial capsule and the cerebrospinal fluid. Tears are seen as gross disruption of the ligament on MRI (Fig. 3).

More commonly, T2 axial sections are obtained and demonstrate a uniform hypointense structure of an intact TL dorsal to the dens. When injured, there is an increase in T2 signal intensity indicative of edema, tearing, or avulsion (Fig. 4).

Alar Ligament Injury

It has been found that 30%–50% of the patients with craniocervical instability have avulsion of the alar ligament (AL), which can best be evaluated in the coronal plane on MRI.[14] This bilateral structure connects the dens to the occipital condyle (Fig. 5).

In one study, the AL was identified using MRI on either side in approximately 80% of healthy patients. Interestingly, it was found that of these healthy patients, 36%–48% had effusion at C1-C2, which in the absence of alar ligament visualization may represent rotational injury.[15] In another study of diverse groups, including healthy volunteers, patients with cervical spine trauma, and cadaveric samples, nearly all alar ligaments could be identified; resection of the ligament on cadaveric samples could also be appreciated as a void on MRI.[16]

Tectorial Membrane Injury

The tectorial membrane (TM) is an extension of the posterior longitudinal ligament, connecting the dorsal aspect of the dens and the vertebral bodies of C2 and C3 to the clivus. Along with the alar ligament, it prevents anterior subluxation of the head on the cervical spine and limits flexion.[17, 18] It appears as a thin, hypointense structure in T2 sequences (Fig. 6).

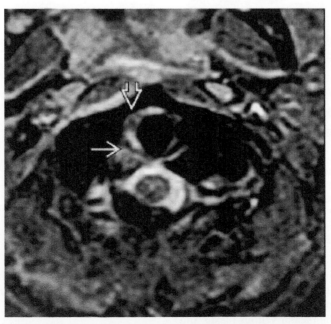

FIG. 3 Axial gradient-echo MRI demonstrating increased signal intensity at the right C1 attachment, representing disruption of the transverse ligament (thin arrow) secondary to the widening of the interval between the dens and lateral mass (thick arrow). (Credit: Ross, J. S., Bendock, B. R., & McClendon Jr, J. (2017). Imaging in Spine Surgery E-Book. Elsevier Health Sciences, Page 162.)

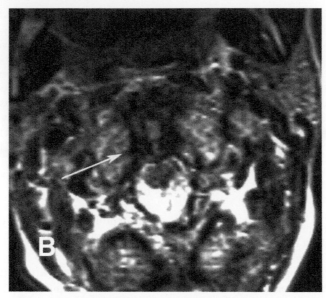

FIG. 4 Increased signal intensity on axial T2 MRI representing injury along transverse ligament (arrow) at left C1 attachment. (Credit: Debernardi A, D'Aliberti G, Talamonti G, Villa F, Piparo M, Cenzato M. Traumatic (type II) odontoid fracture with transverse atlantal ligament injury: a controversial event. World Neurosurg 2013;79(5–6):779–783. doi:10.1016/j.wneu.2012.01.055, Fig. 4B.)

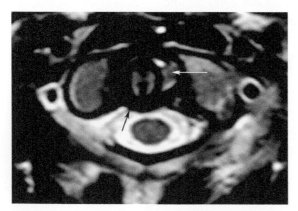

FIG. 5 Axial T2 MRI edematous left alar ligament extending from the dens to the occipital condyle (white arrow). (Credit: Jo, A. S., Wilseck, Z., Manganaro, M. S., & Ibrahim, M. (2018). Essentials of spine trauma imaging: radiographs, CT, and MRI. Semin Ultrasound CT MR, 39(6), 532–550. doi:10.1053/j.sult.2018.10.002, Fig. 5C.)

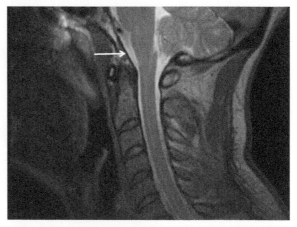

FIG. 6 Sagittal T2 MRI with intact TM, shown as a uniform hypointense band spanning from the tip of the dens to the clivus (arrow).

The tectorial membrane is commonly injured in one of two ways. It can be stripped from the clivus, resulting in retroclival epidural hematoma as a consequence of damage to the basilar venous plexus and dorsal meningeal branch of the meningohypophyseal trunk that reside between the membrane and the clivus. This is more frequently observed in children. In adults, there is a commonly complete or partial disruption of the TM (Fig. 7). The former is visualized as thinning or increased T2 signal within the band, the latter as a discontinuity.[19]

Posterior Complex Soft Tissue

In one series, increased T2 signal within the posterior complex ligaments (capsular joint ligaments and the

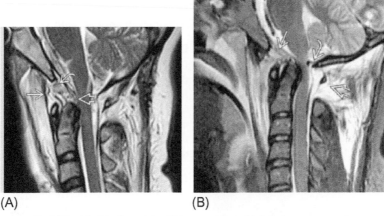

(A)   (B)

FIG. 7 (A) Sagittal T2 MRI with thinning of the TM suggestive of injury, but not complete tear (wide arrow). (B) Sagittal T2 MRI with increased signal intensity within the TM representing disruption of the ligament (thin arrow). (Credit: Ross, J. S., Bendock, B. R., & McClendon Jr, J. (2017). Imaging in Spine Surgery E-Book. Elsevier Health Sciences, Page 160.)

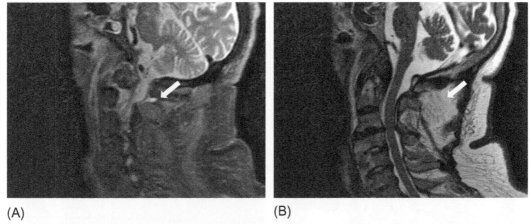

(A)   (B)

FIG. 8 (A) Sagittal STIR MRI of a patient with posterior ligamentous complex injury (white arrow). (B) Sagittal T2 MRI of the same patient with significant posterior ligamentous complex and soft tissue edema (white arrow).

posterior atlantooccipital membrane) and soft tissue was present in all patients with craniocervical trauma (Fig. 8).[2]

While this does not represent gross instability, soft tissue strain or tear may herald bony or ligamentous injury that is associated with instability.

CONGENITAL
Basilar Invagination

Basilar invagination (BI), migration of C2 superiorly, which can cause compression of the cervical spinal cord and brain stem, is typically appreciated and evaluated on

CT scans by comparing the relative position of the odontoid process and McRae's line, a line drawn from basion to opisthion.[20] Basilar invagination is defined as a protrusion of the odontoid greater than 5 mm below this line.[21] MRI is useful for the evaluation of neural structures, such as syrinx, for the purposes of operative planning (Fig. 9).

MRI is specifically useful in assessing the cervicomedullary angle (CMA), the angle between a line parallel to the ventral aspect of the medulla and a line parallel to the ventral upper cervical spinal cord (Fig. 10).[22]

Normal CMA is typically 139.0–175.5°; in patients with basilar invagination, a value of less than 135° is

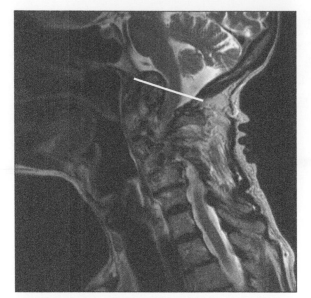

FIG. 9 T2 sagittal MRI showing significant RA pannus resulting in BI with cervical cord/brain stem compression. The white line represents McRae's line extending from basion to opisthion.

associated with neurologic deterioration.[23] Increased CMA postoperatively is associated with better clinical outcomes in patients with BI.[24]

Down Syndrome

Down syndrome is associated with many anomalies of the craniocervical junction. Specifically, one common finding is the flattening of the occipital condyle and C1 facet. This abnormality, which can be appreciated on MRI, allows for anterior and lateral translation of the joint, contributing to overall instability in these patients (Fig. 11).[25]

Chiari I Malformation

Chiari I malformation is defined as herniation of the cerebellar tonsils 3–5 mm below McRae's line. Tonsillar position is measured from McRae's line (opisthion-basion line) to the tonsillar tip in the midsagittal plane. Some authors argue that measurement should be taken in the coronal plane to account for asymmetry of the cerebellar tonsils, which is common in such patients (Fig. 12).[26]

High inter-rater variability has been observed in the measurement of tonsillar herniation, highlighting a need for an alternative diagnostic method.[26]

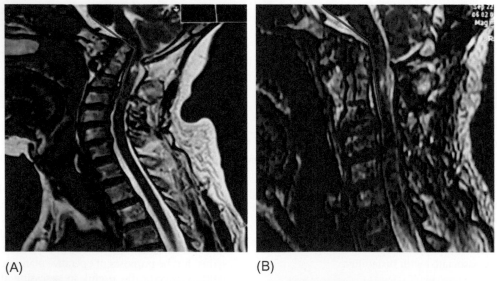

(A)　　　　　　　　　　(B)

FIG. 10 (A) Preoperative T2 sagittal MRI demonstrating the CMA (red angle). (B) Same patient postoperatively, after traction followed by occiput to C2 posterior decompression and fusion. Imaging demonstrates an increased CMA (red angle) on T2 sagittal MRI. (Credit: Guo, X., Han, Z., Xiao, J., Chen, Q., Chen, F., Guo, Q., ... & Ni, B. (2019). Cervicomedullary angle as an independent radiological predictor of postoperative neurological outcome in type a basilar invagination. Sci Rep, 9(1), 1–7. doi:10.1038/s41598-019-55780-w, Fig. 1.)

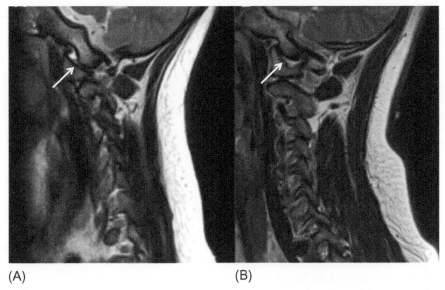

(A)   (B)

FIG. 11 (A) T2 sagittal MRI images showing flattening of the occipital condyle and C1 superior facet seen on T2 sagittal MRI in a patient with Down syndrome (arrow). (B) In comparison, the normal curved shape of the articular facet seen in a patient without Down syndrome (arrow). (Credit: Rodrigues, M., Nunes, J., Figueiredo, S., de Campos, A. M., & Geraldo, A. F. (2019). Neuroimaging assessment in down syndrome: a pictorial review. Insights Imaging, 10(1), 52. doi:10.1186/s13244-019-0729-3, Fig. 13.)

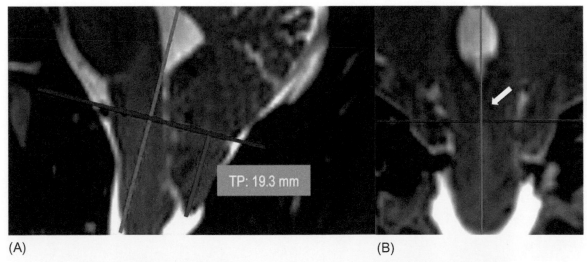

(A)   (B)

FIG. 12 (A, B) T2 MRI in the midsagittal plane (orange) in a patient with Type I Chiari malformation shown with tonsillar herniation measured (red) perpendicular to McRae's line (purple). (Credit: Lawrence, B. J., Urbizu, A., Allen, P. A., Loth, F., Tubbs, R. S., Bunck, A. C., et al. (2018). Cerebellar tonsil ectopia measurement in type I Chiari malformation patients show poor inter-operator reliability. Fluids Barriers CNS, 15(1), 33. doi:10.1186/s12987-018-0118-1, Fig. 1A and B.)

ACQUIRED

Rheumatoid Arthritis

The atlantoaxial joint is the most common joint affected by rheumatoid arthritis (RA).[27] MRI should be used to assess cervical spine stability in patients with RA who have neurologic symptoms or evidence of cervical involvement on radiograph.[28, 29] MRI allows for visualization of structural degeneration, including facet subluxation, dens dislocation, and joint destruction.[27] Occult instability can be visualized with flexion and extension MRI, allowing for appreciation of positional cord compression associated with atlantoaxial instability, which in one study was found to be present in 12% of the cases in flexion position and 12% of the cases in extension position. This functional, or dynamic, MRI is performed by having the patients flex and extend their neck while undergoing MRI.[30, 31] However, it must be noted that radiographs remain the gold standard for assessing unstable atlantoaxial subluxation in these patients, as compared to flexion MRI.[32] Further, MRI is the imaging modality of choice for early evaluation of atlantoaxial involvement, as it can demonstrate early synovial changes (increased synovial volume or contrast enhancement, and indicative of inflammation) and pannus formation, both primarily at the C1-C2 joint, prior to development of overt instability.[27, 33]

In addition to instability, cervicomedullary angle, which can also be assessed on MRI, of less than 135° is associated with cervical myelopathy in patients with RA. Cervical stenosis as a consequence of pannus formation can also be appreciated on MRI (Fig. 13).

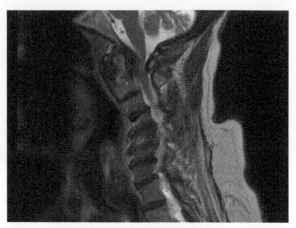

FIG. 13 Sagittal T2 MRI in a patient with RA and formation of a large hypointense pannus (arrow) forming on the odontoid process of C2 causing cervical stenosis.

Pannus regression can be assessed on postoperative T1 contrast MRI as evidence of stability after cervical fusion, whereas increased T2 signal preoperatively within the spinal cord is a predictor of poor postoperative outcome in these patients.[27]

Infection

MRI can be used to evaluate infection throughout the spine. This is of particular importance in the upper cervical spine, where unrecognized compression or instability can have devastating neurologic consequences (Fig. 14).

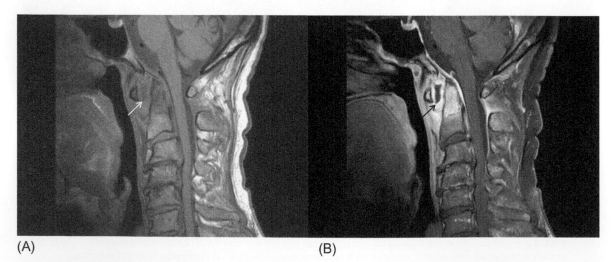

(A)   (B)

FIG. 14 (A) Patient with abscess formation (white arrow) within the atlantodental space causing an increased atlantodental interval. T1 sagittal MRI shows hypo- to isointense signal intensity (black arrow) in the atlantodental space. (B) Postcontrast T1 MRI of the same patient with rim enhancing and hypointense central portion characteristic of abscess.

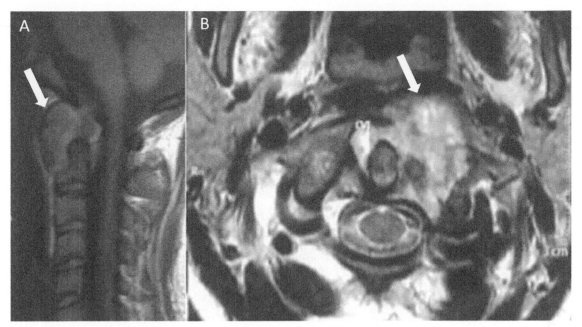

FIG. 15 Tuberculosis infection (A, arrow) causing atlantoaxial dislocation (B, arrow).(Credit: Zou, X., Yang, H., Ge, S., Chen, Y., Ni, L., Zhang, S., ... Ma, X. Y. (2020). Anterior Transoral debridement combined with posterior fixation and fusion for atlantoaxial tuberculosis. World Neurosurg doi:10.1016/j.wneu.2020.02.077, Fig. 2.)

Epidural abscess in the upper cervical spine is rare and can be clinically confused with cervical fracture given similar symptomatology; thus, a postcontrast T1 MRI is essential to differentiate infectious from traumatic pathology.[34] Specifically, tuberculosis can cause destruction and instability in the upper cervical spine although the prevalence varies depending on the patient population (Fig. 15).[28]

reveal dynamic compression of the spinal cord in cases of instability when used in conjunction with flexion and extension radiographs. In the case of trauma, classification schema can be used to guide management in patients with a craniocervical injury. Appropriate use of MRI in patients with known upper cervical pathology or symptoms is critical for the evaluation and management of such patients.

CONCLUSION

MRI of the upper cervical spine, as in the rest of the spinal cord, is a key tool in assessing ligamentous and membranous attachments, joints, and neurologic structures. It is of chief importance in the upper cervical spine, where stability is particularly dependent on soft tissue attachments, and neurologic injury can be especially devastating. This is of particular utility in cases where underlying bony abnormalities may be occult or overlooked by clinicians on CT and radiographic imaging, and it can herald developing instability, revealing underlying joint destruction before overt changes are seen on other imaging modalities. Functional MRI can

REFERENCES

1. Crisco JJ, Oda T, Panjabi MM, Bueff HU, Dvorak J, Grob D. Transections of the C1-C2 joint capsular ligaments in the cadaveric spine. *Spine.* 1991;16:S474–S479.
2. Roy AK, Miller BA, Holland CM, Fountain AJ, Pradilla G, Ahmad FU. Magnetic resonance imaging of traumatic injury to the craniovertebral junction: a case-based review. *Neurosurg Focus.* 2015;38(4):E3. https://doi.org/10.3171/2015.1.focus14785.
3. Debernardi A, D'Aliberti G, Talamonti G, Villa F, Piparo M, Collice M. The craniovertebral junction area and the role of the ligaments and membranes. *Neurosurgery.* 2015;76(Suppl. 1):S22–S32. https://doi.org/10.1227/01.neu.0000462075.73701.d.

4. Muchow RD, Resnick DK, Abdel MP, Munoz A, Anderson PA. Magnetic resonance imaging (MRI) in the clearance of the cervical spine in blunt trauma: a meta-analysis. *J Trauma.* 2008;64(1):179–189. https://doi.org/10.1097/01.ta.0000238664.74117.ac.

5. Ulbrich EJ, Schraner C, Boesch C, et al. Normative MR cervical spinal canal dimensions. *Radiology.* 2014;271(1):172–182. https://doi.org/10.1148/radiol.13120370.

6. Schroeder GD, Hsu WK. Vertebral artery injuries in cervical spine surgery. *Surg Neurol Int.* 2013;4(Suppl. 5):S362–S367. Published 2013 Oct 29 https://doi.org/10.4103/2152-7806.120777.

7. Brolin K, von Holst H. Cervical injuries in Sweden, a national survey of patient data from 1987 to 1999. *Inj Control Saf Promot.* 2002;9(1):40–52. https://doi.org/10.1076/icsp.9.1.40.3318.

8. Dickman CA, et al. Magnetic resonance imaging of the transverse atlantal ligament for the evaluation of atlanto-axial instability. *J Neurosurg.* 1991;75(2):221–227. https://doi.org/10.3171/jns.1991.75.2.0221.

9. Horn EM, Feiz-Erfan I, Lekovic GP, Dickman CA, Sonntag VK, Theodore N. Survivors of occipitoatlantal dislocation injuries: imaging and clinical correlates. *J Neurosurg Spine.* 2007;6(2):113–120. https://doi.org/10.3171/spi.2007.6.2.113.

10. Bellabarba C, et al. Diagnosis and treatment of craniocervical dislocation in a series of 17 consecutive survivors during an 8-year period. *J Neurosurg Spine.* 2006;4(6):429–440. https://doi.org/10.3171/spi.2006.4.6.429.

11. Radcliff K, Kepler C, Reitman C, Harrop J, Vaccaro A. CT and MRI-based diagnosis of craniocervical dislocations: the role of the occipitoatlantal ligament. *Clin Orthop Relat Res.* 2012;470(6):1602–1613. https://doi.org/10.1007/s11999-011-2151-0.

12. Kumar Y, Hayashi D. Role of magnetic resonance imaging in acute spinal trauma: a pictorial review. *BMC Musculoskelet Disord.* 2016;17(1):310. https://doi.org/10.1186/s12891-016-1169-6.

13. Tomycz ND, Chew BG, Chang YF, et al. MRI is unnecessary to clear the cervical spine in obtunded/comatose trauma patients: the four-year experience of a level I trauma center. *J Trauma Acute Care Surg.* 2008;64(5):1258–1263. https://doi.org/10.1097/TA.0b013e3181 66d2bd.

14. Pfirrmann CW, Binkert CA, Zanetti M, Boos N, Hodler J. MR morphology of alar ligaments and occipitoatlantoaxial joints: study in 50 asymptomatic subjects. *Radiology.* 2001;218(1):133–137. https://doi.org/10.1148/radiology.218.1.r01ja36133.

15. Jo AS, Wilseck Z, Manganaro MS, Ibrahim M. Essentials of spine trauma imaging: radiographs, CT, and MRI. *Semin Ultrasound CT MR.* 2018;39(6):532–550. https://doi.org/10.1053/j.sult.2018.10.002.

16. Willauschus WG, Kladny B, Beyer WF, Glückert K, Arnold H, Scheithauer R. Lesions of the alar ligaments. In vivo and in vitro studies with magnetic resonance imaging. *Spine.* 1995;20(23):2493–2498. https://doi.org/10.1097/00007632-199512000-00006.

17. Scott EW, Haid RW, Peace D. Type I fractures of the odontoid process: implications for atlanto-occipital instability: case report. *J Neurosurg.* 1990;72(3):488–492. https://doi.org/10.3171/jns.1990.72.3.0488.

18. Jain N, Verma R, Garga UC, Baruah BP, Jain SK, Bhaskar SN. CT and MR imaging of odontoid abnormalities: a pictorial review. *Indian J Radiol Imaging.* 2016;26(1):108. https://doi.org/10.4103/0971-3026.178358.

19. Fiester P, Soule E, Natter P, Rao D. Tectorial membrane injury in adult and pediatric trauma patients: a retrospective review and proposed classification scheme. *Emerg Radiol.* 2019;26(6):615–622. https://doi.org/10.1007/s10140-019-01710-2.

20. McRae DL. Bony abnormalities in the region of the foramen magnum: correlation of the anatomic and neurologic findings. *Acta Radiol.* 1953;40(2–3):335–354. https://doi.org/10.3109/00016925309176595.

21. Cronin CG, Lohan DG, Mhuircheartigh JN, Meehan CP, Murphy J, Roche C. CT evaluation of Chamberlain's, McGregor's, and McRae's skull-base lines. *Clin Radiol.* 2009;64(1):64–69. https://doi.org/10.1016/j.crad.2008.03.012.

22. Goel A. Treatment of basilar invagination by atlanto-axial joint distraction and direct lateral mass fixation. *J Neurosurg Spine.* 2004;1(3):281–286. https://doi.org/10.3171/spi.2004.1.3.0281.

23. Wang S, Wang C, Passias PG, Li G, Yan M, Zhou H. Interobserver and intraobserver reliability of the cervicomedullary angle in a normal adult population. *Eur Spine J.* 2009;18(9):1349–1354. https://doi.org/10.1007/s00586-009-1112-8.

24. Guo X, Han Z, Xiao J, et al. Cervicomedullary angle as an independent radiological predictor of postoperative neurological outcome in type a basilar invagination. *Sci Rep.* 2019;9(1):1–7. https://doi.org/10.1038/s41598-019-55780-w.

25. Rodrigues M, Nunes J, Figueiredo S, de Campos AM, Geraldo AF. Neuroimaging assessment in down syndrome: a pictorial review. *Insights Imaging.* 2019;10(1):52. https://doi.org/10.1186/s13244-019-0729-3.

26. Lawrence BJ, Urbizu A, Allen PA, et al. Cerebellar tonsil ectopia measurement in type I Chiari malformation patients show poor inter-operator reliability. *Fluids Barriers CNS.* 2018;15(1):33. https://doi.org/10.1186/s12987-018-0118-1.

27. Joaquim AF, Ghizoni E, Tedeschi H, Appenzeller S, Riew KD. Radiological evaluation of cervical spine involvement in rheumatoid arthritis. *Neurosurg Focus.* 2015;38(4):E4. https://doi.org/10.3171/2015.1.FOCUS14664Dhadve.

28. Dhadve RU, et al. Multidetector computed tomography and magnetic resonance imaging evaluation of craniovertebral junction abnormalities. *N Am J Med Sci.* 2015;7(8):362. https://doi.org/10.4103/1947-2714.163644.

29. Mańczak M, Gasik R. Cervical spine instability in the course of rheumatoid arthritis–imaging methods. *Reumatologia.* 2017;55(4):201. https://doi.org/10.5114/reum.2017.69782.

30. Allmann K-H, et al. Functional MR imaging of the cervical spine in patients with rheumatoid arthritis. *Acta Radiol.* 1998;39(5):543–546. https://doi.org/10.1080/02841859809172222.

31. Gupta V, Khandelwal N, Mathuria SN, Singh P, Pathak A, Suri S. Dynamic magnetic resonance imaging evaluation of craniovertebral junction abnormalities. *J Comput Assist Tomogr.* 2007;31(3):354–359. https://doi.org/10.1097/01.rct.0000238009.57307.26.

32. Laiho K, Soini I, Kautiainen H, Kauppi M. Can we rely on magnetic resonance imaging when evaluating unstable atlantoaxial subluxation? *Ann Rheum Dis.* 2003;62(3):254–256. https://doi.org/10.1136/ard.62.3.254.

33. Tehranzadeh J, Ashikyan O, Dascalos J. Magnetic resonance imaging in early detection of rheumatoid arthritis. *Semin Musculoskelet Radiol.* 2003;7(2):79–94. https://doi.org/10.1055/s-2003-41342.

34. Al-Hourani K, Frost C, Mesfin A. Upper cervical epidural abscess in a patient with Parkinson disease: a case report and review. *Geriatr Orthop Surg Rehabil.* 2015;6(4):328–333. https://doi.org/10.1177/2151458515604356.

CHAPTER 4

Upper Cervical Spine: Computed Tomography

ATUL GOEL
Department of Neurosurgery, K.E.M. Hospital and Seth G.S. Medical College, Mumbai, India

INTRODUCTION

The craniovertebral junction is designed to be strong in order to maintain the head on the shoulders. This junction is also supple and mobile to allow for looking at the world in all directions. While mobility and stability are the hallmarks, the architecture is immaculately tuned to provide a wide space for free traversing of critical neural and vascular structures. A large complex of ligaments and bones provide infrastructure to the muscles that power the movements. The human spinal pillar has a Y-shaped configuration. The rostral "V" of the "Y," which is composed of suboccipital bone, atlas, and axis vertebrae, constitutes the craniovertebral junction. The occipitoatlantal joint is the center for stability. The occipitoatlantal joint, by its constitution and by the strength of its ligaments, is one of the strongest joints of the body. The atlantoaxial joint is the center for mobility. The flat and round atlantoaxial articulation that facilitates circumferential movements also makes this joint prone for instability. The term *craniovertebral instability* can be synonymous with *atlantoaxial instability* because, whereas atlantoaxial instability is relatively common, occipitoatlantal instability is significantly infrequent and is rarely identified in cases with severe trauma and in "syndromic" children.

Investigations for Atlantoaxial Instability

Plain radiology was used to investigate and diagnose atlantoaxial dislocation until computer imaging radically changed preoperative investigations. Lateral radiographs with the head in flexion and extension were the most frequently conducted investigation. (Fig. 1) On the basis of this investigation, atlantoaxial dislocation is diagnosed when the atlantodental interval (distance between the posterior limit of anterior arch of atlas and the anterior border of odontoid process) was more than 3 mm on flexion of the head. In children, the atlantodental interval of 3 to 5 mm is sometimes considered to be within the range of normalcy. The dislocation was considered *reducible* when the atlantodental interval returned to normal on head extension; it was considered *irreducible* or fixed or partially reducible when the atlantodental interval did not or incompletely return to normal on head extension.[1,2]

Computer-based imaging: Introduction of computer-based imaging of CT scan and MRI in the later quarter of the previous century has improved the understanding of the craniovertebral junction pathology and has helped in the identification of the optimum format of treatment. 3-D models are the latest introduction in the investigative armamentarium.[3] This investigation aids understanding of the anatomy in the upper cervical spine and in selection of the best site and direction of screw insertion. This investigation is particularly useful in the treatment of complex craniovertebral junction abnormalities.

Atlantoaxial Facetal Instability

A new classification of atlantoaxial dislocation was based on evaluation of the alignment of the facets on lateral profile imaging with the head in neutral position.[4] Visualization of the facets is not always clear in the imaging based primarily on plain radiography. Both CT scan and MRI clearly depict the status of the facets.

Horizontal facetal instability

Anterior atlantoaxial facetal (or type 1) dislocation: The alignment of the facets, weight of the head, and dominance of flexion movements more often result in an anterior facet dislocation of the atlas over the facet of axis (Fig. 2). Such dislocation is characterized by an increase in the atlantodental interval, and can result in the compression of the dural tube and neural structures by the odontoid process. As there is neural compression and deformation, such dislocations are usually associated with acute symptoms.

Atlas of Spinal Imaging. https://doi.org/10.1016/B978-0-323-76111-6.00003-1

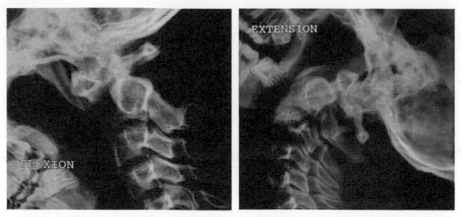

FIG. 1 (A) Lateral flexion cervical spine X-ray showing atlantoaxial dislocation. (B) Lateral extension cervical spine X-ray showing reduction of the atlantoaxial dislocation.

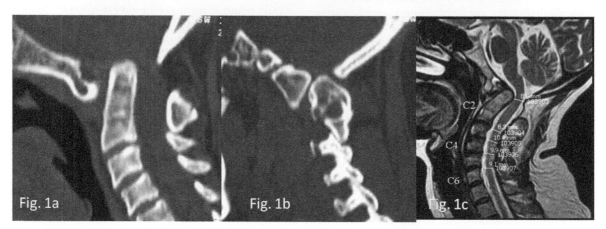

FIG. 2 (A) Computed tomographic (CT) scan showing assimilation of atlas, C2-C3 fusion, basilar invagination, and atlantoaxial instability. (B) Sagittal image of CT scan showing type A atlantoaxial facetal dislocation. (C) Magnetic resonance imaging (MRI) showing the cord compression.

Posterior atlantoaxial (type 2) facetal instability

Posterior atlantoaxial facetal dislocation (type 2) occurs when the facet of the atlas is located posterior to the facet of axis (Fig. 3).

Type 3 facetal instability

Type 3 atlantoaxial facet dislocation is when the facetal surfaces of the atlas and axis are aligned (Figs. 4 and 5). However, other clinical and radiological parameters suggest instability. Instability is confirmed in such cases by an intraoperative observation of the status of the facets on direct manual handling of bones.

Central or axial atlantoaxial instability: In types 2 and 3 atlantoaxial facetal dislocations, the atlantodental interval may be normal or relatively unaffected, and the odontoid process may not displace into the spinal canal or cause neural compression. Such types of atlantoaxial instability are classified as "central or axial" atlantoaxial instability.[5,6] Identification of central atlantoaxial facet instability is based on clinical suspicion and subjective observations. Understanding that central instability occurs in these cases can provide a critical opportunity for curative treatment in the form of a stabilization procedure.

The concept of "central or axial" atlantoaxial instability, wherein there can be atlantoaxial instability, even in the absence of altered atlantodental interval or evidence of neural compression, has expanded the scope of treatment. As neural compression is not early or a primary issue in these cases, the presenting symptoms are usually longstanding. Several commonplace clinical entities like basilar invagination, Chiari formation,

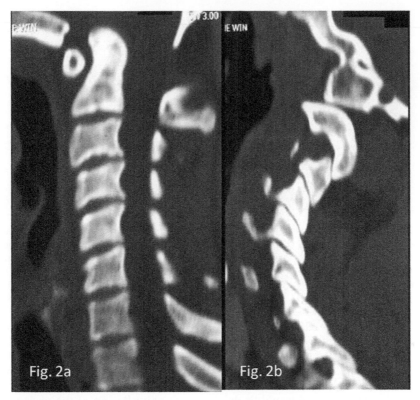

FIG. 3 (A) Sagittal CT scan showing basilar invagination. (B) Sagittal CT scan showing type B atlantoaxial facet dislocation.

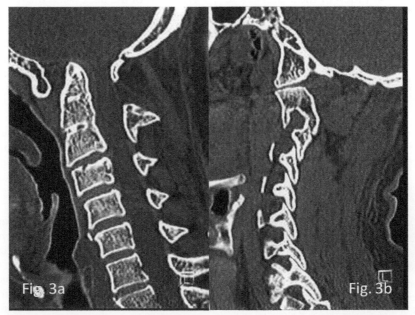

FIG. 4 (A) Sagittal CT scan shows partial assimilation of atlas and C2-C3 fusion. Basilar invagination is present. (B) Sagittal image of the facets showing facets in alignment or type C atlantoaxial facet dislocation.

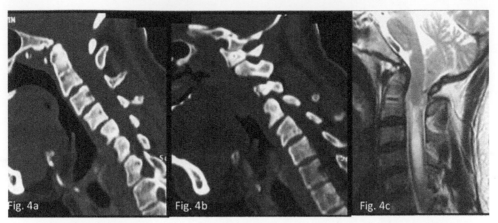

Fig. 4a   Fig. 4b   Fig. 4c

FIG. 5 (A) CT scan shows mild basilar invagination. There is no evidence of any clear atlantoaxial instability as assessed by increased atlantodental interval. (B) Sagittal image of the facets does not show any malalignment. The dislocation in this case is an example of type C facet instability and is identified only during direct surgical handling. (C) Magnetic resonance imaging shows basilar invagination, Chiari malformation, and syringomyelia.

syringomyelia, cervical myelopathy related to cervical spondylosis, and ossified posterior longitudinal ligament can present with pathology related to central or axial atlantoaxial instability.

Lateral atlantoaxial facetal dislocation occurs when the facets of atlas are dislocated lateral to the facets of axis[7] (Fig. 6). Fracture of the anterior and posterior arches of the atlas due to trauma or infection or bifid/trifid constitution of the arches can result in lateral dislocation of the facets of atlas over the facets of axis. Bifid anterior and posterior arches

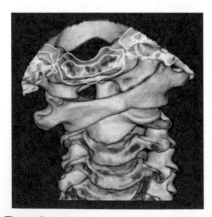

FIG. 6 Three-dimensional reconstruction of CT imaging shows rotatory dislocation. The facet of the atlas is located anterior to the facet of axis on one side and posterior to it on the other side.

of the atlas are frequently associated with atlantoaxial dislocation and basilar invagination.[8] Although it is difficult to measure, the bifidity of the arches can have a dynamic constitution resembling an opened or closed door. The posterior door or bifid opens upon flexion of the neck and accommodates to an extent the abnormal intrusion of the odontoid process into the spinal canal. The door closes upon extension of the neck when the odontoid process returns to its normal position.

Rotatory atlantoaxial dislocation: Depending on the location of the facets, **rotatory atlantoaxial dislocation** can be of various types. The more common type of rotatory dislocation occurs when the facet of atlas is dislocated posterior in relation to the facet of the axis on one side and anterior in its relationship on the contralateral side (Fig. 7). The dislocation can result in painless torticollis in young children.[9] The head is in a "cock robin" position. As there is no pain or neural deficit or symptom, and the main complaint is abnormal neck posture, the management of such cases needs to be precise and based on the understanding of biomechanics of the region.

Vertical mobile Atlantoaxial Dislocation: Vertical mobile atlantoaxial dislocation occurs when the odontoid process moves up or rostrally in relationship to the anterior arch of atlas with flexion of the head and returns to its normal position on neck extension (Fig. 8). The movements of the odontoid process resemble a piston. Ultimately, incompetence of the facet joint is the etiology of vertical atlantoaxial dislocation.[10]

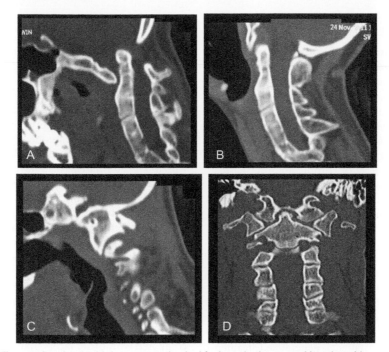

FIG. 7 (A) CT scan showing multiple segmental spinal fusions. In the neutral head position and when head is in extension position, there is no evidence of instability or basilar invagination. (B) CT scan with the head in flexed position showing basilar invagination in the form of vertical or superior migration of the odontoid. (C) CT scan cut through the facets showing no significant malalignment. (D) Coronal image showing a marked neck deformity.

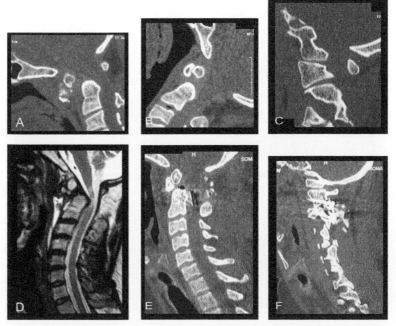

FIG. 8 (A) CT scan with the head in flexion shows atlantoaxial dislocation. Os-odontoideum can be seen. (B) CT scan with the head in extension position showing reduction of the dislocation. (C) Lateral cut of the CT scan passing through the facets. (D) T2-weighted magnetic resonance image showing cord compression. (E) Postoperative CT scan showing atlantoaxial fixation in reduced position. (F) Image showing the implants in the facets of atlas and axis.

Acute and Chronic "Mobile and Reducible" Atlantoaxial Dislocation (Fig. 9)

Acute atlantoaxial dislocation often results from moderate to severe trauma that is associated with sudden mechanical stretch on the ligaments, leading to their disruption or incompetence. In chronic or longstanding atlantoaxial dislocation, the neural structures adapt to and tolerate the abnormal movements of the odontoid process. The exact etiology of chronic atlantoaxial dislocation may also remain uncertain. Although a history of trauma is usually present, the majority of etiologies (particularly in the pediatric age group) are related to developmental defects or genetic syndromes that result in abnormal ligamentous laxity. Compared with patients with a trauma-related acute dislocation, the mobility of the facets is usually significantly higher in patients with chronic dislocation, due to ligamentous laxity.

Atlantoaxial instability related to syndromic affection: It is important to be vigilant in the diagnosis and treatment of spinal abnormalities in patients with genetic syndromes. In pediatric patients, generalized ligamentous laxity, as a result of genetic syndromes, can affect multiple joints. Specifically, in the craniovertebral junction, the atlantoaxial joint is most frequently affected. The occipitoatlantal joint instability is infrequent. The resulting laxity of ligaments also results in rotatory dislocation, usually in young children. Craniovertebral instability has been associated with *Larsen's syndrome, diastrophic dysplasia, Goldenhar's syndrome, Down syndrome, pseudoachondroplasia, Morquio's syndrome, Kniest dysplasia, spondyloepiphyseal dysplasia congenita, 22q11.2 deletion syndrome,* and *fibrodysplasia ossificans progressiva.*[1,11]

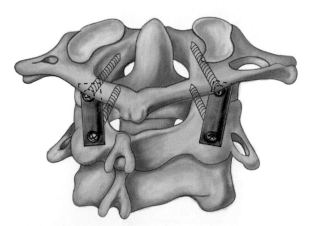

FIG. 9 Line drawing showing the lateral mass plate and screw fixation technique. (Redrawn from: Goel A, Laheri V. Plate and screw fixation for atlanto-axial subluxation. *Acta Neurochir (Wien).* 1994;129(1–2):47–53.)

Of these, instability related to *Down syndrome, as a result of ligamentous laxity,* occurs more often at C1-C2 compared with C0-C1 levels. There can be cervical spine instability at other cervical levels in patients with this syndrome. *Pseudoachondroplasia* and *Morquio's syndrome* have C1-C2 instability because of generalized ligamentous laxity and frequently identified odontoid dysplasia (hypoplasia and os-odontoideum). Patients with *Morquio's syndrome* also have soft tissue glycosaminoglycan deposits that can cause stenosis of the canal and lead to myelopathy.

Atypical C1 and C2 vertebrae: Atlas and axis vertebrae are called *atypical vertebrae* as they have a unique shape and architecture and a characteristic vertebral artery relationship. The facet architecture of the C2 vertebra differs from the facets of all other vertebrae in two important characteristics. Unlike superior facets of all other vertebrae, they do not form a pillar with the inferior facets, being considerably anterior to these. The superior facet is present in proximity to the body when compared with other facets that are located in proximity to the lamina. Two large superior articular facets of axis flank the dens or the odontoid process. Second, the vertebral artery loops medially and is located in the inferior aspect of the superior facet of C2, whereas in other cervical vertebrae, the vertebral artery foramen follows a vertical course and lies within the foramen transversarium. The course of the vertebral artery relative to the inferior aspect of the superior articular facet of the C2 makes it susceptible to injury during transarticular and interfacetal screw implantation techniques.

Surgery for Atlantoaxial Dislocation

The treatment of patients with atlantoaxial instability is a surgical challenge. Clinical outcome after achieving a successful stabilization in these patients is gratifying and can lead to a rapid neurological recovery. The complications of surgery, however, are potentially lethal. The aim of surgery in general is to achieve stability of the atlantoaxial joint and provide an environment optimum for bone fusion. The lateral mass fixation techniques have been identified to be superior and biomechanically stronger to the techniques that involve a fixation of the midline structures such as lamina and arch of atlas.[1,12] The facets of atlas and axis being large in size and the strongest part of the vertebra provide a reliable site for screw purchase for stabilization of the implant and of the region.

Irreducible or Fixed Atlantoaxial Dislocation

The issue of irreducible atlantoaxial dislocation (Fig. 10) has been discussed for over a century.

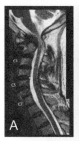
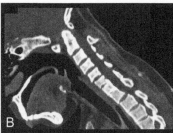
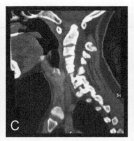
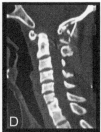
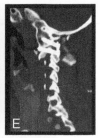

FIG. 10 Images of a 32-year-old female patient (A) T2-weighted MRI showing an "irreducible" atlantoaxial dislocation and cord compression. (B) CT scan with the head in flexed position showing severe atlantoaxial dislocation. (C) CT scan with the head in extension position does not show any reduction in atlantoaxial dislocation. (D) Postoperative CT scan showing realignment of the craniovertebral junction. (E) Postoperative image through the facets showing lateral mass plate and screw fixation.

A number of atlantoaxial dislocations were termed irreducible when dynamic imaging did not show a complete restoration of normal atlantodental interval. Basilar invagination was earlier associated with the presence of irreducible atlantoaxial dislocations. The term *irreducible* or *fixed atlantoaxial dislocation* has therapeutic implications. As the atlantoaxial joint was considered fixed, decompression of the bony structures from either anterior transoral route or posterior foramen magnum decompression formed the basis of treatment. Goel et al. introduced a concept that the so-called irreducible or fixed atlantoaxial dislocations are seldom or never irreducible, fixed, or fused. The joint is pathologically active.[2] Direct manual distraction of facets of atlas and axis and placement of bone graft within it, with or without additional support of metallic spacers, can result in a significant or complete reduction of dislocation. Subsequent atlantoaxial fixation that can sustain the reduction is then performed.

BASILAR INVAGINATION
Radiologic Criteria for Basilar Invagination (Figs. 11–15)
Chamberlain's line
Chamberlain's line is drawn on lateral plain radiograph or lateral sagittal reconstruction images of CT scan or MRI that extends from the hard palate to the opisthion. Basilar invagination was diagnosed when the tip of the odontoid process was at least 2 mm above Chamberlain's line.[12] The analysis of basilar invagination based on Chamberlain's line suggested that the basilar invagination is much more severe in cases with Group B basilar invagination than in patients with Group A basilar invagination.

McRae's line of the foramen magnum.[13]
This is a line drawn on a lateral cervical spine XR, CT scan, or MRI from the anterior to the posterior limits of foramen magnum. In Group A basilar invagination, the odontoid process crosses this line, while in Group B basilar invagination, the odontoid process is usually below this line.

Wackenheim's Clival line
Wackenheim's clival line is a line drawn along the clivus. The tip of the odontoid process is significantly

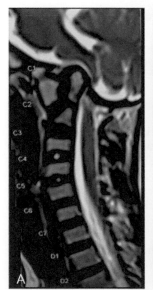
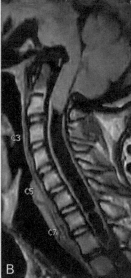

FIG. 11 (A) Sagittal T2-weighted MRI of a case with Group A basilar invagination. Odontoid process is indenting the brainstem. (B) Sagittal T2-weighted MRI of a patient with Group B basilar invagination. There is a Chiari formation and syringomyelia present.

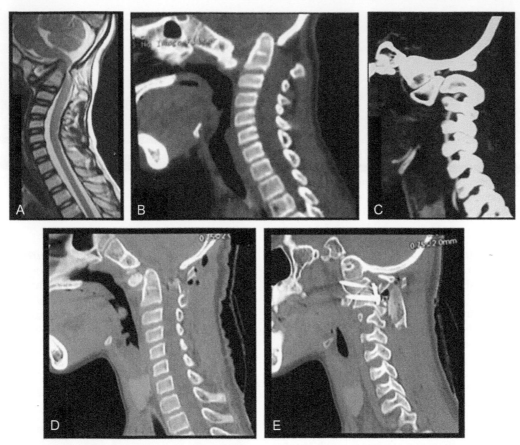

FIG. 12 (A) T2-weighted MRI showing Group A basilar invagination and cord compression. (B) CT scan with the head in flexed position showing severe Group A basilar invagination. (C) CT scan cut through the facets showing Type I atlantoaxial dislocation. (D) Postoperative CT scan showing realignment of the craniovertebral junction. (E) Postoperative image through the facets showing lateral mass plate and screw fixation.

superior to the Wackenheim's clival line in patients with Group A basilar invagination. In patients with Group B basilar invagination, the relationship between the tip of the odontoid process and the lower end of the clivus and the atlantodental and clival-dental interval remained relatively normal. In a majority of these cases, the tip of the odontoid process remained below Wackenheim's clival line.[14] The basilar invagination thus resulted from the rostral positioning of the plane of the foramen magnum in relation to the brainstem.

Platybasia
A line is drawn along the anterior skull base. The angle of this line to the clivus is referred to as the *basal angle*. Reduction of the basal angle is referred to as *platybasia*.

Omega angle (Fig. 14)
Omega angle, or the angulation of the odontoid process from the vertical as described by Klaus et al., serves as a useful guide for the diagnosis of basilar invagination.[15] Goel et al. described a modified omega angle to avoid errors in the measurement of the angle as a result of flexion and extension of the neck.[16] A line was drawn through the center of the base of the axis parallel to the line of the hard palate. As shown in the line drawing, a modified omega angle is the angle subscribed by the odontoid process to this line (Fig. 14). The line of the hard palate was unaffected by the relative movement of the head and the cervical spine during the movement of the neck in these "fixed" craniovertebral anomalies. The omega angle depicted

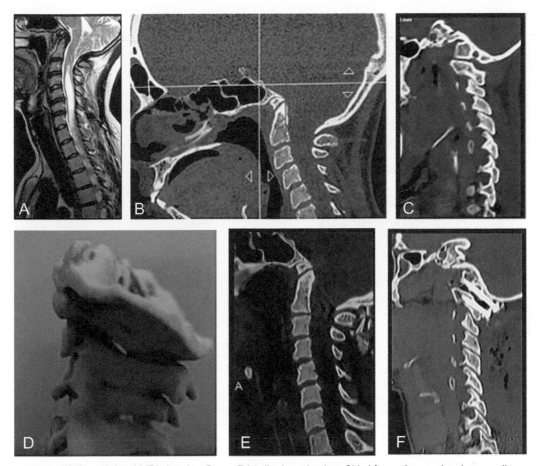

FIG. 13 (A) T2-weighted MRI showing Group B basilar invagination, Chiari formation, and syringomyelia. (B) CT scan showing severe Group B basilar invagination and assimilation of the atlas. (C) CT scan cut through the facets showing the facets in alignment. (D) 3D printed model of the patient. (E) Postoperative CT scan. (F) Postoperative image through the facets showing lateral mass plate and screw fixation.

the direction of displacement of the odontoid process. The omega angle was severely reduced in patients with Group A basilar invagination, whereas it was much larger in patients with Group B basilar invagination. The reduction in the omega angle demonstrated that in patients with Group A basilar invagination, the odontoid process had tilted toward the horizontal and was posteriorly angulated. Conversely, odontoid process was near vertical and superiorly migrated in patients with Group B basilar invagination.

Neck size (Fig. 14)
The cervical height was measured from the tip of the odontoid process to the midpoint of the base of the C7 vertebral body. Direct physical measurement of the neck length can be a useful parameter. The parameter of direct physical measurement of the neck length from inion to the tip of the C7 spinous process is also useful.[17]

Os-Odontoideum: (Fig. 9)
Abnormalities of the odontoid process are relatively rare. Os-odontoideum is among the more frequently encountered anomalies of the odontoid process. Giacomini first described os-odontoideum in 1886. By original definition, it refers to an independent odontoid process of bone that is separated from its base at the site of attachment to the body of axis. Our

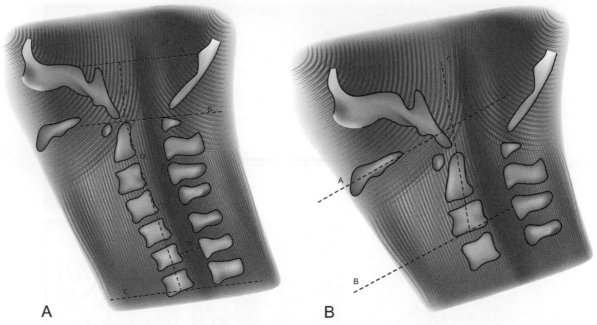

A   B

FIG. 14 (A) Illustration of the cervical spine which shows measurements of the posterior fossa and neck height. With the patient in a neutral head position, a horizontal line (line A) is drawn connecting the tuberculum sellae to inion. Line B is drawn parallel to line A and coursed over the tip of the odontoid process. Line C is drawn parallel to line B and coursed over the midpoint of the base of the C7 vertebra. The distance between lines A and B is considered to be the posterior cranial fossa height, and the distance between lines B and C is considered to be neck height. (B) This illustration reveals the Goel's modified omega angle. Line A is drawn along the line of hard palate. Line B is a line that is drawn parallel to line A. It passes through the midpoint of inferior surface of body of C3 vertebra. Line C is a line drawn from the midpoint of inferior surface of body of C3 vertebra and passes through the tip of the odontoid process. The angle between lines B and C is considered to be the modified omega angle. (Redrawn from: Goel A, Shah A. Reversal of longstanding musculoskeletal changes in basilar invagination after surgical decompression and stabilization. *J Neurosurg Spine*. 2009;10(3):220–227.)

analysis identifies that the odontoid process separation is more often not exactly at the probable site of junction of the odontoid process with the body of axis.[18] We identified os-odontoideum as a condition where a "significant" part of the odontoid process is separated from the rest of the odontoid process and body of C2. The separated part of the odontoid process has a smooth inferior border and has no anatomic continuity or functional congruence with the remaining part of the odontoid process or the body of axis. Os-odontoideum can sometimes mimic trauma-related fracture at the base of the odontoid process. Irregular edges of the fractured segments and a history of significant trauma help distinguish

fracture of odontoid process from os-odontoideum. Os-terminale and ossification or osteophyte formation in the region of apical ligament are other odontoid process-related alterations.

CONCLUSION

The atlantoaxial joint is the most mobile joint of the body. It's flat and round articular surfaces that allow circumferential movements also subject it to enhanced risk of instability. Modern computer-based imaging has assisted in understanding subtleties of the craniovertebral junction. 3-D models are the outcome of the latest advances in radiographic techniques.

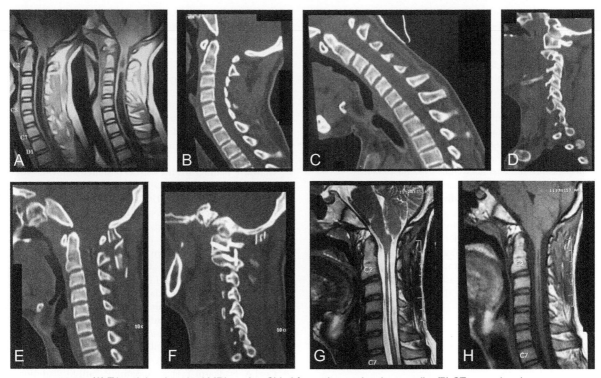

FIG. 15 (A) T1 weighted sagittal MRI sowing Chiari formation and syringomyelia. (B) CT scan showing no craniovertebral junction bone anomaly. (C) CT scan with the head in flexion showing no change in the atlantodental interval. (D) CT scan with the cut passing through the facets showing Type 2 facetal instability. (E) Post-operative CT scan. (F) Postoperative CT scan showing the implants. (G) Post-operative T2 weighted MRI showing marked resolution of the Chiari formation and syringomyelia. (H) Post-operative T1 weighted MRI.

REFERENCES

1. Goel A, Laheri VK. Plate and screw fixation for atlanto-axial dislocation.(Technical report). *Acta Neurochir.* 1994;129:47–53.
2. Goel A, Kulkarni AG, Sharma P. Reduction of fixed atlantoaxial dislocation in 24 cases: technical note. *J Neurosurg Spine.* 2005;2:505–509.
3. Goel A, Jankharia B, Shah A, Sathe P. Three-dimensional models: an emerging investigational revolution for craniovertebral junction surgery. *J Neurosurg Spine.* 2016;25(6):740–744.
4. Goel A. Goel's classification of atlantoaxial 'facetal' dislocation. *J Craniovertebr Junction Spine.* 2014;5:15–19.
5. Goel A. A review of a new clinical entity of ' atlantoaxial instability': expanding horizons of craniovertebral junction surgery. *Neurospine.* 2019;16(2):186–194.
6. Goel A. Central or axial atlantoaxial instability: expanding understanding of craniovertebral junction. *J Craniovertebr Junction Spine.* 2016;7(1):1–3.
7. Goel A, Shah A. Lateral atlantoaxial facetal dislocation in craniovertebral region tuberculosis: report of a case and analysis of an alternative treatment. *Acta Neurochir.* 2010;152:709–712.
8. Goel A, Nadkarni T, Shah A, Ramdasi R, Patni N. Bifid anterior and posterior arches of atlas: surgical implication and analysis of 70 cases. *Neurosurgery.* 2015;77(2):296–305 [discussion 305-6].
9. Goel A, Shah A. Atlantoaxial facet locking: treatment by facet manipulation and fixation. Experience in 14 cases. *J Neurosurg Spine.* 2011;14:3–9.
10. Goel A, Shah A, Rajan S. Vertical and mobile atlanto-axial dislocation. Clinical article. *J Neurosurg Spine.* 2009;11:9–14.

11. Goel A. Occipitocervical fixation: is it necessary? *J Neurosurg Spine.* 2010;13(1):1–2.
12. Goel A, Desai K, Muzumdar D. Atlantoaxial fixation using plate and screw method: a report of 160 treated patients. *Neurosurgery.* 2002;51:1351–1357.
13. McRae DL. Bony abnormalities in the region of foramen magnum: correlation of anatomic and neurologic findings. *Acta Radiol.* 1953;40:335–354.
14. Thiebaut F, Wackenheim A, Vrousos C. New median sagittal pneumostratigraphical findings concerning the posterior fossa. *J Radiol Electrol Med Nucl.* 1961;42:1–7.
15. Klaus E. Rontgendiagnostik der platybasic und basilaren impression. *Fortscher Rontgenstr.* 1957;86:460–469.
16. Goel A, Bhatjiwale M, Desai K. Basilar invagination: a study based on 190 surgically treated cases. *J Neurosurg.* 1998;88:962–968.
17. Goel A, Shah A. Reversal of longstanding musculoskeletal changes in basilar invagination after surgical decompression and stabilization. *J Neurosurg Spine.* 2009;10:220–227.
18. Goel A, Patil A, Shah A, Dandpat S, Rai S, Ranjan S. Os-odontoideum: analysis of 190 surgically treated cases. *World Neurosurg.* 2020;134:e512–e523.

FURTHER READING

19. Gupta S, Goel A. Quantitative anatomy of the lateral masses of the atlas and axis vertebrae. *Neurol India.* 2000;48:120–125.
20. Cacciola F, Phalke U, Goel A. Vertebral artery in relationship to C1-C2 vertebrae: an anatomical study. *Neurol India.* 2004;52:178–184.
21. Pilcher LS. Atlo-axoid fracture-dislocation. *Ann Surg.* 1910;51:208–211.
22. Foerster O. *Die Leitungsbahnen des Schmerzgefuhls und die ChirurgischeBehandlung der Schmerzzustande.* Berlin: Urban and Schwarzenberg; 1927.
23. Gallie WE. Fractures and dislocations of cervical spine. *Am J Surg.* 1939;46:495–499.
24. Brooks AL, Jenkins EB. Atlanto-axial arthrodesis by the wedge compression method. *J Bone Joint Surg Am.* 1978;60:279–284.
25. Dickman CA, Sonntag VK, Papadopoulos SM, et al. The interspinous method of posterior atlantoaxial arthrodesis. *J Neurosurg.* 1991;74:190–198.
26. Goel A. Letter: occipitocervical fixation: a single surgeon's experience with 120 patients. *Neurosurgery.* 2017;80(6):E263–E264.
27. Jeanneret B, Magerl F. Primary posteriorfusions C1-2 in odontoid fractures: indications, technique and results of transarticular screw fixation. *J Spinal Disord.* 1992;5:464–475.
28. Shah A, Serchi E. Management of basilar invagination: a historical perspective. *J Craniovertebr Junction Spine.* 2016;7(2):96–100.
29. Menezes AH. Primary craniovertebral anomalies and hindbrain herniation syndrome (Chiari I): database analysis. *Pediatr Neurosurg.* 1995;23:260–269.
30. Virchow R. *BeitragezurphysischenAnthropologie der Deutschen, mitbesondererBerucksichtigung der Friesen.* Berlin: Abhandlungen de KoniglichenAkademie der Wissenschaften; 1876.
31. Grawitz P. BeitragzurLehre von der basilaren Impression des Schadels. *Arch Pathol Anat Physiol Klin Med.* 1880;80:449.
32. Von Torklus D, Gehle W. *The Upper Cervical Spine: Regional Anatomy, Pathology, and Traumatology. A Systematic Radiological Atlas and Textbook.* New York: Grune & Stratton; 1972:1–98.
33. Chamberlain WE. Basilar impression (platybasia). A bizarre developmental anomaly of the occipital bone and upper cervical spine with striking and misleading neurologic manifestations. *Yale J Biol Med.* 1939;11:487–496.
34. Goel A, Sathe P, Shah A. Atlantoaxial fixation for basilar invagination without obvious atlantoaxial instability (group B basilar invagination): outcome analysis of 63 surgically treated cases. *World Neurosurg.* 2017;99:164–170.
35. Goel A. Instability and basilar invagination. *J Craniovertebr Junction Spine.* 2012;3:1–2.
36. Goel A, Nadkarni T, Shah A, Sathe P, Patil M. Radiologic evaluation of basilar invagination without obvious atlantoaxial instability (group B basilar invagination): analysis based on a study of 75 patients. *World Neurosurg.* 2016;95:375–382.
37. Goel A. Is atlantoaxial instability the cause of Chiari malformation? Outcome analysis of 65 patients treated by atlantoaxial fixation. *J Neurosurg Spine.* 2015;22:116–127.
38. Goel A, Jain S, Shah A. Radiological evaluation of 510 cases of basilar invagination with evidence of atlantoaxial instability (group a basilar invagination). *World Neurosurg.* 2018;110:533–543.
39. Goel A. Is Chiari malformation nature's protective "airbag"? Is its presence diagnostic of atlantoaxial instability? *J Craniovertebr Junction Spine.* 2014;5:107–109.
40. Goel A, Prasad A, Shah A, Gore S, Dharurkar P. Voice quality affection as a symptom of Chiari formation. *World Neurosurg.* 2019;121:e296–e301.
41. Goel A, Kaswa A, Shah A. Atlantoaxial fixation for treatment of Chiari formation and syringomyelia with no craniovertebral bone anomaly: report of an experience with 57 cases. *Acta Neurochir Suppl.* 2019;125:101–110.

Clinical Correlations to Specific Phenotypes and Measurements With Classification Systems

PETER R. SWIATEK[a] • ERIC J. SANDERS[a] • ERIK B. GERLACH[a] •
RICHARD W. NICOLAY[a] • MICHAEL H. MCCARTHY[b]
[a]Northwestern Memorial Hospital, Department of Orthopaedic Surgery, Chicago, IL, United States,
[b]Indiana Spine Group, Carmel, IN, United States

INTRODUCTION

Trauma to the upper cervical spine can result in a spectrum of pathology, ranging from benign to catastrophic. Upper cervical spine fractures account for nearly 70% of all cervical injuries in elderly adults and more than 35% of cervical injuries in young adults resulting in significant neurologic damage, chronic pain, and serious disability.[1] Proper diagnosis, stabilization, and definitive management of upper cervical spine injuries are critical to avoid short- and long-term mortality and morbidity. Over the last several decades, numerous classification schemes have been developed to assist clinicians and surgeons in proper medical and surgical decision-making. This chapter aims (1) to present the various classification systems for describing upper cervical spine injuries, (2) to discuss the clinical correlates associated with each classification, specifically management of upper cervical spine injuries, and (3) to critique the classification based upon literature review.

Understanding the clinical implications of upper cervical spine injuries requires a robust understanding of the craniovertebral junction and upper cervical spine anatomy (Fig. 1). The atlantooccipital joint is ellipsoid or kidney bean in shape and consists of the occipital condyles superiorly and the superior facet of C1 lateral mass inferiorly. The joint is supported by ligamentous craniocervical structures connecting the borders of the foramen magnum with the arches of the atlas.[2] The ligamentous anatomy of this joint is critical in maintaining stability and can be divided into intrinsic and extrinsic structures.

The extrinsic ligaments include the anterior atlantooccipital membrane, which is the broad and dense continuation of the anterior longitudinal ligament (ALL) and the posterior atlantooccipital ligament, which is a broad and thin continuation of the ligamentum flavum.[3] The intrinsic ligaments originate from the posterior aspect of the anterior ring of C1 and the odontoid process with three layers of ligamentous structures providing the bulk of support to the craniovertebral articulation. The apical and alar ligaments, commonly referred to as the odontoid ligaments, form the anteriormost layer. The apical ligament is a relatively weak midline structure extending from the odontoid process to the anterior margin of the foramen magnum. The alar ligaments are a pair of thick cord-like structures extending anterolaterally from the odontoid process to the occipital condyles to limit extreme atlantoaxial rotation. In the middle lay the transverse ligament, which connects the posterior odontoid of C2 to the anterior arch of C1. Most posterior in this ligamentous bundle is the tectorial membrane, which is a broad, strong band-like continuation of the posterior longitudinal ligament (PLL) connecting the odontoid body to the anterior foramen magnum. These intrinsic ligaments provide the primary constraint to extreme flexion (i.e., bony atlantooccipital articulation), extension (i.e., tectorial membrane), rotation and lateral flexion (i.e., alar ligaments), and distraction (i.e., tectorial membrane and alar ligaments).[3]

OCCIPITAL CONDYLE FRACTURE

Introduction

In 1817, Sir Charles Bell provided the first scientific report of a patient with an occipital condyle fracture (OCF). Per his account, a man fell backward off a 5-ft wall, striking his head. The man recovered in

A

B

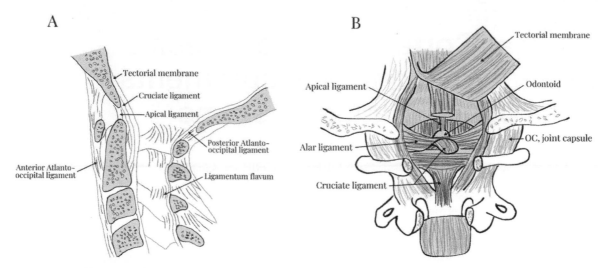

FIG. 1 Ligaments of the upper cervical spine. (A) Illustration showing a posterior view of the ligaments of the craniovertebral junction. (B) Illustration showing a sagittal view of the ligaments of the craniovertebral junction. (Source: Illustrated by Erik Gerlach. Modified from Karam YR, Traynelis VC. Occipital condyle fractures. *Neurosurgery*. 2010. https://doi.org/10.1227/01.NEU.0000365751.84075.66.)

the hospital, seeming to have experienced only a minor concussion. However, when he was preparing to leave the hospital, he turned his head in gathering his belongings and lost consciousness and died. The autopsy revealed a displaced occipital condyle fragment compressing the medulla oblongata.[4] Historically, the presence of occipital condyle fractures has been difficult to diagnose owing to the low visibility on plain radiographic imaging of the skull and cervical spine.[5, 6] Now, however, with the increased availability of computed tomography (CT) and widespread use of CT in the standard trauma protocols for suspected craniocervical injury, we know that OCF injuries are more common than once thought. Although the exact prevalence of OCF is unknown, the incidence is estimated to be up to 16% among patients suffering severe craniocervical injury[7] and between 0.1% and 0.4% of all trauma patients.[8, 9] Additionally, more than 20% of patients with OCF injuries have associated cervical spine injuries, primarily at C1 and C2.[3] Despite the rarity of OCF injuries, prompt evaluation, identification, and management of these injuries are imperative, as delayed diagnosis and treatment may be catastrophic.

Clinical presentation of patients with occipital condyle fractures is variable and largely dependent upon severity and presence of concomitant vascular, cranial, or brain stem injury. Other than a history of trauma, general high cervical neck pain, or loss of consciousness,[10] patients may suffer lower cranial nerve injury known as Collet-Sicard syndrome.[11, 12] Symptoms

include difficulty swallowing and hoarseness (CN XI or glossopharyngeal nerve and CN X or vagus nerve), difficulty shrugging shoulders (CN XI or cranial nerve), or difficulty chewing or talking due to tongue weakness (CN XII or hypoglossal nerve).[11] Occasionally, the presence of retropharyngeal hematoma, often seen on advanced imaging, may be the only indication that a craniovertebral insult has occurred.[6] A number of classifications have been devised to describe and categorize occipital condyle fractures based upon fracture morphology, soft tissue injury, or pattern of instability.

Anderson-Montesano Classification

In 1988, Paul Anderson and Pasquale Montesano devised an OCF classification based upon fracture morphology, pertinent anatomy, and biomechanics of OCF injuries in a total of 26 patients (Fig. 2).[10] Their classification is as follows:

- **Type I:** Impacted occipital condyle fracture
  - Results from axial loading of the skull onto C1 and compression of the condyle onto the superior facet of the C1 lateral mass
  - Occipital condyle demonstrates comminution with little or no displacement
  - Ipsilateral alar likely intact given minimal fragment displacement
  - **Generally a stable injury** if intact contralateral alar ligament and tectorial membrane with minimal or no displacement of ipsilateral condyle fragments

A   **B**   **C**

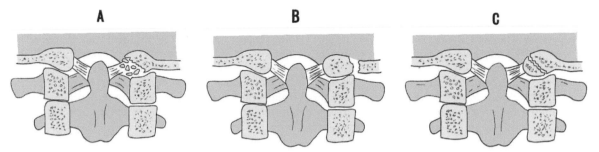

FIG. 2 Anderson-Montesano classification. Illustration demonstrating (A) Type I, (B) Type II, and (C) Type III occipital condyle fracture according to Anderson and Montesano. (Source: Illustrated by Erik Gerlach. Modified from Karam YR, Traynelis VC. Occipital condyle fractures. *Neurosurgery*. 2010. https://doi.org/10.1227/01.NEU.0000365751.84075.66.)

- **Type II:** Basilar skull fracture that exits through occipital condyle(s)
  - Results from a direct blow to the skull
  - Occipital condyle demonstrates fracture line exiting into the foramen magnum
  - Fragment is generally nondisplaced or minimally displaced
  - Alar ligament likely intact given minimal or no displacement of condyle fragment
  - **Generally a stable injury** if intact contralateral alar ligament and tectorial membrane with minimal or no displacement of condyle fragment
- **Type III:** Avulsion fracture of occipital condyle
  - Results from excessive occipitocervical rotation or lateral bending
  - Occipital condyle demonstrates fractured fragment displaced toward odontoid tip indicating occipitocervical dissociation
  - Ipsilateral alar ligament is compromised, and contralateral alar ligament and tectorial membrane are loaded
  - **Generally an unstable injury** given the incompetent ipsilateral alar ligament complex which leads to overloading of the contralateral alar ligament and tectorial membrane

Tuli et al. Classification

Although the Anderson-Montesano classification of OCF injuries is touted as the first major classification that associates fracture pattern with instability, the extent to which it accurately predicted stability and directed treatment strategy is controversial. In 1997, Tuli et al. attempted to address these shortcomings by introducing a new classification scheme based upon the degree of ligamentous injury based upon CT and overall occipital-atlantoaxial instability as determined by X-ray and MRI.[13] They retrospectively reviewed 3 cases

from their home institution and 96 cases reported in the literature to devise three specific endpoints of their treatment algorithm. The Tuli et al. classification is as follows:
- **Type I:** Stable, nondisplaced occipital condyle fracture
  - Diagnosed with CT only, no XR or MRI required
  - No immobilization required
- **Type II:** Displaced, stable occipital condyle fracture
  - CT/XR without evidence of O-C1-C2 instability*
  - Hard collar required
- **Type III:** Displaced, unstable occipital condyle fracture
  - CT/XR with evidence of O-C1-C2 instability*
  - Halo vest or surgical fixation required
- *Criteria of O-C1-C2 instability as derived from biomechanical analyses of spinal instability by White and Panjabi include any one of the following[13–15]:
  - CT/XR criteria of O-C1-C2 instability
    - > 8-degree axial rotation of O-C1 to one side
    - > 1 mm of O-C1 translation
    - > 7 mm of overhang of C1 on C2
    - > 45 degrees of axial rotation of C1-C2 to one side
    - > 4 mm of C1-C2 translation
    - < 13 mm distance between the posterior body of C2 to C1 posterior ring
    - Avulsed transverse ligament
  - MR evidence of ligamentous disruption

When comparing the Tuli et al. classification to the Anderson-Montesano classification, it is clear that additional imaging and more stringent criteria for ligamentous instability offer a more specific indication of ligamentous injury. In their retrospective review of 24 patients with OCF injuries, Byström et al. compared multiple OCF classification schemes. They noted certain difficulties with the Anderson-Montesano classification, specifically differentiating Type I versus Type III categorization for three of their patients. Additionally, of the seven patients who were determined to have unstable OCF injuries by Anderson-Montesano, only one of the seven was determined to have unstable OCF patterns by Tuli et al.[16] Although both the Anderson-Montesano and Tuli et al. classifications provide a framework for understanding occipital condyle fractures and risk of ligamentous instability, they are not generally used by spine surgeons. There is disagreement in the literature regarding the definition of fracture displacement, criteria for instability, and management recommendations for stable nondisplaced OCF injuries and of bilateral OCF injuries.[9, 17, 18]

Some suggest that the Anderson-Montesano and Tuli et al. classification schemes are more useful for academic purposes and less important for determining treatment. In their retrospective review of 106 OCFs, Maserati et al. concluded that detailed classification of OCF injuries, beyond the identification of craniocervical misalignment on CT (i.e., O-C1 interval > 2.0 mm[19, 20]), does not affect the clinical decision-making process. They suggest that OCF injuries showing disruption of the O-C1 joint or neural compression should be treated with fusion surgery, while all others could be treated with a rigid cervical orthosis.[9]

OCCIPITOCERVICAL INSTABILITY AND DISLOCATION

Introduction

Instability at the occipitocervical junction portends a serious risk of severe neurologic morbidity and mortality if left undiagnosed and untreated. Although commonly associated with traumatic atlantooccipital dislocation (AOD), more indolent conditions and disorders such as inflammatory arthropathy, rheumatoid arthritis, neoplasm, and infection may lead to instability at the occipitocervical junction.[21-24] Patients may present with acute neurologic changes, following trauma, or with more progressive neurologic changes and craniocervical deformity, seen in atraumatic cases of instability.[21, 25] Following traumatic injury, AOD often results in an incongruent association between one or both occipital condyles and the paired C1 lateral mass. The most sensitive method for diagnosing traumatic AOD has traditionally been the measurement of the basion axial-basion dens interval on computed tomography (CT).[26] In addition to O-C1 joint dislocation, more than half (~ 55%) of the cases of AOD are associated with atlantoaxial injury, instability, or frank dislocation.[26] MRI may be indicated for the identification of

ligamentous disruption and rotational instability of the upper cervical spine. For atraumatic conditions, such as rheumatoid arthritis, CT and MRI may be equally as important for diagnosing O-C1 instability, as RA patients with occipitocervical instability who are treated conservatively generally suffer a poor outcome.[27, 28] With respect to classification schemes, occipitocervical instability has primarily been described in association with trauma.

Traynelis Classification

In 1986, Traynelis et al. published a simple classification for AOD based upon a review of 17 patients who survived more than 48 hours after AOD injury.[29] Type of injury is based primarily upon radiographic and CT findings of displacement or dislocation of the occiput relative to the atlas (Fig. 3). Thresholds for defining the degree of displacement were previously published. Powers et al. discuss the relationship among four bony landmarks of the occipitocervical spine, specifically the ratio of the basion (B) to C1 posterior arch distance (C) and the opisthion (O) to the C1 anterior arch distance (A) (Fig. 3A1).[30] A "Powers ratio" greater than 1.0 is indicative of AOD and is most sensitive for detecting anterior dislocations.[31] In rare instances, such as patients with congenital anomalies,[32] a posterior dislocation injury,[33] or a pure distraction injury,[34] the Powers ratio may be less than 1.0 despite the presence of AOD. The Traynelis classification accounts for horizontal displacement as measured by the distance between the mandible to the anterior arch of the atlas and the mandible to the anterior aspect of the odontoid. The standard measurements for each relationship are 2 mm and 10 mm, respectively (Fig. 3A2).[35] Lastly, Traynelis et al. included an assessment of longitudinal distraction measured from the occipital condyle to the superior facet of C1 (occipital-C1 interval or CCI). A gap greater than 5 mm in pediatric patients[19, 34] and greater than 2 mm in adult patients indicated AOD.[20] Using these parameters, Traynelis classified AOD as follows (Fig. 3B):

- **Type I:** Anterior displacement of the occiput relative to C1
- **Type II:** Longitudinal distraction of the occiput relative to C1
- **Type III:** Posterior displacement of the occiput relative to C1

Historically, the purpose of this classification served to describe the type of AOD and to suggest which types of injury may improve with axial traction. Traynelis et al. proposed that longitudinal traction in a Type II AOD may not be indicated, as it would only exacerbate, rather than reduce, the original injury. Instead, the group suggested

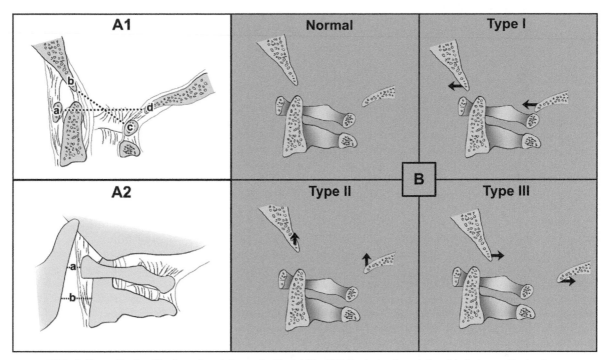

FIG. 3 Traynelis classification of occipitocervical instability. (A1) illustrates the relationship between the basion (b) and posterior arch of C1 (c) and the relationship between the anterior arch of C1 (a) and the opisthion (o). (A2) demonstrates the relationship between the posterior border of the mandible and anterior arch of C1 (a) and the odontoid (b). (B) shows the normal relationship between the occiput relative to C1. Type I is anterior displacement. Type 2 is longitudinal traction. Type 3 is posterior displacement. (Source: Illustrated by Erik Gerlach and Richard Nicolay. Modified from Traynelis VC, Marano GD, Dunker RO, Kaufman HH. Traumatic atlanto-occipital dislocation. Case report. *J Neurosurg*. 1986. https://doi.org/10.3171/jns.1986.65.6.0863.)

that longitudinal traction is best used in cases of Type I or Type III AOD injuries. At the time, case reports suggested that cervical traction safely reduced bony structures, restored alignment, and decompressed the cord, resolving major neurologic deficits in Type I and Type III injuries—injuries in which the primary displacement was not longitudinal.[29] More recent literature, however, recommends against cervical traction and instead suggests immediate immobilization, followed by halo fixation and/or occipitocervical fusion. Cervical traction has been shown to increase the risk of neurologic deterioration by nearly 10% in cases of AOD.[36] Aside from the questionable indications for cervical traction, Traynelis' classification has additionally been critiqued for not accounting for coronal or rotational occipitocervical malalignment. Additionally, without a detailed examination of the ligamentous structures, head positioning during imaging could result in "normal" radiographic parameters despite ligamentous compromise. Lastly, the classification system does not address the severity of the injury.[22]

Harborview Classification of Craniocervical Injury

In 2006, Bellabarba et al. published a new, three-stage classification system that accounts for potential upper cervical ligamentous instability and injury severity.[22] Their group retrospectively analyzed 17 consecutive cases of patients surviving AOD between 1994 and 2002 and found a significant delay between time of presentation and time of proper diagnosis of AOD. This lag time led was associated with a delay to surgical fixation and worse neurologic outcomes compared to those treated acutely. The classification leverages MRI data to determine ligamentous strain or disruption and anatomic measurement, such as the BAI and BDI to determine displacement. Harborview classification of craniocervical injury is as follows:

- **Stage 1:** Stable, minimally or nondisplaced
  - MRI evidence of injury to craniocervical osseoligamentous stabilizers
  - Craniocervical alignment within 2 mm of normal

- Distraction of ≤ 2 mm on provocative traction radiography
- For example, unilateral alar ligament injuries, partial ligamentous strains
- **Stage 2:** Unstable, partially or complete spontaneously reduced
  - MRI evidence of injury to craniocervical osseoligamentous stabilizers
  - Craniocervical alignment within 2 mm of normal
  - Distraction of > 2 mm on provocative traction radiography
- **Stage 3:** Unstable, displaced, or unreduced
  - Craniocervical malalignment of > 2 mm on static radiography

Stage 1 injuries typically can be treated nonoperatively, while Stage 2 and 3 injuries require rigid internal fixation. One criticism of the classification is that no patients in the author' series suffered a Stage 1 injury. Therefore, a direct comparison of these diagnostic parameters is not feasible.[26, 37] Another criticism of the Harborview classification is the inclusion of dynamic traction radiography in the diagnostic criteria, particularly for distinguishing between Stage 1 and Stage 2 injury.[26] Data in support of using dynamic traction radiography come primarily from biomechanical studies using cadaver models. Child et al. found that craniocervical traction reliability evaluates instability and requires only 5–10 pounds of traction.[38] Although dynamic traction may be considered the gold standard for diagnosing craniocervical instability, the safety and utility of dynamic traction radiography have not been well studied clinically in the context of acute spine trauma. Additionally, several authors recommend against acute traction given the possibility of further neurologic deterioration.[29, 36, 39]

C1 FRACTURES
Introduction
Fractures of the first cervical vertebra (C1) or atlas are of low incidence and relatively low risk of neurologic injury when occurring in isolation, comprising 2%–13% of all cervical spine fractures and up to 25% of C1-C2 complex injuries.[40–44] The distinct osseous and ligamentous anatomy of the atlas renders it a highly mobile, articular ring of the craniovertebral junction (CVJ), facilitating approximately half of the flexion-extension and rotational motion of the cervical axis. This motion occurs at the atlantooccipital and atlanto-axial complexes, respectively. As an integral component to CVJ stability, unique consideration is required in the context of injury and fracture. Atlas fractures most often

are the result of an axial load—impact of occipital condyle on atlas ring—with variable secondary vectors of forward flexion, extension, and lateral bending.[43, 45–47] Albeit risk of neurologic deficit is rare in isolated atlas injuries, appraisal of fracture stability determines the risk of unacceptable cervical dysfunction, delayed deformity, and contributes to treatment selection.

Jefferson, Landells and Van Peteghem, Gehweiler, Levine and Edwards Classification
No single accepted classification of atlas fractures exists. Sir Geoffrey Jefferson, as published in 1919, provided the first complied description of atlas fractures and theorized mechanisms of failure.[46] In a review of 46 atlas fractures—derived from 2 personal cases, 2 dry museum specimens, and 42 published case-reports—Jefferson deduced an anatomical description of atlas fracture patterns, "sites of fracture of the atlas ring." Later to be attributed as the first atlas fracture classification scheme, Jefferson described the following patterns:

- **Type I:** Posterior arch in isolation
- **Type II:** Anterior arch in isolation
- **Type III:** One or more fractures including both arches
- **Type IV:** Lateral mass or masses in isolation
- **Type V:** Lateral mass or masses and posterior arch

Jefferson's classification is as notated in Table IV of his original publication, and various iterations of his classification exist in the literature.[46] What is most commonly referred to as a "Jefferson's fracture" is a Jefferson Type III, also known as an atlas burst fracture given the predominant axial mechanism and pattern of fragment dispersion (Fig. 4). Classifications since Jefferson's initial description are numerous and include those of Landells and Van Peteghem, Gehweiler et al., and Levine and Edwards. Each system restructures Jefferson's descriptions with the variable addition of transverse process fractures and primary pattern modifications.[41, 48–50] Regional preference of classifications is prevalent with Landells and Van Peteghem's reaching proclivity in the United States and Gehweiler's being most commonly reported in European literature. In a review of 35 atlas fractures, Landells and Van Peteghem proposed their three-part classification consolidating Jefferson's descriptions:

- **Type I:** Confined to a single arch, either anterior or posterior.
- **Type II:** One or more fractures including both arches.
- **Type III:** Lateral mass with fracture extension, if present, limited to one arch.[41]

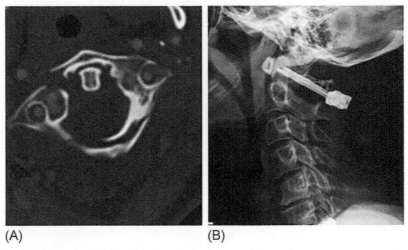

(A)   (B)

FIG. 4 Jefferson's fracture. (A) CT axial reformat of a Jefferson's burst fracture of the C1 vertebra characterized by the disruption of the anterior and posterior arch. (B) Postoperative radiographs of C1 osteosynthesis. (Source: No permission required.)

Lateral mass fractures with the involvement of both arches would satisfy the criterion of Landells and Van Peteghem Type II. Landells and Van Peteghem reported an overall C2 fracture incidence of 4.7% among 750 cervical spine injuries comprised of 45.7% Type I, 37.1% Type II, and 17.1% Type III variants. Overall, the variability of prevalence exists among atlas fracture literature with burst fractures, posterior arch, and lateral mass variants accounting for 20%–30% of all fracture descriptions.[50, 51] The Jefferson and Landells and Van Peteghem classifications are simultaneously exhibited within Fig. 5.[41] Gehweiler's five-part classification is more analogous to Jefferson's descriptions with the supplement of transverse process fractures and transverse atlantal ligament assessment:

- **Type I:** Anterior arch in isolation
- **Type II:** Posterior arch in isolation
- **Type IIIa:** Anterior and posterior arch with the integrity of the transverse atlantal ligament
- **Type IIIb:** Anterior and posterior arch with the disruption of the transverse atlantal ligament
- **Type IV:** Lateral mass in isolation
- **Type V:** Transverse process in isolation[50, 52]

Description of transverse atlantal ligament (TAL) integrity provides management implications contingent on the nature of the ligamentous disruption. TAL assessment, classification, and management considerations will be discussed in the following sections. Although better known for their descriptive contributions to C2 "Hangman" fractures, Levine and Edwards provide the final atlas fracture classification to be discussed. Their proposed primary classification types are as follows:

- **Type I:** Posterior arch in isolation
- **Type II:** Lateral mass in isolation, unless Type VII
- **Type III:** Anterior and posterior arch fractures
- **Type IV:** Avulsion fracture from the anterior arch
- **Type V:** Transverse process fracture
- **Type VI:** Anterior arch fracture, not an avulsion etiology
- **Type VII:** Comminuted unilateral intra-articular lateral mass fracture[49]

Levine and Edwards "Type IV" injuries in contrast to "Type VI" are generally of horizontal morphology and may have incomplete involvement of the anterior arch from longus coli avulsion. In aggregation, these taxonomic arrangements describe most atlas fracture patterns or variants thereof aside from behavioral distinct sagittal lateral mass fractures as described by Bransford et al.[51] Aside from Gehweiler "Type IIIb" injuries, the discussed classifications provide limited practicality for distinction in management. Validation studies are suitably deficient, and their use is limited to descriptive purposes. Table 1 displays each classification organized by anatomic location of fracture for ease of comparison. The AOSpine Upper Cervical Spine Trauma classification details fractures and ligamentous injuries of the entire occipito-atlantoaxial complex (O-C2), and its application and utility will be discussed in the coming sections. In the absence of a ubiquitously accepted fracture classification system, the determination of atlas

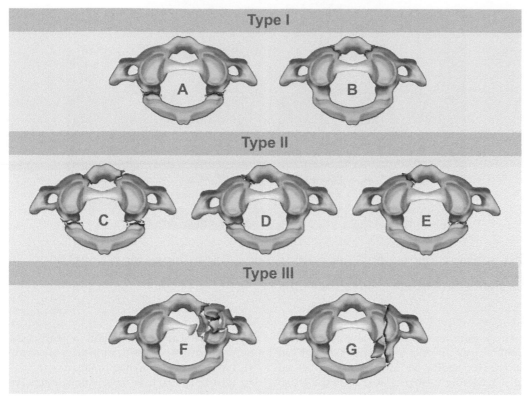

FIG. 5 Landells and Van Peteghem classification of atlas fractures. (A, B) Landells and Van Peteghem "Type I." Posterior arch (Jefferson "Type I") and anterior arch (Jefferson "Type II"), respectively. (C, D, E) Landells and Van Peteghem "Type II" and Jefferson "Type III." One or more fractures of anterior and posterior arch. (F, G) Landells and Van Peteghem "Type III." Lateral mass (Jefferson "Type IV") and lateral mass with posterior arch extension (Jefferson "Type V"), respectively. (Source: Illustrated by Richard Nicolay. Modified from Dickman CA, Greene KA, Sonntag VKH. Injuries involving the transverse Atlantal ligament: classification and treatment guidelines based upon experience with 39 injuries. *Neurosurgery*. 1996;38(1):44–50. https://doi.org/10.1097/00006123-199601000-00012.)

TABLE 1
Atlas Fracture Classifications by Anatomic Location.

Anatomic Location	Jefferson	Landells et al.	Gehweiler	Levine et al.
Posterior arch	I	I	II	I
Anterior arch	II	I	I	IV (avulsion), VI
Anterior arch, posterior arch	III	II	IIIa, IIIb (TAL disruption)	III
Lateral mass	IV	III	IV	II, VII (comminuted)
Lateral mass + arch	VI (posterior)	III (either)	IV	II, VII (comminuted)
Transverse process			V	V

Roman numeral denotation indicates classification type. Posterior arch fracture, Jefferson "Type I."
Source: No permission required, modified as required.

fracture stability using imaging-based standards guides evaluation and treatment considerations.

Assessing Atlas Stability, Dickman Classification of Transverse Atlantal Ligament Injury

The mechanics of force distribution and atlas failure under axial overload were first described in Jefferson's original publication, "the direction of this force is a horizontal one, and the net result of the crush of the atlas is, therefore, a lateral spread, a separation of the two lateral masses from one another, and a consequent tension fracture at one or more of the weak points in the atlas ring."[46] In the sagittal plane, the atlas is an osseous ring comprised of two lateral articular masses connected by anterior and posterior osseous arches. Each lateral mass is in articular congruity with the occipital condyles and superior axial articular facets. The anterior arch additionally articulates with the C2 dens. In coronal cross section, the C1 lateral masses form apex medial, wedge-shaped articular pillars that under axial load disseminate force in a tensile, centripetal distribution throughout the contiguous C1 ring. Osseous integrity is accordingly paramount for load distribution and stability under axial load. Fractures at a singular point in the ring or at a solitary arch are otherwise generally stable from displacement due to residual ring continuity. Under the context of anterior and posterior arch fractures (Jefferson Type III burst fracture), atlas stability and resistance to lateral mass dispersion are reliant on transverse atlantal ligament (TAL) integrity. The TAL inserts on the medial tubercle of each lateral mass forming a ligamentous sling dorsal to the C2 dens, serving as restraint to anterior subluxation of C1 relative to C2 and lateral mass dispersion in the event of burst pattern fractures. Although the atlantodens relationship relies on multiple myoligamentous and ligamentous stabilizers, the TAL is biomechanically the most significant ligamentous restraint to burst fracture displacement. In the context of isolated atlas fractures, assessing the integrity of the TAL is axiomatic to determining atlantoaxial stability.[40, 53]

As with all cervical injuries, evaluation requires radiographic assessment. Evaluation of the atlas compels at minimum AP open-mouth odontoid and lateral cervical radiographs. Coronal and sagittal computerized tomography (CT) reformats, respectively, are higher resolution substitutes. Flexion-extension radiographs are used at some institutions depending on concern for gross instability, mechanism of injury, and patient presentation. The atlantodental interval (ADI) should be assessed on lateral cervical radiographs or sagittal CT reformats. ADI is the distance from the posterior cortex of the anterior alar arch to the anterior cortex of the dens. Radiographic values < 3 mm in adults and < 5 mm in skeletally immature adolescents have been traditionally accepted to indicate an intact TAL. Values greater than these findings indicate possible TAL disruption and further evaluation.[42, 54] Increased utilization of magnetic resonance imaging (MRI) has demonstrated that up to 82% of TAL injuries with associated atlas fractures may have ADI less than 3 mm with an average of ADI assessment of 1.8 mm according to Perez et al.[55] The use of ADI on flexion-extension radiographs has similarly shown a 25% false-negative detection rate of TAL injury.[56] Further evidence is likely required before ADI can be recommended as an absolute criterion. Lack of ADI diastasis does not rule out injury; however, its presence requires high suspicion of TAL disruption.

Posterior arch fractures may be identified on lateral radiographs. As an axial injury in hyperextension, posterior arch fractures can be associated with 50% prevalence of injuries elsewhere in the cervical spine.[43, 49] Thorough evaluation for injury at other levels is warranted.[48] Assessment of lateral films should additionally include appraisal of the retropharyngeal soft tissue shadow. Measurement is assessed from the ventral aspect of the anterior vertebral body to the soft tissue-air interface of the trachea. Evidence has shown a limited detection rate for injury with a sensitivity of 14.4% at C2 according to Hiratzka et al.; however, many recommend a value > 7 mm at C2 may indicate the possibility of anterior arch fractures or other concomitant upper cervical anterior pathology.[48, 49, 51, 57, 58] Further assessment with tomography would be indicated.

Assessment of the lateral mass alignment of C1-C2 is visualized on open-mouth odontoid radiographs or coronal CT reformats. Lateral mass displacement (LMD) is the combined distance from the lateral margin of C2 to the lateral margin of the C1 lateral mass (Fig. 6). LMD as an indication of TAL injury was first described by Spence et al. in 1970 using cadaveric models.[59] In assessment of the biomechanical force and lateral mass excursion required for TAL rupture in 10 cadaver specimens, "Spence's rule" defines > 6.9 mm of combined LMD as indicative of TAL incompetency. Heller et al. later determined that AP open-mouth odontoid radiographs have an inherent magnification of 18%; therefore, LMD threshold of 8.1 mm should be used in radiographs with magnification.[60] Dickman et al. and others have since demonstrated the limited diagnostic sensitivity of Spence's LMD threshold as compared to MR interpretation of TAL injury. In a

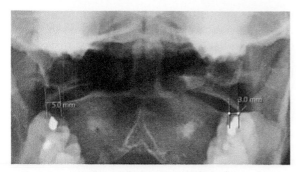

FIG. 6 AP open-mouth odontoid demonstrating measurement of lateral mass displacement (LMD). LMD is assessed from the lateral aspect of C2 articular body to the lateral aspect of C1 lateral mass. This demonstrates an LMD of 8 mm. "Rule of Spence" suggests LMD > 6.9 mm as indicative of TAL injury. (Source: Permission not required.)

study of 23 atlas fractures, only 39% would have been diagnosed as TAL incompetent, rendering underdiagnosis or false-negative rate of 61% in TAL-disrupted atlas fractures.[56, 61] Further studies have shown Spence's and Heller's LMD criterion (6.9–8.1 mm) to result in 50%–90% under-diagnosis of TAL failure as compared to MR evaluation.[55, 56, 61–63] In skeletally immature adolescents less than 7 years old, pseudospread of the C1-C2 lateral borders can mimic a burst fracture due to a physiologically widened LMD.[64] Further evaluation on axial CT is recommended as pending clinical suspicion.

Dickman's classification of TAL injury provides functional delineation of the healing and management characteristics of TAL injury subtypes (Fig. 7).

- **Type IA:** Intratendinous or midsubstance TAL rupture
- **Type IB:** Disruption at the osteoperiosteal interface of TAL insertion
- **Type IIA:** Comminuted fracture of the lateral mass resulting in loss of TAL integrity

- **Type IIB:** Avulsion of the medial tubercle resulting in loss of TAL integrity[65–69]

Type I injuries indicate ligamentous disruption of the TAL without fracture or osseous injury to the C1 lateral mass. Most clinicians approach Type I injuries under the assumption that they lack the capacity to heal tendon-tendon disruption and require surgical stabilization. Instability following conservative management of an atlas burst fracture may indicate the under-diagnosis of a Type 1 injury. MR assessment is required for diagnosis. Lack of agreement in intervention exists with the general consensus being surgical management with C1-2 fusion or isolated C1 cross-linked constructs.[52, 70] As common to other atlas injuries, concomitant upper cervical spine pathology often dictates treatment. Type II injuries are secondary to fracture and osseous failure of the TAL to lateral mass connection. Evidence suggests a 74%–85.7% rate of stable outcome in Type II disruptions with nonoperative management. Close follow-up for evidence of instability is required.[56, 62]

Similar to ADI assessment critiques, lack of LMD diastasis does not rule out injury but its presence requires high suspicion of TAL disruption. In observation of current evidence, the traditional criterion of LMD and ADI thresholds cannot be recommended as stand-alone clinical guidelines for defining TAL disruption and atlas stability. The presence of LMD and ADI diastasis remains significant as to their specificity of potential TAL injury in the correct clinical context. At this time, MR assessment of TAL integrity is recommended. Further studies are required to determine CT-guided criteria for TAL disruption without MR evaluation.[63, 71] Evidence of flexion, extension CT reformats is of limited clinical purpose at this time but may prove useful in patient care settings without expeditious access to MRI.[71] Recognition of TAL injury is critical for the prevention of impaired outcomes secondary to late atlantoaxial instability. Evidence of its disruption is hallmark to diagnosing atlas instability.

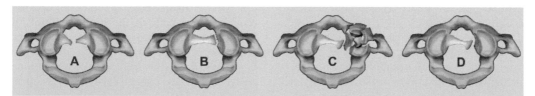

FIG. 7 Dickman classification of transverse atlantal ligament (TAL) injuries. (A) "Type 1a" intratendinous TAL disruption. (B) "Type 1b" disruption at the TAL osteoperiosteal interface. (C) "Type 2a" comminuted fracture of the lateral mass resulting in loss of TAL integrity. (D) "Type 2b" avulsion of the medial tubercle resulting in loss of TAL integrity. (Source: Illustrated by Richard Nicolay. Modified from Dickman CA, Greene KA, Sonntag VKH. Injuries involving the transverse Atlantal ligament: classification and treatment guidelines based upon experience with 39 injuries. *Neurosurgery*. 1996;38(1):44–50. https://doi.org/10.1097/00006123-199601000-00012.)

Unstable Lateral Mass Fracture Variant

Sagittal unilateral lateral mass fractures are at risk of instability patterns and displacement analogous to atlas burst fractures. As viewed on axial CT reformats, the injury is characterized by sagittal disruption of the lateral mass with an otherwise intact alar ring. Bransford et al. identified this injury with relative incidence of 11% among atlas fractures, describing injury sequela of progressive cock-robin coronal deformity, limitations of rotary motion, and inhibitory discomfort. All surviving patients required deformity correction with occipitocervical fusion.[51] This pattern consists of vertical disruption of the C1 lateral articular pillar peripheral to TAL insertion, creating unrestrained lateral articular fragment(s). Under axial occipital condyle load, the lateral mass fragments extrude peripherally with occipital condyle subsidence to the superior axial facet. Cognizance of this unstable variant may allow for earlier intervention with motion sparing techniques rather than more invasive deformity correction measures.[67, 72] Identification may be apparent on AP open-mouth odontoid views with unilateral displacement of the lateral mass and coronal occiput angulation. Further delineation is recommended on axial and sagittal CT reformats, and concomitant evaluation of TAL integrity is additionally required.[51, 53]

C2 ODONTOID FRACTURES

Introduction

Fractures of the odontoid process have historically been challenging to classify due to the complexity of the anatomy, the biomechanical characteristics of the upper cervical spine, and difficulty in predicting the most appropriate treatment methods.[73] The odontoid bone consists of the tip, neck, and body. The tip is mostly cortical bone and serves as the insertion site for the apical and alar ligaments. The neck is also comprised of primarily cortical bone, forming part of the articulation with the atlas on its anterior aspect and an insertion site for the transverse ligament posteriorly. Lastly, the base is composed of primarily cancellous bone and forms the junction between the neck of the odontoid process and the body of C2. Importantly, blood is supplied to the odontoid superiorly and inferiorly, leaving the odontoid neck as a watershed zone of poor vascularity.[74] Therefore, the neck is at increased risk of injury during traumatic events. Given that the C1-C2 complex primarily allows lateral rotation and relatively constrains flexion, extension, and lateral bending, different directions of force or trauma will generate unique patterns of injury. For example,

trauma causes excessive lateral bending is most likely to produce a transverse fracture while excessive flexion or extension will produce a fracture with a sagittal fracture pattern. Extreme lateral rotation stresses the ligamentous attachments on the odontoid and produces avulsion fracture of the tip.[75]

Given the complexity of odontoid fractures, multiple groups have devised classification schemes to effectively characterize the many fracture patterns. Althoff et al.,[76] Anderson and D'Alonzo,[77] De Mourgues et al.,[78] and Schatzker[79] classify odontoid fractures by position of the fracture; Roy-Camille et al. classify odontoid fractures by direction of the fracture line;[80] and Korres et al.[75] classify the fractures by the anatomy of the odontoid process. This chapter focuses on the classic Anderson and D'Alonzo classification, still commonly favored today among clinicians.

Anderson and D'alonzo Classification

In the early 1970s, Schatzker et al. proposed a two-type classification system of odontoid fractures based upon the presence of fracture above or below the odontoid's accessory ligament.[79] In 1974, Anderson and D'Alonzo published their three-type classification systems with the intention of providing more prognostic information regarding the likelihood of bony union based upon fracture location (Fig. 8).[77] Their classification is as follows:

- **Type I:** Oblique fractures through the odontoid tip due to avulsion of the alar ligament
- **Type II:** Fracture through the odontoid neck at the junction of the body and axis
- **Type III:** Fracture extending into the body of the axis

Of all odontoid fractures, Type II fractures are considered the unstable and are at the highest risk of nonunion, especially in the cases of severely comminuted or displaced fractures in older patients with osteoporosis.[81, 82] Therefore, immobilization has been shown to be imperative for true Type II odontoid fractures—often requiring collar or halo immobilization versus anterior[83] or posterior[84] fixation. The limitations of the Anderson and D'Alonzo classification were the ambiguity in distinguishing Type II odontoid fractures from Types III fractures and limited consideration for various fracture characteristics such as fracture trajectory, comminution, or displacement.[82] In 2005, Grauer et al. devised a subtype classification of Type II odontoid fractures that included an associated treatment recommendation:

- **Type IIA:** Nondisplaced or minimally displaced (< 1 mm) odontoid neck fracture
  - Management is external immobilization

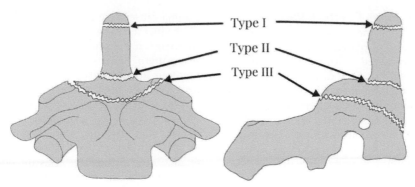

FIG. 8 Anderson and D'Alonzo classification. (A) Type 1 injuries involve the tip of the odontoid (B). Type II injuries involve the waist or base of the odontoid. (C) Type III injuries extend into the body of C2. (Source: Illustrated by Erik Gerlach. Modified from Grauer JN, Shafi B, Hilibrand AS, et al. Proposal of a modified, treatment-oriented classification of odontoid fractures. *Spine J.* 2005. https://doi.org/10.1016/j.spinee.2004.09.014.)

- **Type IIB:** Displaced (> 1 mm) odontoid neck fracture with an anterosuperior to posteroinferior fracture trajectory
  - Management is anterior odontoid screw in patients with adequate bone stock
  - Using the odontoid screw preserves much of the atlantoaxial lateral rotation compared to posterior fixation
- **Type IIC:** Displaced or comminuted odontoid neck fracture with an anteroinferior to posterosuperior fracture trajectory
  - Management is posterior fixation

Of the five spine surgeons that classified odontoid fractures based upon the aforementioned classification, Grauer et al. found interrater agreement in 70% of cases, suggesting moderate agreement and reproducibility of this subtype classification system.[82] Nevertheless, the Anderson and D'Alonzo classification of odontoid fractures still receives criticism for lack of clarification between Type II neck fractures and Type III body fractures.[73]

Several other classification systems characterize odontoid fractures based upon the position of the fracture. Althoff describes four patterns. In the first type, the fracture passes through the neck. In the second type, the fracture passes through the superior aspect of the body. The third type involves the lateral masses, and the fourth type passes through the body of the axis. Pseudarthrosis rate is highest for the first type, a pure neck fracture, and second type, superior aspect body (64% vs. 55%, respectively).[76] De Mourgues describes only two types of fractures, including through the base of the odontoid with 100% union rates and those through the neck with 50% union rates.[78] Lastly, Roy-Camille characterized odontoid fractures into three

types based upon the direction of the fracture line. Type A demonstrates posterosuperior to anteroinferior trajectory; Type B demonstrates anterosuperior to posteroinferior; and Type C is purely transverse.[80]

C2 HANGMAN'S FRACTURES
Introduction

First described by Wood-Jones in 1913 as the *ideal lesion produced by judicial hanging*,[85] the "hangman's fracture" describes a C2 fracture involving bilateral fractures of the pars interarticularis with or without anterior spondylolisthesis of the axis on C3.[86] These injuries result from excessive cervical hyperextension or axial loading and are typically associated with high-energy mechanisms, such as a motor vehicle accidents or trauma. The eponym is derived from placing the knot of a noose anteriorly leading to a hyperextension moment during execution. These fractures are typically classified by Effendi et al.[87] and modified by Levine and Edwards.[88] Different from "typical" hangman's fracture involving bilateral fractures of the pars interarticularis, atypical hangman's fracture involves fracture of only one side of the neural arch and typically one other structure, such as posterior C2 vertebral body.[89] The literature aimed at specifically characterizing atypical hangman's fracture is limited, but modifications of the traditional Levine and Edwards Classification have been proposed.[90]

Levine and Edwards Classification of Hangman's Fractures

In the 1981 retrospective review of 131 patients suffering traumatic injury to the C2, Effendi et al. classified acute injuries of the axial ring into three categories based upon radiographic displacement and stability.[87]

Shortly after, Levin and Edwards proposed a modification to the traditional classification based upon the mechanism of injury and more detailed patterns of stability.[88] The Levine and Edwards classification of hangman's fracture is as follows:

- **Type I:** Nondisplaced or minimal horizontal displacement (< 3 mm)
  - Mechanism: Hyperextension and axial loading
  - Disc: C2/3 disc intact
  - Stability: Fracture considered stable
  - Treatment: Halo vest orthosis vs. rigid cervical collar with high rates of union[91, 92]
- **Type II:** Vertical fracture line, horizontal displacement > 3 mm, angulation > 11 degrees
  - Mechanism: Hyperextension, axial loading, and rebound flexion
  - Disc: C2/3 disc incompetent, ALL may be injured, PLL usually disrupted
  - Stability: Fracture generally considered unstable
  - Treatment: Reduction and halo vest orthosis vs. surgical fixation depending upon displacement[93, 94]
- **Type IIa:** Horizontal fracture line, no horizontal displacement, angulation > 11 degrees
  - Mechanism: Flexion-distraction
  - Disc: C2/3 disc intact
  - Stability: Fracture considered unstable
  - Treatment: Reduction without traction, compression halo immobilization vs. surgical fixation depending upon displacement[93, 95]
    - Traction may increase displacement at the fracture site[96]
- **Type III:** Displacement > 3 mm, angulation > 11 degrees, and facet subluxation/dislocation
  - Mechanism: Flexion-compression
  - Disc: Generally incompetent
  - Stability: Fracture considered unstable
  - Treatment: Surgical reduction of facet dislocation and surgical fixation

Atypical Hangman's Fractures

One of the limitations of the Levine and Edwards classification is the lack of inclusion of atypical hangman's fractures, which are a variant of Type I and Type II fractures. These injuries are unique in that they are typically unilateral (i.e., single pars interarticularis affect) and involve injury to an additional bony element, such as the posterior cortex of the vertebral body. Different from Type I and Type II fractures, the atypical hangman's fracture is also thought to carry a higher risk of neurologic injury.[97] Some authors have reported these C2 fractures as a distinct subtype

of hangman's fracture,[89, 98, 99] while others consider them in the broader context of C2 body or otherwise miscellaneous fractures.[87] In 2017, Li et al. proposed a new classification for atypical hangman's fractures based upon their review of 46 patients with atypical C2 fracture patterns.

- **Type A1:** Posterior C2 body fracture, contralateral fracture of pars interarticularis
- **Type A2:** Posterior C2 body fracture, contralateral fracture of lamina
  - Highest incidence of neurologic deficit[90]
- **Type B1:** Bilateral posterior C2 body fractures
- **Type B2:** Bilateral posterior C2 body fractures, with one oblique and the contralateral fracture vertical

Given the novelty of any classification system for atypical hangman's fractures, most authors typically recommend the traditional Levine and Edwards classification be applied for guidance in treatment recommendations.[89, 90, 97] Further studies with a greater number of patients will be required to further develop and validate classification systems for atypical hangman's fractures.

AOSPINE CLASSIFICATION OF UPPER CERVICAL SPINE INJURIES
Introduction

The AOSpine Upper Cervical Classification System (UCCS) was proposed by the AOSpine Knowledge Forum to standardize upper cervical spine injury classifications into a comprehensive system of prognostic value that offers universal communication and agreement among practitioners in injury severity and treatment.[100] This system was developed under expert consensus following the AOSpine subaxial spine (C3–C7) classification system, AOSpine thoracolumbar (T1–L5) classification system, and AOSpine sacral (S1–S5, including coccyx) classification system under the intent of creating an inclusive, practical classification with the reproducibility requisite for high intra- and interobserver reliability in clinical and research practice. It condenses prior Upper Cervical Spine Trauma (UCST) classifications into the standard AO nomenclature of—A, B, C—injury morphology descriptions as localized to anatomic level of injury (I–III). As with prior classification systems, morphology is based on radiographic examination. Neurologic (N0–NX), case-specific (M1–M4) modifiers indicating neurologic status and nuances of patient-specific treatment considerations, respectively, should be applied to each classification as indicated. Sequence of classification description is in order of the four criteria: (1) level of injury, (2) morphology of injury, (3) neurologic status modifier, and (4) case-specific modifiers.[100–103]

Location and Morphology of Injury

Levels of injury within the Upper Cervical Classification System are divided into three regions:

- **Region I:** Occipital condyle "OC" and craniocervical "O-C1" joint complex
- **Region II:** Atlas "C1" ring and "C1-2" joint complex
- **Region III:** Axis "C2" and "C2-3" joint complex

The abbreviations annotated with apostrophes are used to describe the level of involvement. The three regions are uniformly subdivided into the A, B, and C injury morphologies comparable to the AOSpine subaxial, thoracolumbar, and sacral classifications.[101–103]

- **Type A:** Osseous injury only
- **Type B:** Tension band or ligamentous injury
- **Type C:** Translation injury

Type A injuries are fractures—e.g., osseous only. Type A morphology does not involve ligamentous disruption, tension band failure, or disc involvement. Injuries are generally considered stable with the basis of treatment falling under conservative therapy. An isolated anterior ring fracture of the atlas is classified as "C1 Type A." Type B injuries are either ligamentous disruption or tension band failure with implicated ligamentous disruption, with or without osseous injury. No translation of vertebral levels may be present, and alignment of the spinal axis is preserved. An atlas burst fracture with TAL injury is classified as "C1 Type B." Type B injuries are either stable or unstable depending on specific injury morphology with conservative or surgical management often being appropriate. Type C injuries are translational disruptions hallmarked by translational displacement of a vertebral level. Translation may be of any direction—anterior, posterior, lateral, or vertical. These injuries describe the separation of anatomic integrity with disruption of the spinal axis. Type C does not include angular distraction or osseous fragment displacement, and these are best described by Type A or Type B depending on the injury. Type C injuries are unstable, and management is often surgical. Any associated Type A or Type B injury is specified separately after Type C designation to preserve injury hierarchy.[100, 101]

Modifiers

Neurologic modifiers are graded (NO–NX). Six neurologic statuses exist and are consistent among all AOSpine classifications:

- **N0:** Neurologically intact
- **N1:** Transient neurological deficit

- **N2:** Radicular symptoms
- **N3:** Incomplete spinal cord injury or any degree of cauda equina injury
- **N4:** Complete spinal cord injury
- **NX:** Cannot be examined

The NX designation may be secondary to loss of consciousness, altered mental status, coexisting state of injury, or any condition that prevents the completion of an examination. The supplementary designation "+" is given to any injury with continued radiographic cord compression in the setting of an incomplete neurological deficit or nerve injury, e.g., "N3 +."[100, 101]

Case-specific clinical modifiers are used to describe patient-specific or injury-specific conditions intended to supplement clinical decision-making. The following modifiers are specific to the Upper Cervical Classification System:

- **M1:** Injuries at high risk for nonunion with nonoperative treatment (e.g., odontoid waist fracture in the elderly individual, C2 Type A, M1)
- **M2:** Injury with significant potential for instability (e.g., atlas burst fracture with ligamentous TAL disruption, C1 Type B, M2)
- **M3:** Patient-specific factors affecting treatment (e.g., medial comorbidities, ankylosing spondylitis, smoking history)
- **M4:** Vascular injury or abnormality affecting treatment (e.g., vertebral artery injury)

The use of modifiers communicates the potential need for unique consideration of patient-specific factors that may alter treatment selection. The AOSpine classification systems including their classification system visual aids and introductory videos can be found on the AOSpine website (https://aospine.aofoundation.org/) (Fig. 9).[100, 101, 104]

Validation Studies

Evidence-based validation of the AO UCCS remains limited to a single investigation at the time of authorship. Maeda et al. assessed intra- and interobserver reliability of site (I, II, III), morphology (A, B, C), and treatment recommendations. Their study reported moderate to almost perfect kappa values with experienced reviewers in higher agreement. Intraobserver reliability of (K 0.751–0.999) substantial/almost perfect and interobserver reliability of (K 0.585–0.863) moderate to almost perfect was consistently higher in site and morphology identification than treatment recommendations.[100] The AO UCCS offers promise as a universal form of communication and agreement among surgeons with further validation required prior to stand-alone use in treatment guidance.

AO Spine Upper Cervical Classification System

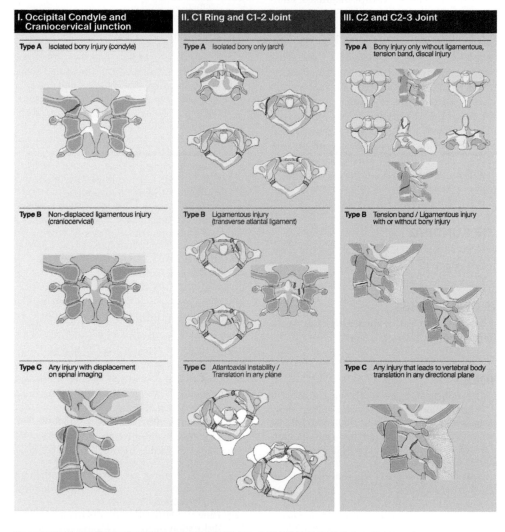

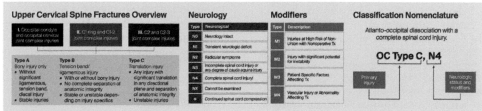

Further information:
www.aospine.org/classification

FIG. 9 AOSpine upper cervical classification system. (Source: Creative Commons Attribution-NonCommercial-No Derivatives (CC BY-NC-ND).)

CONCLUSIONS

Upper cervical spine fractures and ligamentous insults are serious injuries with the potential for catastrophic consequences if mismanaged. Prompt diagnosis, characterization, prognosis, and intervention are necessary for ensuring the best possible outcome for a patient with an upper cervical spine injury. The classification systems discussed in the chapter provide a framework for characterizing upper cervical spine injuries. Despite the evolution of classification systems, no one system entirely describes all possible injury patterns or perfectly dictates that best treatment strategy for a given fracture. Further research into the clinical correlations between various classification schemes, treatment protocols, and prognostic indicators is necessary to optimize the management of patients with upper cervical spine injuries.

SOURCE OF FUNDING

The authors received no outside funding for the work presented in this chapter.

CONFLICT OF INTEREST

The authors have no conflicts of interest related to the subject matter presented in this chapter.

REFERENCES

1. Daffner RH, Goldberg AL, Evans TC, Hanlon DP, Levy DB. Cervical vertebral injuries in the elderly: a 10-year study. *Emerg Radiol.* 1998. https://doi.org/10.1007/BF02749124.
2. Kayalioglu G. The vertebral column and spinal meninges. In: *The Spinal Cord;* 2009. https://doi.org/10.1016/B978-0-12-374247-6.50007-9.
3. Alcelik I, Manik KS, Sian PS, Khoshneviszadeh SE. Occipital condylar fractures. *J Bone Joint Surg Br.* 2006. https://doi.org/10.1302/0301-620x.88b5.16598.
4. Bell C. *Surgical observations: quarterly report of cases in surgery treated in the Middlesex Hospital.* vol. 1; 1817:469–470.
5. Chugh S, Kamian K, Depreitere B, Schwartz ML. Occipital condyle fracture with associated hypoglossal nerve injury. *Can J Neurol Sci.* 2006. https://doi.org/10.1017/S0317167100005229.
6. Karam YR, Traynelis VC. Occipital condyle fractures. *Neurosurgery.* 2010. https://doi.org/10.1227/01.NEU.0000365751.84075.66.
7. Bloom AI, Neeman Z, Slasky BS, et al. Fracture of the occipital condyles and associated craniocervical ligament injury: incidence, CT imaging and implications. *Brain Lang.* 1997. https://doi.org/10.1016/s0009-9260(97)80273-5.
8. Malham GM, Ackland HM, Jones R, Williamson OD, Varma DK. Occipital condyle fractures: incidence and clinical follow-up at a level 1 trauma centre. *Emerg Radiol.* 2009. https://doi.org/10.1007/s10140-008-0789-z.
9. Maserati MB, Stephens B, Zohny Z, et al. Occipital condyle fractures: clinical decision rule and surgical management. Clinical article. *J Neurosurg Spine.* 2009. https://doi.org/10.3171/2009.5.SPINE08866.
10. Anderson PA, Montesano PX. Morphology and treatment of occipital condyle fractures. *Spine (Phila Pa 1976).* 1988. https://doi.org/10.1097/00007632-198807000-00004.
11. Utheim NC, Josefsen R, Nakstad PH, Solgaard T, Roise O. Occipital condyle fracture and lower cranial nerve palsy after blunt head trauma - a literature review and case report. *J Trauma Manag Outcomes.* 2015. https://doi.org/10.1186/s13032-015-0024-3.
12. Collet F. Sur un novueau syndrome paralytique pharyngo-larynge par blessure de guerre (hemiplegie glosso-laryngo-scapulo-pharyngee). *Lyon Med.* 1915;124:121–129.
13. Tuli S, Tator CH, Fehlings MG, Mackay M. Occipital condyle fractures. *Neurosurgery.* 1997. https://doi.org/10.1097/00006123-199708000-00006.
14. White A, Panjabi M. *Clinical Biomechanics of the Spine.* 2nd ed. Lippincott Williams & Wilkins; 1990:752 pp. ISBN-10: 0397507208, ISBN-13: 978-0397507207.
15. Panjabi MM, White AA. Basic biomechanics of the spine. *Neurosurgery.* 1980. https://doi.org/10.1227/00006123-198007000-00014.
16. Byström O, Jensen TS, Poulsen FR. Outcome of conservatively treated occipital condylar fractures - a retrospective study. *J Craniovertebr Junction Spine.* 2017. https://doi.org/10.4103/jcvjs.JCVJS_97_17.
17. Hanson JA, Deliganis AV, Baxter AB, et al. Radiologic and clinical spectrum of occipital condyle fractures: retrospective review of 107 consecutive fractures in 95 patients. *Am J Roentgenol.* 2002. https://doi.org/10.2214/ajr.178.5.1781261.
18. Aulino JM, Tutt LK, Kaye JJ, Smith PW, Morris JA. Occipital condyle fractures: clinical presentation and imaging findings in 76 patients. *Emerg Radiol.* 2005. https://doi.org/10.1007/s10140-005-0425-0.
19. Pang D, Nemzek WR, Zovickian J. Atlanto-occipital dislocation. *Neurosurgery.* 2007. https://doi.org/10.1227/01.neu.0000290897.77448.1f.
20. Pang D, Nemzek WR, Zovickian J. Atlanto-occipital dislocation—part 2. *Neurosurgery.* 2007. https://doi.org/10.1227/01.neu.0000303196.87672.78.
21. Nockels RP, Shaffrey CI, Kanter AS, Azeem S, York JE. Occipitocervical fusion with rigid internal fixation: long-term follow-up data in 69 patients. *J Neurosurg Spine.* 2007. https://doi.org/10.3171/SPI-07/08/117.
22. Bellabarba C, Mirza SK, West GA, et al. Diagnosis and treatment of craniocervical dislocation in a series of 17 consecutive survivors during an 8-year period. *J Neurosurg Spine.* 2006. https://doi.org/10.3171/spi.2006.4.6.429.
23. Sanpakit S, Mansfield FL, Liebsch NJ. Role of onlay grafting with minimal internal fixation for occipitocervical fusion in oncologic patients. *J Spinal Disord.* 2000. https://doi.org/10.1097/00002517-200010000-00003.

24. Arunkumar MJ, Rajshekhar V. Outcome in neurologically impaired patients with craniovertebral junction tuberculosis: results of combined anteroposterior surgery. *J Neurosurg.* 2002. https://doi.org/10.3171/spi.2002.97.2.0166.

25. Deutsch H, Haid RW, Rodts GE, Mummaneni PV. Occipitocervical fixation: long-term results. *Spine (Phila Pa 1976).* 2005. https://doi.org/10.1097/01.brs.0000154715.88911.ea.

26. Horn EM, Feiz-Erfan I, Lekovic GP, Dickman CA, Sonntag VKH, Theodore N. Survivors of occipitoatlantal dislocation injuries: imaging and clinical correlates. *J Neurosurg Spine.* 2007. https://doi.org/10.3171/spi.2007.6.2.113.

27. Marks JS, Sharp J. Rheumatoid cervical myelopathy. *Q J Med.* 1981. https://doi.org/10.1097/00004728-198402000-00059.

28. Matsunaga S, Sakou T, Onishi T, et al. Prognosis of patients with upper cervical lesions caused by rheumatoid arthritis: comparison of occipitocervical fusion between C1 laminectomy and nonsurgical management. *Spine (Phila Pa 1976).* 2003. https://doi.org/10.1097/00007632-200307150-00019.

29. Traynelis VC, Marano GD, Dunker RO, Kaufman HH. Traumatic atlanto-occipital dislocation. Case report. *J Neurosurg.* 1986. https://doi.org/10.3171/jns.1986.65.6.0863.

30. Powers B, Miller MD, Kramer RS, Martinez S, Gehweiler JA. Traumatic anterior atlanto-occipital dislocation. *Neurosurgery.* 1979. https://doi.org/10.1227/00006123-197901000-00004.

31. Hall GC, Kinsman MJ, Nazar RG, et al. Atlanto-occipital dislocation. *World J Orthod.* 2015. https://doi.org/10.5312/wjo.v6.i2.236.

32. Pang D, Wilberger JE. Traumatic atlanto-occipital dislocation with survival: case report and review. *Neurosurgery.* 1980. https://doi.org/10.1227/00006123-198011000-00017.

33. Woodring JH, Selke ACDE. Traumatic atlantooccipital dislocation with survival. *Am J Neuroradiol.* 1981. https://doi.org/10.1227/00006123-198011000-00017.

34. Kaufman RA, Dunbar JS, Botsford JA, McLaurin RL. Traumatic longitudinal atlanto-occipital distraction injuries in children. *Am J Neuroradiol.* 1982;3(4):415–419.

35. Dublin AB, Marks WM, Weinstock D, Newton TH. Traumatic dislocation of the atlanto-occipital articulation (AOA) with short-term survival. With a radiographic method of measuring the AOA. *J Neurosurg.* 1980. https://doi.org/10.3171/jns.1980.52.4.0541.

36. Theodore N, Aarabi B, Dhall SS, et al. The diagnosis and management of traumatic atlanto-occipital dislocation injuries. *Neurosurgery.* 2013. https://doi.org/10.1227/NEU.0b013e31827765e0.

37. Kasliwal MK, Fontes RB, Traynelis VC. Occipitocervical dissociation—incidence, evaluation, and treatment. *Curr Rev Musculoskelet Med.* 2016. https://doi.org/10.1007/s12178-016-9347-6.

38. Child Z, Rau D, Lee MJ, et al. The provocative radiographic traction test for diagnosing craniocervical dissociation: a cadaveric biomechanical study and reappraisal of the pathogenesis of instability. *Spine J.* 2016. https://doi.org/10.1016/j.spinee.2016.03.057.

39. Radcliff K, Kepler C, Reitman C, Harrop J, Vaccaro A. CT and MRI-based diagnosis of craniocervical dislocations: the role of the occipitoatlantal ligament. *Clin Orthop Relat Res.* 2012. https://doi.org/10.1007/s11999-011-2151-0.

40. Kakarla UK, Chang SW, Theodore N, Sonntag VKH. Atlas fractures. *Neurosurgery.* 2010;66(suppl 3):60–67. https://doi.org/10.1227/01.NEU.0000366108.02499.8F.

41. Landells C, Van Peteghem PK. Fractures of the atlas: classification, treatment and morbidity. *Spine (Phila Pa 1976).* 1988;13(5):450–452.

42. Oda T, Panjabi M, Crisco J, Oxland T, Katz L, Nolt L. Experimental study of atlas injuries II: relevance to clinical diagnosis and treatment. *Spine (Phila Pa 1976).* 1991;16(10S):S466–S473.

43. Gebauer M, Goetzen N, Barvencik F, et al. Biomechanical analysis of atlas fractures: a study on 40 human atlas specimens. *Spine (Phila Pa 1976).* 2008;33(7):766–770. https://doi.org/10.1097/BRS.0b013e31816956de.

44. Greene KA, Dickman CA, Marciano FF, Drabier JB, Hadley MN, Sonntag VKH. Acute axis fractures: analysis of management and outcome in 340 consecutive cases. *Spine (Phila Pa 1976).* 1997;22(16):1843–1852. https://doi.org/10.1097/00007632-199708150-00009.

45. Sköld G. Fractures of the arches of the atlas: a study of their causation. *Z Rechtsmed.* 1983;90(4):247–258. https://doi.org/10.1007/bf02116199.

46. Jefferson G. Fracture of the atlas vertebra. Report of four cases, and a review of those previously recorded. *Br J Surg.* 1919;7(27):407–422. https://doi.org/10.1002/bjs.1800072713.

47. Proubasta I, Sancho R, Alonso J, Palacia A. Horizontal fracture of the anterior arch of the atlas. *Spine (Phila Pa 1976).* 1987;12(6):615–618.

48. Levine A, Edwards C. Traumatic lesions of the occipitoatlantoaxial complex. *Clin Orthop Relat Res.* 1989;(239):53–68.

49. Levine AM, Edwards CC. Fractures of the atlas. *J Bone Joint Surg Ser A.* 1991;73(5):680–691. https://doi.org/10.2106/00004623-199173050-00006.

50. Gehweiler JA, Duff DE, Martinez S, Miller MD, Clark WM. Fractures of the atlas vertebra. *Skelet Radiol.* 1976;1(2):97–102. https://doi.org/10.1007/BF00347414.

51. Bransford RJ, Falicov A, Ngyuen Q, Chapman J. Unilateral C-1 lateral mass sagittal split fracture: an unstable Jefferson fracture variant. *J Neurosurg Spine.* 2009;10(5):466–473.

52. Kandziora F, Chapman JR, Vaccaro AR, Schroeder GD, Scholz M. Atlas fractures and atlas osteosynthesis: a comprehensive narrative review. *J Orthop Trauma.* 2017;31(suppl. 4):S81–S89. https://doi.org/10.1097/BOT.0000000000000942.

53. Bransford RJ, Alton TB, Patel AR, Bellabarba C. Upper cervical spine trauma. *J Am Acad Orthop Surg.* 2014;22(11):718–729. https://doi.org/10.5435/JAAOS-22-11-718.

54. Fielding JW, Van Cochran BG, Lawsing JF, Hohl M. Tears of the transverse ligament of the atlas. A clinical and biomechanical study. *J Bone Joint Surg Ser A.* 1974;56(8):1683–1691. https://doi.org/10.2106/00004623-197456080-00019.

55. Perez-Orribo L, Snyder LA, Kalb S, et al. Comparison of CT versus MRI measurements of transverse atlantal ligament integrity in craniovertebral junction injuries. Part 1: a clinical study. *J Neurosurg Spine.* 2016;24(6):897–902. https://doi.org/10.3171/2015.9.SPINE13808.

56. Dickman CA, Greene KA, Sonntag VKH. Injuries involving the transverse Atlantal ligament: classification and treatment guidelines based upon experience with 39 injuries. *Neurosurgery.* 1996;38(1):44–50. https://doi.org/10.1097/00006123-199601000-00012.

57. Hiratzka JR, Yoo JU, Ko JW, et al. Traditional threshold for retropharyngeal soft-tissue swelling is poorly sensitive for the detection of cervical spine injury on computed tomography in adult trauma patients. *Spine (Phila Pa 1976).* 2013;38(4). https://doi.org/10.1097/BRS.0b013e31827f0dc3.

58. Templeton PA, Young JW, Mirvis SE, Buddemeyer EU. The value of retropharyngeal soft tissue measurements in trauma of the adult cervical spine. Cervical spine soft tissue measurements. *Skelet Radiol.* 1987;16(2):98–104. https://doi.org/10.1007/bf00367755.

59. Spence KF, Decker S, Sell KW. Bursting atlantal fracture associated with rupture of the transverse ligament. *J Bone Joint Surg Am.* 1970;52(3):543–549. https://doi.org/10.2106/00004623-197052030-00013.

60. Heller JG, Viroslav S, Hudson T. Jefferson fractures: the role of magnification artifact in assessing transverse ligament integrity. *J Spinal Disord.* 1993;6(5):392–396.

61. Dickman C, Mamourian A, Sontag VKH, Drayer B. Magnetic resonance imaging of the transverse atlantal ligament for the evaluation of atlantoaxial instability. *J Neurosurg.* 1991;75(2):221–227.

62. Liu P, Zhu J, Wang Z, et al. "Rule of Spence" and Dickman's classification of transverse atlantal ligament injury revisited: discrepancy of prediction on atlantoaxial stability based on clinical outcome of nonoperative treatment for atlas fractures. *Spine (Phila Pa 1976).* 2019;44(5):E306–E314. https://doi.org/10.1097/BRS.0000000000002877.

63. Radcliff KE, Sonagli MA, Rodrigues LM, Sidhu GS, Albert TJ, Vaccaro AR. Does C_1 fracture displacement correlate with transverse ligament integrity? *Orthop Surg.* 2013;5(2):94–99. https://doi.org/10.1111/os.12034.

64. Suss RA, Zimmerman RD, Leeds NE. Pseudospread of the atlas: false sign of Jefferson fracture in young children. *Am J Roentgenol.* 1983;140(6):1079–1082. https://doi.org/10.2214/ajr.140.6.1079.

65. Kesterson L, Benzel E, Orrison W, Coleman J. Evaluation and treatment of atlas burst fractures (Jefferson fractures). *J Neurosurg.* 1991;75(2):213–220. https://doi.org/10.3171/jns.1991.75.2.0213.

66. Hadley MN, Dickman CA, Browner CM, Sonntag VKH. Acute traumatic atlas fractures: management and long term outcome. *Neurosurgery.* 1988;23(1):31–35. https://doi.org/10.1227/00006123-198807000-00007.

67. Ruf M, Melcher R, Harms J. Transoral reduction and osteosynthesis C1 as a function-preserving option in the treatment of unstable Jefferson fractures. *Spine (Phila Pa 1976).* 2004;29(7):823–827. https://doi.org/10.1097/01.brs.0000116984.42466.7e.

68. Rajasekaran S, Soundararajan DCR, Shetty AP, Kanna RM. Motion-preserving navigated primary internal fixation of unstable C1 fractures. *Asian Spine J.* 2020;(February). https://doi.org/10.31616/asj.2019.0189.

69. Hein C, Richter H-P, Rath SA. Atlantoaxial screw fixation for the treatment of isolated and combined unstable Jefferson fractures - experiences with 8 patients. *Acta Neurochir (Wien).* 2002;144(11):1187–1192. https://doi.org/10.1007/s00701-002-0998-2.

70. Shatsky J, Bellabarba C, Nguyen Q, Bransford RJ. A retrospective review of fixation of C1 ring fractures-does the transverse atlantal ligament (TAL) really matter? *Spine J.* 2016;16(3):372–379. https://doi.org/10.1016/j.spinee.2015.11.041.

71. Perez-Orribo L, Kalb S, Snyder LA, et al. Comparison of CT versus MRI measurements of transverse atlantal ligament integrity in craniovertebral junction injuries. Part 2: a new CT-based alternative for assessing transverse ligament integrity. *J Neurosurg Spine.* 2016;24(6):903–909. https://doi.org/10.3171/2015.9.SPINE13807.

72. Bohm H, Kayser R, El Saghir H, Heyde C. Direct osteosynthesis of instable Gehweiler type III atlas fractures. Presentation of a dorsoventral osteosynthesis of instable atlas fractures while maintaining function. *Unfallchirurg.* 2006;109(9):754–760. https://doi.org/10.1007/s00113-006-1081-x.

73. Korres DS, Chytas DG, Markatos KN, Efstathopoulos NE, Nikolaou VS. The "challenging" fractures of the odontoid process: a review of the classification schemes. *Eur J Orthop Surg Traumatol.* 2017. https://doi.org/10.1007/s00590-016-1895-3.

74. Schiff DCM, Parke WW. The arterial supply of the odontoid process. *J Bone Joint Surg Ser A.* 1973. https://doi.org/10.2106/00004623-197355070-00012.

75. Korres DS. Fractures of the odontoid process. In: *The Axis Vertebra*; 2013. https://doi.org/10.1007/978-88-470-5232-1_6.

76. Althoff B. Fracture of the odontoid process. An experimental and clinical study. *Acta Orthop Scand Suppl.* 1979. https://doi.org/10.3109/ort.1979.50.suppl-177.01.

77. Anderson LD, D'Alonzo RT. Fractures of the odontoid process of the axis. *J Bone Joint Surg Ser A.* 1974. https://doi.org/10.2106/00004623-197456080-00017.

78. De Mourgues G, Fischer LP, Bejui J, et al. Fracture of the odontoid process. *Rev Chir Orthop Reparatrice Appar Mot.* 1981;67:783–790 [in French].

79. Schatzker J, Rorabeck CH, Waddell JP. Fractures of the dens (odontoid process). An analysis of thirty-seven cases. *J Bone Joint Surg Ser B.* 1971. https://doi.org/10.1302/0301-620X.53B3.392.

80. Roy-Camille R, Bleynie JF, Saillant G, Judet T. Odontoid process fractures associated with fractures of the pedicles of the axis (author's transl). *Rev Chir Orthop Reparatrice Appar Mot.* 1979.

81. Vaccaro AR, Madigan L, Ehrler DM. Contemporary management of adult cervical odontoid fractures. *Orthopedics.* 2000. https://doi.org/10.3928/0147-7447-20001001-11.

82. Grauer JN, Shafi B, Hilibrand AS, et al. Proposal of a modified, treatment-oriented classification of odontoid fractures. *Spine J.* 2005. https://doi.org/10.1016/j.spinee.2004.09.014.

83. Geisler FH, Cheng C, Poka A, Brumback RJ, Cooper PR, Hadley MN. Anterior screw fixation of posteriorly displaced type II odontoid fractures. *Neurosurgery.* 1989. https://doi.org/10.1227/00006123-198907000-00006.

84. Coyne TJ, Fehlings MG, Wallace MC, Bernstein M, Tator CH. C1-c2 posterior cervical fusion: long-term evaluation of results and efficacy. *Neurosurgery.* 1995. https://doi.org/10.1227/00006123-199510000-00012.

85. Wood-Jones F. The ideal lesion produced by judicial hanging. *Lancet.* 1913. https://doi.org/10.1016/S0140-6736(01)47782-8.

86. Schneider RC, Livingston KE, Cave AJ, Hamilton G. "Hangman's fracture" of the cervical spine. *J Neurosurg.* 1965. https://doi.org/10.3171/jns.1965.22.2.0141.

87. Effendi B, Roy D, Cornish B, Dussault RG, Laurin CA. Fractures of the ring of the axis. A classification based on the analysis of 131 cases. *J Bone Joint Surg Ser B.* 1981. https://doi.org/10.1302/0301-620x.63b3.7263741.

88. Levine AM, Edwards CC. The management of traumatic spondylolisthesis of the axis. *J Bone Joint Surg Ser A.* 1985. https://doi.org/10.2106/00004623-198567020-00007.

89. Samaha C, Lazennec JY, Laporte C, Saillant G. Hangman's fracture: the relationship between asymmetry and instability. *J Bone Joint Surg Ser B.* 2000. https://doi.org/10.1302/0301-620X.82B7.10408.

90. Li G, Zhong D, Wang Q. A novel classification for atypical hangman fractures and its application. *Medicine (United States).* 2017. https://doi.org/10.1097/MD.0000000000007492.

91. Grady MS, Howard MA, Jane JA, Persing JA. Use of the Philadelphia collar as an alternative to the halo vest in patients with C-2, C-3 fractures. *Neurosurgery.* 1986. https://doi.org/10.1227/00006123-198602000-00006.

92. Coric D, Wilson JA, Kelly DL. Treatment of traumatic spondylolisthesis of the axis with nonrigid immobilization: a review of 64 cases. *J Neurosurg.* 1996. https://doi.org/10.3171/jns.1996.85.4.0550.

93. Vaccaro AR, Madigan L, Bauerle WB, Blescia A, Cotler JM. Early halo immobilization of displaced traumatic spondylolisthesis of the axis. *Spine (Phila Pa 1976).* 2002. https://doi.org/10.1097/00007632-200210150-00009.

94. Suchomel P, Hradil J, Barsa P, et al. Surgical treatment of fracture of the ring of axis - "Hangman's fracture". *Acta Chir Orthop Traumatol Cechoslov.* 2006.

95. Ryken TC, Hadley MN, Aarabi B, et al. Management of isolated fractures of the axis in adults. *Neurosurgery.* 2013. https://doi.org/10.1227/NEU.0b013e318276ee40.

96. Gornet ME, Kelly MP. Fractures of the axis: a review of pediatric, adult, and geriatric injuries. *Curr Rev Musculoskelet Med.* 2016. https://doi.org/10.1007/s12178-016-9368-1.

97. Starr JK, Eismont FJ. Atypical hangman's fractures. *Spine (Phila Pa 1976).* 1993. https://doi.org/10.1097/00007632-199310001-00005.

98. Burke JT, Harris JH. Acute injuries of the axis vertebra. *Skelet Radiol.* 1989. https://doi.org/10.1007/BF00361422.

99. Benzel EC. Conservative treatment of neural arch fractures of the axis: computed tomography scan and X-ray study on consolidation time. *World Neurosurg.* 2011. https://doi.org/10.1016/j.wneu.2010.09.036.

100. Maeda FL, Formentin C, de Andrade EJ, et al. Reliability of the new AOSpine classification system for upper cervical traumatic injuries. *Neurosurgery.* 2020;86(3):E263–E270. https://doi.org/10.1093/neuros/nyz464.

101. AOSpine Upper Cervical Classification System. *YouTube;* 2018. https://www.youtube.com/watch?v=KyUYfa_JMb4&feature=youtu.be. Accessed 7 April 2020.

102. Vaccaro AR, Koerner JD, Radcliff KE, et al. AOSpine subaxial cervical spine injury classification system. *Eur Spine J.* 2016;25(7):2173–2184. https://doi.org/10.1007/s00586-015-3831-3.

103. Vaccaro AR, Oner C, Kepler CK, et al. AOSpine thoracolumbar spine injury classification system: fracture description, neurological status, and key modifiers. *Spine (Phila Pa 1976).* 2013;38(23):2028–2037. https://doi.org/10.1097/BRS.0b013e3182a8a381.

104. Divi SN, Schroeder GD, Oner FC, et al. AOSpine—spine trauma classification system: the value of modifiers: a narrative review with commentary on evolving descriptive principles. *Global Spine J.* 2019;9(1 suppl):77S–88S. https://doi.org/10.1177/2192568219827260.

CHAPTER 6

Subaxial Cervical Spine Plain Radiographs

GARRETT K. HARADA[a] • KAYLA L. LEVERICH[a] • ZAKARIAH K. SIYAJI[a] •
PHILIP K. LOUIE[a,b] • HOWARD S. AN[a]
[a]Department of Orthopaedic Surgery, Rush University Medical Center, Chicago, IL, United States
[b]Department of Neurosurgery, Virginia Mason Medical Center, Seattle, WA, United States

INTRODUCTION

The subaxial cervical spine refers to cervical vertebrae located below the "axis" (C2) and is a critical distinction due to inherent biomechanical differences from vertebral levels more cephalad and caudad.[1] Responsible for the majority of cervical range of motion, vertebrae ranging from C3 to C7 contribute roughly 70 of flexion, 40 of extension, 30 of lateral bending, and 45 of rotation to either side.[2] Furthermore, in the native cervical spine, C3–C7 (specifically, the facet joints) is responsible for about two-thirds of the total axial load imposed by the cranium. The remaining load is then distributed among cervical intervertebral discs.[2] These relationships are held in a close equilibrium that is ultimately dependent upon a precise sagittal alignment, where the global cervical lordosis (i.e., C2–C7 curvature), sagittal vertical axis (SVA), T1 slope (T1S), and various other radiographic parameters cohesively interact.[3,4]

However, in the setting of various pathologies, these biomechanical relationships are frequently disrupted, often resulting in a redistribution of axial loading and diminished capacity to maintain native range of motion.[2] Ultimately, these findings stress the importance of making appropriate radiographic measurements in the cervical spine, as the magnitude of radiographic disturbance is associated with disease prognosis and may help guide surgical management. As such, the present chapter will discuss the importance of critical subaxial radiographic measures, with particular emphasis placed on the clinical relevance and technique required to accurately perform these assessments.

SPECIFIC RADIOGRAPHIC PARAMETERS

While indications for specific radiographic measures may differ based upon the presenting situation, certain assessments can be made routinely in a clinical evaluation of the cervical spine. Broadly speaking, these measures assess the overall alignment and sagittal balance of the cervical spine in relation to adjacent vertebrae, intervertebral discs, and neighboring soft tissues. In select situations, such as those seen in traumatic cervical spine injuries, supplementation of these general measures may require assessments of overall stability, as this information may help guide subsequent surgical planning. Moreover, postoperatively, radiographic assessment is particularly important, as this allows adequate visualization of osseous fusion and inspection of instrumentation and may help the practitioner assess for known complications after a cervical procedure. Overall, a collective understanding of the radiographic techniques involved in the evaluation of the cervical spine is an invaluable asset to the spine surgeon's armamentarium and is necessary for proper patient management. All measures are made using standing lateral views of the cervical spine unless otherwise specified.

General Cervical Spine
Contour lines
Contour lines for the cervical spine are simple drawings that roughly outline the path of the anterior/posterior vertebral bodies, orientation of the lamina, and the spinous processes. As such, these lines are named the anterior vertebral line, posterior vertebral line, spinolaminar line, and posterior spinal line, respectively. They are frequently used to make quick assessments of

Atlas of Spinal Imaging. https://doi.org/10.1016/B978-0-323-76111-6.00002-X

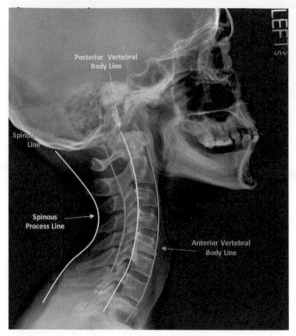

FIG. 1 Cervical spine contour lines. Lateral radiograph of the cervical spine demonstrating contour lines.

overall cervical alignment, where disruption in a given line (defined as ≥ 3 mm translation in adults, ≥ 5 mm in children) raises suspicion of bony or ligamentous injury.[5,6] To make these measurements (Fig. 1):

- Anterior vertebral line
  - Start at the anterior border of the dens
  - Draw a line following the anterior edge of each vertebral body from C2 to C7, passing through the corners of the corresponding anterior endplates
- Posterior vertebral line
  - Start at the posterior border of the dens
  - Draw a line following the posterior edge of each vertebral body from C2 to C7, passing through the corners of the corresponding posterior endplates
  - This will roughly map the anterior border of the spinal canal
- Spinolaminar line
  - Start at the anterior border of the C2 spinous process base (or the anterior edge of the posterior arch of C1, if visible)
  - Draw a line following the anterior margin of the base of each spinous process, extending to C7
  - This will roughly map the posterior border of the spinal canal

- Posterior spinal line
  - Start at the tip of the C2 spinous process
  - Draw a line caudally, connecting the tips of spinous processes from C2 to C7

Some common pitfalls or issues that arise when interpreting and measuring contour lines include pseudosubluxation and concurrence of diffuse degenerative pathology (e.g., osteophytes). Pseudosubluxation is defined as the physiologic translation of one cervical vertebra relative to another, possibly causing a disruption in contour lines.[7,8] This is traditionally seen in pediatric patients under the age of 7 at C2–C3 or C3–C4 due to underdeveloped cervical paraspinal muscles.[8] Similarly, degenerative cervical spine pathology may make tracing contours difficult, as there may be structural changes that obstruct natural anatomy. In these situations, care should be taken to pass through the approximate location of the native endplate corners, and avoid incorporation of osteophytes or other degenerative changes that may obscure native structures.

In general, contour lines serve as a relatively simple assessment tool that has the greatest utility in trauma settings. Disruptions or step-offs of contour lines may suggest the presence of a fracture or malalignment of the vertebral column. Specifically, step-offs observed upon inspection of anterior or posterior vertebral lines may suggest spondylolisthesis, while disruptions of the spinolaminar or posterior spinal lines may indicate a spinous process fracture (i.e., "Clay Shoveler's" fracture).[9] However, as these conditions are often diagnosed without the need for such measures, contour line assessment is perhaps best reserved for occult injuries with supplementation with more advanced imaging modalities. Despite this, some studies have suggested further utility for such measures. In 1999, Seybold et al. noted that the posterior vertebral line may be used to assess the integrity of the odontoid, noting that step-offs ≥ 3 mm should be used as a threshold for subsequent computed tomography (CT) evaluation to rule out occult fractures.[10] More recently, in 2016, Oshima et al. demonstrated that the spinolaminar line at the level of C2–C3 can be used in reference to axis (C1) to screen for C1 spinal stenosis.[11] However, with the increased use of CT and magnetic resonance imaging (MRI) studies, contour lines currently see limited clinical use and are often less sensitive than other radiographic assessments.

C2–C7 lordosis

C2–C7 lordosis measures the overall curvature of the cervical spine and is a critical assessment in determining overall sagittal alignment. At present, there are four

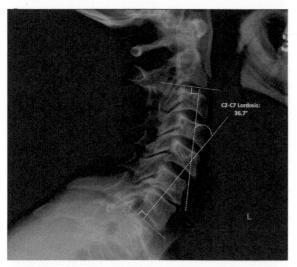

FIG. 2 C2–C7 cervical lordosis assessments. Cobb angle measurement of the sagittal curvature from C2 to C7.

reliable metrics used to assess cervical lordosis: (1) Cobb angle, (2) Ishihara's index, (3) Harrison's C2–C7 posterior tangent method, and (4) the modified Toyama method.[12-18] Note that the following methods are often simplified by modern radiographic annotation tools, and specific methods may vary between different software interfaces (Fig. 2).

- Cobb angle
  - Draw a line along the inferior endplate of C2
  - Draw a perpendicular line intersecting this first line
  - Draw a line along the inferior endplate of C7
  - Draw a second perpendicular line intersecting this second line
  - The angle formed by the intersection of the two perpendicular lines is the Cobb angle measurement for cervical lordosis
  - By convention, lordotic angles are mathematically negative (−), while kyphotic measures are positive (+)
  - Normal values: − 20 to − 40 degrees
- Ishihara's index
  - Draw a straight line connecting the posterior inferior corner of C2 to the posterior inferior corner of C7
  - Draw a perpendicular line connecting this first line to the posterior inferior corner of C3
  - Repeat for C4–C6
  - Take the sum of the length of the lines drawn from C3 to C6 and divide by the length of the line connecting C2 and C7

- Lines from C3 to C6 are considered positive (+) if they travel from anterior to posterior in order to intersect the line drawn from C2 to C7, while those traveling from posterior to anterior are negative (−)
- Harrison's posterior tangent
  - Draw a line tangent to the posterior border of C2
  - Repeat for C7
  - The angle formed by the intersection of these two lines generates the C2–C7 lordosis
  - By convention, lordotic angles are mathematically positive (+), while kyphotic measures are negative (−)
- Modified Toyama method
  - Draw a line from the posterior inferior corner of C2 to the posterior superior corner of C7
  - Kyphotic curves are identified if the posterior walls of the vertebral bodies from C3 to C6 are posterior to this line
  - Lordotic curves are present if the posterior walls of C3–C6 lie anterior to this line
  - Straight curves are present if the posterior walls of C3–C6 lie on this line

Currently, there is significant debate over which technique is the most appropriate for routine clinical use. While each method has demonstrated high intra- and interobserver reliability in various studies, the selection of a given approach is likely best dictated by the treating clinician's needs.[19] In many instances, assessment of the precise angle of curvature helps guide surgical management, and as such, Cobb angle measurements or Harrison's posterior tangent may be more useful. However, in 2017, Donk et al. highlighted some of the shortcomings of these angle measurement techniques, noting in particular that lordotic angles under Harrison's posterior tangent method may present with grossly kyphotic alignments.[18] Here, they suggest the modified Toyama approach may be a better assessment, though emphasize that this technique is limited due to lack of clear quantification techniques. This suggests that there may be some utility in combining multiple techniques to achieve the most accurate assessment of cervical lordosis.

Irrespective of the technique employed, lordosis measures are currently one of the most clinically significant metrics in the radiographic evaluation of the cervical spine. Both anterior and posterior cervical procedures have that tendency to drastically affect lordosis measures secondary to manipulation of intervertebral disc spaces through the use of various interbody implants and/or utilization of posterior decompression. These techniques may inherently be kyphogenic due to iatrogenic damage of various supporting structures and may lead to postoperative losses in lordosis. Studies have identified many patients treated with an isolated cervical decompression who develop eventual deterioration.[20] Similarly, loss of cervical lordosis, whether iatrogenic or not, has been associated with worse health-related quality of life (HRQOL) scores.[21] Such reports have made radiographic assessments of lordosis integral to cervical spine standard of care and are frequently used to guide sagittal corrections in operative management.

Sagittal vertical axis (SVA)

Like cervical lordosis, SVA is another key measure in assessing sagittal alignment of the cervical spine. However, rather than measuring overall curvature, SVA calculates the anterior or posterior translation of C2 relative to the base of the subaxial cervical spine (Fig. 3). The cervical SVA (at times referred to as the "C2–C7 SVA") is held in contrast to the SVA used for global sagittal alignment, a measure that uses the C7 vertebral body as a reference for larger spinal deformities (Fig. 3).

- Sagittal vertical axis
  - Draw an "X" over the body of C2 by connecting a line from the posterior inferior corner of C2 to the anterior superior border, and a second line from the posterior anterior corner of C2, to the posterior superior border
  - Draw a vertical axis line through the center of this "X," perpendicular to the inferior edge of the entire film

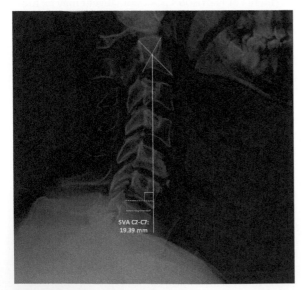

FIG. 3 Sagittal vertical axis (SVA) of the cervical spine.

- Draw an orthogonal line from this axis line connecting the posterior superior corner of C7
- Normal values: ≤20 mm

Clinically, the connection between SVA and C2–C7 lordosis has only been recently established, with studies suggesting these two measures interact harmoniously in determining sagittal balance.[22] Specifically, with increasing cervical SVA, compensatory suboccipital hyperextension and subaxial cervical flexion are believed to ensue in order to preserve horizontal gaze.[23] Moreover, the evidence surrounding large positive shifts in SVA is arguably greater than that of C2–C7 lordosis, with multiple studies suggesting measures over 40 mm are highly associated with worse disability and HRQOL scores.[24–26] This understanding has subsequently been implemented in further studies, suggesting that large cervical SVA measures may be more or less amenable to certain approaches. For instance, Kato et al. demonstrated that cervical myelopathy patients with larger C2–C7 SVA measures (≥35 mm) had greater incidences of neck pain following decompression than those with smaller SVA values.[26] Realizing this, Miyamoto et al. go on to suggest such patients may be better treated with a concurrent correction of sagittal malalignment through a posterior instrumented fusion.[27] In any case, this illustrates the importance of taking regular SVA measures when making assessments of sagittal balance, and to consider their use in further clinical decision-making.

T1 slope (T1S)

T1S serves as another measurement to assess sagittal balance of the cervical spine and has been associated with other parameters such as C2–C7 lordosis and SVA.[28–30] While all three measures may not be routinely performed for all patients, in some circumstances, utilization of multiple sagittal assessments may provide the most holistic view of a patient's cervical alignment and propensity for unfavorable radiographic change. While the T1 slope is thought to be relatively constant, age, posture, and degenerative change may lead to variations over time, ultimately leading to associated changes in sagittal alignment (Fig. 4).[30]

- T1 slope
  - Draw a horizontal axis through the posterior superior corner of the T1 vertebral body
  - Draw a line tangent to the superior endplate of T1
  - The acute angle formed by the intersection of these lines represents the T1 slope
  - Normal values: about 25 ± 5 degrees[31,32]

Acquisition of the T1 slope measures is dependent upon the obtained field of radiographic exposure. Frequently, radiographs may be positioned more

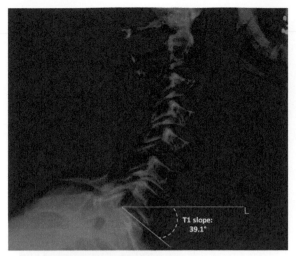

FIG. 4 T1 slope of the cervical spine.

cephalad than intended, leading to poor visualization of the T1 vertebral body. Moreover, variations in patient anatomy such as interference from shoulder contours and neck/truncal obesity may obscure clear boundaries. Though such factors less frequently prevent measurability of C2–C7 lordosis or SVA, clinicians aiming to collect the T1 slope should be aware of these common pitfalls.

However, much like SVA, the T1 slope is a third measurement that closely relates to other radiographic sagittal parameters. In a retrospective review of radiographic images, Park et al. demonstrated that as C2–C7 lordosis increases, the T1 slope also increases.[4] They suggest that the T1 slope may indicate the maximal lordotic curvature a patient may obtain from surgical correction. In addition, some evidence suggests that the magnitude of the T1 slope may be a risk factor for the development of various cervical spine pathologies. Jun et al. noted that high T1 slope was significantly associated with the development of degenerative cervical spondylolisthesis when measured on CT images.[3] Having a low T1 slope, however, has also been associated with increased risks of degenerative cervical spondylotic myelopathy.[33] Collectively, these findings emphasize the clinical value of the T1 slope, though the full utility of this measure continues to evolve.

Disc height

Measurements of intervertebral disc height on radiographs face numerous logistical challenges, as degree of radiographic magnification and slight adjustments in patient positioning may prevent an accurate

assessment.[34] As such, there have been numerous attempts at techniques for accurate measures of disc height, though each is known to have distinct limitations (Fig. 5).[35-38]

- Endplate-to-endplate disc height
  - Draw a line from the edge of one vertebral endplate to the adjacent endplate, spanning the intervertebral disc space
  - The size of this line is the endplate-to-endplate disc height
- Distortion-compensated Roentgen analysis (DCRA)[39]
  - Mark the four corners of two adjacent vertebral bodies
  - Identify a plane bisecting each vertebral body between the marked points
  - Identify a third plane lying equidistant from the first two planes bisecting the intervertebral disc space
  - Draw a perpendicular line from a marked point on the cephalad vertebral body to the third plane
  - Repeat for the caudal vertebral body
  - The sum of the distances of these perpendicular lines is the disc height with reference to the marked points
  - Note: Measured distances from anterior points measure the anterior disc height, and measured distances from posterior points measure the posterior disc height. Points may be placed in the middle of each endplate for a middle disc height as well.
- Modified DCRA[35]
  - Mark the four corners of two adjacent vertebral bodies as above
  - Draw a line connecting the anterior points
  - Draw a second line connecting the posterior points
  - Identify the midpoint of both lines and draw a third line connecting the two
  - This line now serves as a plane to draw perpendicular lines to the marked points
  - The sum of the distances measures the disc height, as above

Due to inconsistencies with alignment on lateral radiographs of the cervical spine, a high degree of measurement error has been documented with disc height assessments. For example, when vertebral endplates are misaligned in the sagittal plane, measures from endplate-to-endplate may largely overestimate the actual disc height. Furthermore, when using the DCRA approach, changes in vertebral body morphology may drastically affect the placement of measurement planes, leading to poor estimates as well. The modified DCRA approach is a relatively recent adaptation

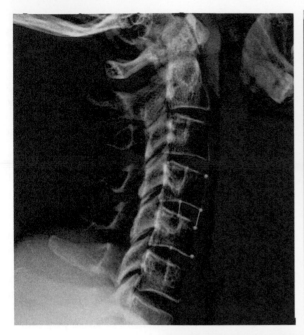
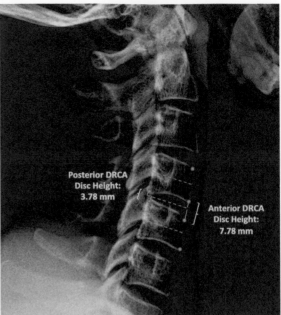
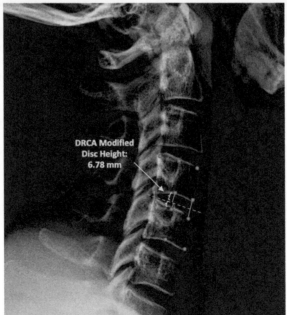

FIG. 5 Endplate-to-endplate height measurements. Disc height measurement technique using edges of vertebral cortices. Distortion-compensated Roentgen analysis (DCRA) disc height measurements. Lateral radiographs of the sagittal lateral cervical spine demonstrating the DCRA technique for disc height measurement.

by Allaire et al. and has demonstrated a high degree of inter- and intra-observer reliability within their study.[35] However, this technique requires further validation in the clinical setting before its use can be effectively determined. As such, the clinical utility of disc height measurements is currently being investigated. At present, its use is largely being applied to radiographic assessments of outcomes after cervical total disc replacement.[40]

Spondylolisthesis

Spondylolisthesis is defined as the anterior, posterior, or lateral translation (or "slip") of one vertebral body relative to an adjacent level. While etiologies for spondylolisthesis vary, techniques for assessing this condition are consistent and are based upon simple measurement techniques. However, when spondylolisthesis is present, further assessment is warranted to determine the stability (or lack thereof) of a given slip. Such techniques will be discussed separately in this chapter (Fig. 6).

- Distance technique
  - Identify potential spondylolistheses by grossly examining the alignment of the vertebral bodies
    - This can be assisted through the use of cervical contour lines
  - At a suspected level, identify the disc space and corresponding endplates
  - Starting at the posterior edge of either endplate, draw a line parallel to this endplate toward the adjacent vertebral body's endplate edge
  - The measured size of this line defines the translation of one vertebra relative to the adjacent
  - Normal values: < 2 mm[41]

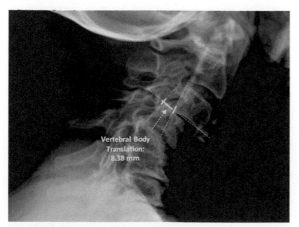

FIG. 6 Spondylolisthesis assessment. Lateral radiograph of the sagittal cervical spine demonstrating C3–C4 spondylolisthesis.

- Meyerding classification technique
  - As above, identify a potentially spondylolisthetic level through gross examination
  - Measure the entire width of the caudal "normally aligned" vertebral endplate
  - As with the distance technique, measure the magnitude of spondylolisthesis between the two adjacent vertebrae
  - Divide this distance by the total distance of the "normal" endplate
  - This value defines the percentage of translation relative to an adjacent normal level to generate Meyerding grades:
    - Grade I: ≤ 25%
    - Grade II: 25%–50%
    - Grade III: 50%–75%
    - Grade IV: 75%–100%
    - Grade V: > 100%

Proper assessment of spondylolisthesis typically extends beyond identification and classification on a single film. When spondylolisthesis is identified, typically a flexion-extension film is indicated to determine the stability of the affected level(s). When obtained, if repeating spondylolisthesis measures lead to an increase > 3 mm, then surgical fixation is that instability may lead to progression of the slip, increasing the risk for catastrophic neurologic compromise.[42] If no change in measured spondylolisthesis occurs with flexion or extension, then serial monitoring may be performed using routine radiographic examination to determine the future progression of pathology. Increases seen at this time would necessitate repeating flexion-extension measurements as well.

Torg-Pavlov ratio

The Torg-Pavlov ratio is a tool used to assess cervical canal stenosis on lateral radiographs. Historically, cervical stenosis was diagnosed using gross measurement techniques with various cutoffs.[43,44] However, in a series of two articles published in 1986 and 1987, Joseph Torg and Helene Pavlov highlighted the high inter- and intra-observer error associated with this method and instead developed a ratio of the canal width relative to the cervical vertebral body width.[43,44] This method has since replaced traditional measurement techniques in clinical practice (Fig. 7).

- Torg-Pavlov ratio
  - Measure the width of a desired vertebral body by measuring from the middle of the anterior border to the middle of the posterior border
  - Measure the width of the spinal canal from the middle of the posterior vertebral body border to the middle of the spinous process, posteriorly

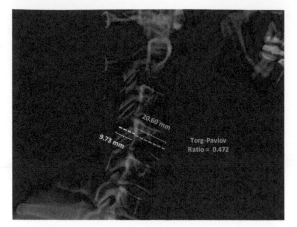

FIG. 7 Torg-Pavlov ratio. Lateral cervical spine radiograph demonstrating the technique for the Torg-Pavlov ratio.

- Divide the length of the spinal canal by the length of the width of the vertebral body
- Normal values: Ratio ≥ 0.8

Since its conception, the Torg-Pavlov ratio has seen application in numerous settings, the most recent of which includes its utility in risk stratification and/or prediction of patients for various cervical spine outcomes. In 2001, Yue et al. identified that the Torg-Pavlov ratio was significantly lower in patients with cervical spondylotic myelopathy compared to healthy controls.[45] Similarly, in 2013, Aebli et al. demonstrated that patients with a Torg-Pavlov ratio of 0.7 or lower were at greater risk for spinal cord injury after minor trauma.[46] However, when compared to sagittal diameter and area measures on MRI, Prasad et al. noted there is a poor relationship between MRI measures and this ratio.[47] Further, Blackley et al. performed a similar analysis utilizing CT and found the same poor association.[48] Given this, Fehlings et al. posit that the best technique for assessing spinal canal compromise may best be performed on midsagittal CT reconstructions and/or T2-weighted MRI.[49–51] Their technique suggests measuring the anteroposterior distance between the furthest posterior vertebral body and the posterior arch (Di), followed by the distance between the midvertebral body level and anterior edge of the posterior arch of the first unaffected cranial and caudal vertebrae (Da and Db, respectively). The degree of spinal cord compromise is then calculated using $(1 - Di)/[(Da + Dab)/2] \times 100$.

Chin-brow to vertical angle (CBVA)

CBVA measurements are used in particularly niche situations where concerns about a patient's horizontal gaze are prevalent. Such considerations are usually taken

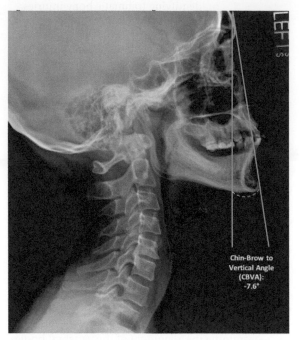

FIG. 8 Chin-brow to vertical angle. Lateral radiograph of the cervical spine and skull demonstrating the chin-brow to vertical angle technique.

when a given patient presents with large kyphotic deformities and/or ankylosis of the cervical spine (Fig. 8).

- Chin-brow to vertical angle
  - Draw a line tangent to the patient's chin and forehead
  - Draw a second vertical axis line intersecting the first
  - The acute angle formed by the intersection of these lines is the CBVA
  - Normal values: -5 to 17 degrees
    - Values outside of this range constitute a loss of horizontal gaze[52]

Loss of horizontal gaze is typically a large concern in patients with end-stage ankylosing spondylitis (AS). As ankylosis progresses to the cervical spine, AS patients will typically see a progressive increase in CBVA measures due to increasing cervical kyphosis. These patients will often compensate for such changes by flexing at the knees and extending at the hip, in an effort to maintain horizontal gaze.[52,53] In a retrospective study of 303 patients, Lafage et al. demonstrated that CBVA measures were correlated with low Oswestry Disability Index (ODI) scores between -4.7 and 17.7 degrees.[54] These values have since been used to assist in dictating corrective cervical osteotomies for such patients.

However, Yan et al. demonstrated perturbances of other cervical sagittal parameters when CBVA was <−1.5 or >5.8 degrees, suggesting theoretical risks of even slight CBVA shifts.[55] To this point, CBVA measures should be considered in any patient with rigid cervical deformity, with consideration for cervical osteotomy to restore appropriate alignment. Despite evidence from Lafage et al. highlighting −4.7 to 17.7 degrees as "normal," patients have been shown to tolerate ± 10 degrees of CBVA reasonably well after surgery.[54,56,57]

Prevertebral soft tissue shadows

Assessment of prevertebral soft tissues is also made possible on lateral radiographs of the cervical spine and may assist in the diagnosis of occult hemorrhage in nasopharyngeal, retropharyngeal, or retrotracheal spaces.[58] Unfortunately, these measures are highly variable and nonspecific, and all abnormal measures should be further evaluated through further examination or advanced imaging (Fig. 9).

- Nasopharyngeal soft tissue shadow
  - Identify the anterior arch of C1
  - Draw a line from the anterior border of the anterior arch of C1 to the posterior edge of the upper pharynx shadow
  - The distance of this line is equal to the width of the nasopharyngeal soft tissue
  - Normal values: < 10 mm (adult)

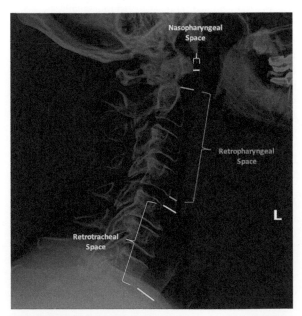

FIG. 9 Prevertebral soft tissue shadows. Zones delineating prevertebral soft tissue shadows.

- Retropharyngeal soft tissue shadow
  - Identify the anterior border of any vertebral body from C2 to C4
  - Draw a line from the anterior border of the chosen level to the posterior edge of the lower pharynx shadow
  - The distance of this line is equal to the width of the retropharyngeal soft tissues
  - Normal values: < 5–7 mm
- Retrotracheal soft tissue shadow
  - Identify the anterior border of any vertebral body from C5 to C7
  - Draw a line from the anterior border of the chosen level to the posterior edge of the tracheal shadow
  - Normal values: < 14 mm (children), < 22 mm (adult)

Despite the wide application of such measures in clinical practice, some studies have highlighted the issues with soft tissue shadow variability between age-groups, gender, injury type, and vertebral level. In a case series of 30 hospitalized patients with cervical spine injuries, Penning examined the widening of prevertebral soft tissue shadows based upon the vertebral level and injury, noting that measurements drastically differed in each scenario. They suggest that the upper limit of normal for a given soft tissue shadow measure should be specific to the level examined, taking into account differences in posture.[59] Since the original thresholds have been described in 1958 by Wholey et al., numerous studies have since reported slightly different results. Across these studies, mean values for all soft tissue shadows differed by a max of 2.15 mm, suggesting that the true value of prevertebral soft tissues likely falls within a relatively large variance.[59–63]

Traumatic Cervical Spine

The traumatic cervical spine offers many unique challenges regarding management, making a careful radiographic assessment critical for guiding appropriate therapy. While many of the aforementioned techniques are also useful in the evaluation of the traumatic cervical spine, the following measures have limited application outside of this setting. Moreover, other imaging modalities such as computed tomography (CT) or magnetic resonance imaging (MRI) may be preferred to rule out occult fractures and/or to surrounding soft tissues.[64] Nevertheless, plain radiographs may offer sufficient visualization to diagnose many injuries to cervical vertebrae and its various articulations.

Vertebral body height loss

Vertebral body height measure is a well-defined technique that assesses the overall morphology at various

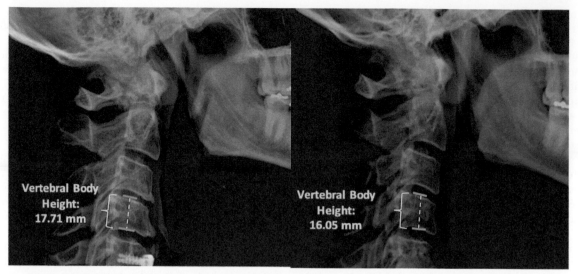

FIG. 10 Vertebral height loss. Lateral cervical spine radiographs demonstrating technique for measuring vertebral height loss.

zones (anterior, middle, or posterior). While some conditions are known to cause "wedging" of vertebral bodies (a progressive loss of vertebral height moving from posterior to anterior), in the traumatic setting, height loss typically indicates a compression fracture.[65,66] At present, there are two major methods for assessing vertebral body height loss (Fig. 10):

- Vertebral body height loss
  - Method 1
    - Identify the cervical vertebra with suspected height loss
    - Draw a line along the length of the posterior vertebral body, from endplate-to-endplate
    - Repeat this process for the anterior border
    - Divide the length of the anterior line by the length of the posterior line and multiply by 100
    - This yields a percentage equal to the height loss moving from posterior to anterior
    - Normal values: 20%–25% mild compression fracture, 25%–40% moderate, >40% severe[65]
  - Method 2
    - Identify the cervical vertebra with suspected height loss, as well as the unaffected levels immediately cephalad and caudad
    - As above, measure the anterior border length for all three levels
    - Divide the length of the suspect level by the average of the neighboring levels and multiply by 100

- This yields a value equal to the percentage decrease in height, relative to the "normal" heights of neighboring cervical vertebrae[49]

Assessing vertebral body height is considered a routine measurement in the surveillance of identified vertebral body compression fractures. This is performed to verify stability and/or identify the progression of a fractured vertebral level. However, Mikula et al. noted that height loss, while a fairly sensitive marker, does not effectively rule out compression fracture when absent on imaging.[66] As most vertebral compression fractures are treated conservatively, patients with progression and subsequent neurologic compromise are indicated for vertebroplasty or kyphoplasty. Seo et al. demonstrated that assessments of endplate integrity should also be considered with vertebral height measures, as patients with posterior vertebral height loss and violation of both endplates were significantly more likely to present with future spinal canal compromise.[67]

Facet fracture

Diagnosis of facet fractures in the cervical spine represents a type of injury that is better visualized on CT. However, many facet fractures may be identified on plain radiography with careful assessment. At present, the following technique has yet to be validated in clinical practice or tested for reliability (Fig. 11).

- Facet fracture
  - Measure the length of the first unaffected cephalad vertebral facet articulation (A)

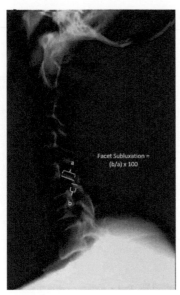

FIG. 11 Cervical facet fractures and subluxation/dislocation. Lateral cervical spine radiograph demonstrating the technique and formula for facet subluxation at C5–C6.

- Measure the length of the intact facet at the adjacent affected level (B)
- Calculate the percentage of the remaining intact facet relative to the unaffected facet ($B/A \times 100$)[49]

Facet subluxation/dislocation

Depending upon the severity, facet subluxations and/or dislocations are usually readily apparent on radiographic imaging due to distinct changes in normal cervical anatomy. They are often accompanied by a concurrent anterolisthesis of the cephalad vertebra and may also have evidence of concurrent fracture. As with the technique outlined for facet fractures, this approach for quantification of facet subluxation/dislocation has yet to be validated as well.

- Facet subluxation/dislocation
  - Measure the length of the inferior articular facet at the affected articulation (A)
  - Measure the length of the corresponding superior articular facet (B)
  - Calculate the percentage of facet opposition ($B/A \times 100$)[68]

Postoperative Cervical Spine

Postoperative radiographic assessment of the cervical spine is necessary to evaluate the integrity of attempted fusion, evaluate instrumentation and various implants, and monitor the incidence of adverse postoperative outcomes. Such films are routinely taken at scheduled postoperative visits and require an intimate understanding of appropriate measurement techniques to successfully evaluate the cervical spine. As in traumatic settings, general cervical spine measurements are also used in the evaluation of the postoperative cervical spine, though additional measures are frequently indicated based upon the antecedent procedure.

Fusion/pseudarthrosis

With most spine surgery procedures, osseous fusion tends to be a primary objective for the practitioner. Given this importance, the past few decades have seen a proliferation of various techniques to assist in fusion and include variations in instrumentation, innovations in grafting technique, and use of bone morphogenetic protein.[69–71] Despite this, assessment of postoperative fusion on radiographs has remained unchanged and is a relatively simple process, requiring few technical measures (Fig. 12).

- Assessment of fusion/pseudarthrosis
  - Identify the operative levels needing evaluation
  - Inspect films for evidence of intervertebral bony bridging, suggestive of fusion progression
  - In questionable cases, a flexion/extension view may be ordered and inspected for immobility or <3 degrees of intervertebral position change using the Cobb angle measurements (see C2–C7 lordosis)

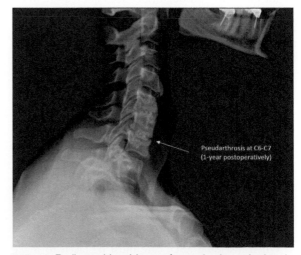

FIG. 12 Radiographic evidence of nonunion/pseudarthrosis. Lateral radiograph of the cervical spine demonstrating postsurgical fusion at C5–C6 and an anterior pseudarthrosis at C6–C7 1 year postoperatively.

- If uncertainty still remains, a CT is indicated for further evaluation
- In cases involving the use of an interbody, the above criteria in addition to the following may be used[72]:
  - Lack of a lucent area surrounding the implant
  - Minimal loss of disc height
  - No evidence of instrument, bone graft, or vertebral fracture
  - No sclerosis observed in graft and/or adjacent vertebrae

Complete fusion is typically observed at 6–9 months postoperatively.[73] At this time, patients without evidence of fusion and/or evidence of an unstable fusion are said to have radiographic evidence of a nonunion (pseudarthrosis). Patients with pseudarthrosis may present with pain and/or radicular symptoms at the affected level months to years after the index procedure, though some may remain asymptomatic.[74] Revision surgery is indicated for pseudarthrosis when no other etiology is found for a patient's recurrent symptoms.

Adjacent segment degeneration (ASD)

ASD is a common complication seen after cervical spine surgery, occurring at an incidence of roughly 2% per year following a given procedure.[75,76] While the onset of ASD is not necessarily imminently accompanied by symptoms, adjacent-level changes threaten sagittal alignment, leading to losses in cervical lordosis and/or SVA, and may cause further consequences if missed by the clinician. Although ASD does not require intervention unless patients present with gross symptomatology, identification of these features on radiographs may identify patients at greater risk for this outcome (Fig. 13).

- Assessment of adjacent segment degeneration
  - Identify the levels proximal and distal to a previously operated segment
  - Examine these levels for any of the following by making comparisons to previous radiographs:
    - New or enlarged adjacent-level vertebral body osteophytes
    - Anterior longitudinal ligament calcification
    - Spondylolisthesis with displacement ≥ 2 mm
    - Disc space narrowing greater than 30% of the preoperative height
    - New or worsening endplate sclerosis

When assessing ASD, care must be taken to make appropriate comparisons between films. Specifically, as ASD is defined as the *new* development of adjacent-level pathology, follow-up films should be compared to preoperative cervical spine films. This allows an

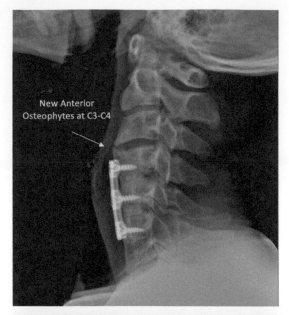

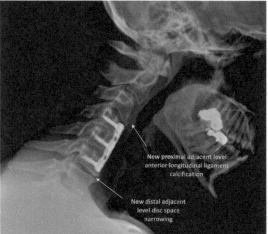

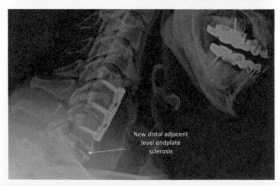

FIG. 13 Adjacent segment degeneration. Lateral cervical spine radiographs demonstrating criteria for defining adjacent segment degeneration (ASD).

appropriate assessment of new radiographic findings attributable to iatrogenic interventions.

Radiographic ASD remains a significant complication after cervical spine surgery, with a reported incidence as high as 2.79%–2.9% per year after a procedure.[75,77] Though such outcomes may largely be asymptomatic, many patients may develop the adjacent-level disease, requiring reoperation. Current evidence suggests that the various factors associated with ASD include older age, length of fusion, and preexisting adjacent-level degenerative pathology.[75–79]

Subsidence

Subsidence is a known consequence of many cervical procedures, though the clinical significance of this phenomenon remains uncertain. Many theoretical risks surround subsidence, however, and include potential neurologic compromise secondary to postoperative migration of graft/fusion constructs. With the growing popularity of interbody use in cervical spine surgery, concerns surrounding subsidence have increased, and with it increases the number of radiographic techniques used to assess this finding (Fig. 14).[80]

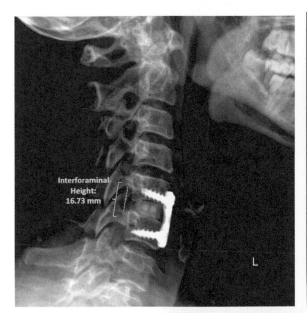
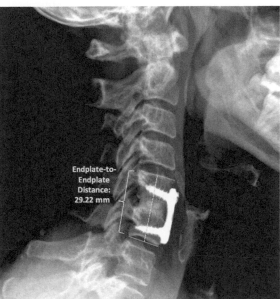
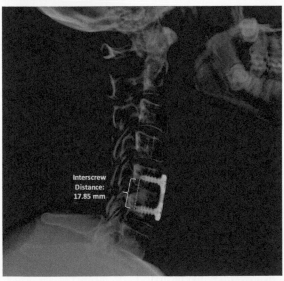

FIG. 14 Subsidence assessments. Lateral cervical spine radiograph demonstrating criteria for subsidence.

- Interscrew distance
  - Identify the tips of two adjacent screws at an instrumented level
  - Measure the distance between the tips of both screws to calculate the interscrew distance
  - This measure is then subtracted from a previous measure to determine change in interscrew distance to determine subsidence
  - Normal values: <2–3 mm
- Endplate-to-endplate distance
  - Identify the anterior, middle, and/or posterior superior endplate edge of a target level
  - Identify the corresponding anterior, middle, and/or posterior inferior endplate edge of the adjacent level
  - Measure the distance between both endplates to calculate the anterior, middle, and/or posterior endplate-to-endplate distance
  - When measuring endplate-to-endplate distance at the L5–S1 level, measurements are drawn from the superior endplate of L5 to the superior endplate of S1
  - These values are then subtracted from previous endplate-to-endplate distances to calculate subsidence
  - Normal values: <2–3 mm
- Interforaminal height
  - Identify the inferior vertebral notch of a cephalad neural foramina
  - Identify the corresponding superior vertebral notch of the caudad level
  - Measure the distance from the top of the inferior notch to the bottom of the superior notch to calculate interforaminal height
  - This value is then subtracted from a previous interforaminal height measure to determine subsidence
  - Normal values: <2–3 mm

CONCLUSION

Given the prevalence of cervical spine procedures in modern spine surgery, an understanding of appropriate imaging techniques is an invaluable addition to the surgeon's diagnostic armamentarium. As demonstrated, the methods outlined here are not only useful for routine clinical practice, but have applications in research as well. While other methods have yet to be subjected to rigorous reliability and validation assessments, the sheer volume of techniques speaks to the importance of imaging assessments and highlights the amount of information provided through plain radiographs. As such, it is both extremely likely that the techniques outlined here will see continued use in cervical spine surgery and that new approaches will emerge in the years to come.

REFERENCES

1. Swartz EE, Floyd RT, Cendoma M. Cervical spine functional anatomy and the biomechanics of injury due to compressive loading. *J Athl Train.* 2005;40(3):155–161.
2. Tan LA, Riew KD, Traynelis VC. Cervical spine deformity-part 1: biomechanics, radiographic parameters, and classification. *Neurosurgery.* 2017;81(2):197–203.
3. Jun HS, Kim JH, Ahn JH, et al. T1 slope and degenerative cervical spondylolisthesis. *Spine (Phila Pa 1976).* 2015;40(4):E220–E226.
4. Park JH, Cho CB, Song JH, Kim SW, Ha Y, Oh JK. T1 slope and cervical sagittal alignment on cervical CT radiographs of asymptomatic persons. *J Korean Neurosurg Soc.* 2013;53(6):356–359.
5. Brady WJ, Moghtader J, Cutcher D, Exline C, Young J. ED use of flexion-extension cervical spine radiography in the evaluation of blunt trauma. *Am J Emerg Med.* 1999;17(6):504–508.
6. Harris Jr JH, Carson GC, Wagner LK. Radiologic diagnosis of traumatic occipitovertebral dissociation: 1. Normal occipitovertebral relationships on lateral radiographs of supine subjects. *AJR Am J Roentgenol.* 1994;162(4):881–886.
7. Cattell HS, Filtzer DL. Pseudosubluxation and other normal variations in the cervical spine in children. A study of one hundred and sixty children. *J Bone Joint Surg Am.* 1965;47(7):1295–1309.
8. Ghanem I, El Hage S, Rachkidi R, Kharrat K, Dagher F, Kreichati G. Pediatric cervical spine instability. *J Child Orthop.* 2008;2(2):71–84.
9. Matar LD, Helms CA, Richardson WJ. "Spinolaminar breach": an important sign in cervical spinous process fractures. *Skelet Radiol.* 2000;29(2):75–80.
10. Seybold EA, Dunn EJ, Jenis LG, Sweeney CA. Variation in the posterior vertebral contour line at the level of C-2 on lateral cervical roentgenograms: a method for odontoid fracture detection. *Am J Orthop (Belle Mead, NJ).* 1999;28(12):696–701.
11. Oshima Y, Kelly MP, Song KS, et al. Spinolaminar line test as a screening tool for C1 stenosis. *Global Spine J.* 2016;6(4):370–374.
12. Guo G-M, Li J, Diao Q-X, et al. Cervical lordosis in asymptomatic individuals: a meta-analysis. *J Orthop Surg Res.* 2018;13(1):147.
13. Harrison DD, Janik TJ, Troyanovich SJ, Holland B. Comparisons of lordotic cervical spine curvatures to a theoretical ideal model of the static sagittal cervical spine. *Spine (Phila Pa 1976).* 1996;21(6):667–675.
14. Harrison DE, Haas JW, Cailliet R, Harrison DD, Holland B, Janik TJ. Concurrent validity of flexicurve instrument measurements: sagittal skin contour of the cervical spine compared with lateral cervical radiographic measurements. *J Manip Physiol Ther.* 2005;28(8):597–603.

15. Harrison DD, Harrison DE, Janik TJ, et al. Modeling of the sagittal cervical spine as a method to discriminate hypolordosis: results of elliptical and circular modeling in 72 asymptomatic subjects, 52 acute neck pain subjects, and 70 chronic neck pain subjects. *Spine (Phila Pa 1976).* 2004;29(22):2485–2492.

16. Ishihara A. Roentgenographic studies on the mobility of the cervical column in the sagittal plane. *Nihon Seikeigeka Gakkai Zasshi.* 1968;42(11):1045–1056.

17. Ishihara A. Roentgenographic studies on the normal pattern of the cervical curvature. *Nihon Seikeigeka Gakkai Zasshi.* 1968;42(11):1033–1044.

18. Donk RD, Fehlings MG, Verhagen WIM, et al. An assessment of the most reliable method to estimate the sagittal alignment of the cervical spine: analysis of a prospective cohort of 138 cases. *J Neurosurg Spine.* 2017;26(5):572–576.

19. Donk RD, Arnts H, Verhagen WIM, Groenewoud H, Verbeek A, Bartels RHMA. Cervical sagittal alignment after different anterior discectomy procedures for single-level cervical degenerative disc disease: randomized controlled trial. *Acta Neurochir.* 2017;159(12):2359–2365.

20. McAllister BD, Rebholz BJ, Wang JC. Is posterior fusion necessary with laminectomy in the cervical spine? *Surg Neurol Int.* 2012;3(suppl 3):S225–S231.

21. Youn MS, Shin JK, Goh TS, Kang SS, Jeon WK, Lee JS. Relationship between cervical sagittal alignment and health-related quality of life in adolescent idiopathic scoliosis. *Eur Spine J.* 2016;25(10):3114–3119.

22. Matsubayashi Y, Chikuda H, Oshima Y, et al. C7 sagittal vertical axis is the determinant of the C5–C7 angle in cervical sagittal alignment. *Spine J.* 2017;17(5):622–626.

23. Patwardhan AG, Havey RM, Khayatzadeh S, et al. Postural consequences of cervical sagittal imbalance: a novel laboratory model. *Spine (Phila Pa 1976).* 2015;40(11):783–792.

24. Roguski M, Benzel EC, Curran JN, et al. Postoperative cervical sagittal imbalance negatively affects outcomes after surgery for cervical spondylotic myelopathy. *Spine.* 2014;39(25):2070–2077.

25. Tang JA, Scheer JK, Smith JS, et al. The impact of standing regional cervical sagittal alignment on outcomes in posterior cervical fusion surgery. *Neurosurgery.* 2012;71(3):662–669. discussion 669.

26. Kato M, Namikawa T, Matsumura A, Konishi S, Nakamura H. Effect of cervical sagittal balance on laminoplasty in patients with cervical myelopathy. *Global Spine J.* 2017;7(2):154–161.

27. Miyamoto H, Maeno K, Uno K, Kakutani K, Nishida K, Sumi M. Outcomes of surgical intervention for cervical spondylotic myelopathy accompanying local kyphosis (comparison between laminoplasty alone and posterior reconstruction surgery using the screw-rod system). *Eur Spine J.* 2014;23(2):341–346.

28. Vital JM, Senegas J. Anatomical bases of the study of the constraints to which the cervical spine is subject in the sagittal plane. A study of the center of gravity of the head. *Surg Radiol Anat.* 1986;8(3):169–173.

29. Wang ZL, Xiao JL, Mou JH, Qin TZ, Liu P. Analysis of cervical sagittal balance parameters in MRIs of patients with disc-degenerative disease. *Med Sci Monit.* 2015;21:3083–3088.

30. Guo Q, Deng Y, Wang J, et al. Influence of the T1-slope on sagittal alignment of the subaxial cervical spine after posterior atlantoaxial fusion in os odontoideum. *Clin Neurol Neurosurg.* 2016;149:39–43.

31. Janusz P, Tyrakowski M, Glowka P, Offoha R, Siemionow K. Influence of cervical spine position on the radiographic parameters of the thoracic inlet alignment. *Eur Spine J.* 2015;24(12):2880–2884.

32. Xing R, Liu W, Li X, Jiang L, Yishakea M, Dong J. Characteristics of cervical sagittal parameters in healthy cervical spine adults and patients with cervical disc degeneration. *BMC Musculoskelet Disord.* 2018;19(1):37.

33. Sun J, Zhao HW, Wang JJ, Xun L, Fu NX, Huang H. Diagnostic value of T1 slope in degenerative cervical spondylotic myelopathy. *Med Sci Monit.* 2018;24:791–796.

34. Pope MH, Hanley EN, Matteri RE, Wilder DG, Frymoyer JW. Measurement of intervertebral disc space height. *Spine.* 1977;2(4):282–286.

35. Allaire BT, DePaolis Kaluza MC, Bruno AG, et al. Evaluation of a new approach to compute intervertebral disc height measurements from lateral radiographic views of the spine. *Eur Spine J.* 2017;26(1):167–172.

36. Amonoo-Kuofi HS. Morphometric changes in the heights and anteroposterior diameters of the lumbar intervertebral discs with age. *J Anat.* 1991;175:159–168.

37. Agius R, Galea R, Fava S. Bone mineral density and intervertebral disc height in type 2 diabetes. *J Diabetes Complicat.* 2016;30(4):644–650.

38. Abu-Leil S, Floman Y, Bronstein Y, Masharawi Y. A morphometric analysis of all lumbar intervertebral discs and vertebral bodies in degenerative spondylolisthesis. *Eur Spine J.* 2016;25(8):2535–2545.

39. Frobin W, Brinckmann P, Biggemann M, Tillotson M, Burton K. Precision measurement of disc height, vertebral height and sagittal plane displacement from lateral radiographic views of the lumbar spine. *Clin Biomech (Bristol, Avon).* 1997;12(suppl 1):S1–S63.

40. Peng CW, Quirno M, Bendo JA, Spivak JM, Goldstein JA. Effect of intervertebral disc height on postoperative motion and clinical outcomes after Prodisc-C cervical disc replacement. *Spine J.* 2009;9(7):551–555.

41. Lee C, Woodring JH, Rogers LF, Kim KS. The radiographic distinction of degenerative slippage (spondylolisthesis and retrolisthesis) from traumatic slippage of the cervical spine. *Skelet Radiol.* 1986;15(6):439–443.

42. Simmonds AM, Rampersaud YR, Dvorak MF, Dea N, Melnyk AD, Fisher CG. Defining the inherent stability of degenerative spondylolisthesis: a systematic review. *J Neurosurg Spine.* 2015;23(2):178–189.

43. Torg JS, Pavlov H, Genuario SE, et al. Neurapraxia of the cervical spinal cord with transient quadriplegia. *J Bone Joint Surg Am.* 1986;68(9):1354–1370.

44. Pavlov H, Torg JS, Robie B, Jahre C. Cervical spinal stenosis: determination with vertebral body ratio method. *Radiology.* 1987;164(3):771–775.
45. Yue WM, Tan SB, Tan MH, Koh DC, Tan CT. The Torg-Pavlov ratio in cervical spondylotic myelopathy: a comparative study between patients with cervical spondylotic myelopathy and a nonspondylotic, nonmyelopathic population. *Spine (Phila Pa 1976).* 2001;26(16):1760–1764.
46. Aebli N, Wicki AG, Ruegg TB, Petrou N, Eisenlohr H, Krebs J. The Torg-Pavlov ratio for the prediction of acute spinal cord injury after a minor trauma to the cervical spine. *Spine J.* 2013;13(6):605–612.
47. Prasad SS, O'Malley M, Caplan M, Shackleford IM, Pydisetty RK. MRI measurements of the cervical spine and their correlation to Pavlov's ratio. *Spine (Phila Pa 1976).* 2003;28(12):1263–1268.
48. Blackley HR, Plank LD, Robertson PA. Determining the sagittal dimensions of the canal of the cervical spine. The reliability of ratios of anatomical measurements. *J Bone Joint Surg Br.* 1999;81(1):110–112.
49. Bono CM, Vaccaro AR, Fehlings M, et al. Measurement techniques for lower cervical spine injuries: consensus statement of the Spine Trauma Study Group. *Spine (Phila Pa 1976).* 2006;31(5):603–609.
50. Fehlings MG, Rao SC, Tator CH, et al. The optimal radiologic method for assessing spinal canal compromise and cord compression in patients with cervical spinal cord injury. Part II: results of a multicenter study. *Spine (Phila Pa 1976).* 1999;24(6):605–613.
51. Rao SC, Fehlings MG. The optimal radiologic method for assessing spinal canal compromise and cord compression in patients with cervical spinal cord injury. Part I: An evidence-based analysis of the published literature. *Spine (Phila Pa 1976).* 1999;24(6):598–604.
52. Diebo BG, Challier V, Henry JK, et al. Predicting cervical alignment required to maintain horizontal gaze based on global spinal alignment. *Spine.* 2016;41(23):1795–1800.
53. Nemani VM, Derman PB, Kim HJ. Osteotomies in the cervical spine. *Asian Spine J.* 2016;10(1):184–195.
54. Lafage R, Challier V, Liabaud B, et al. Natural head posture in the setting of sagittal spinal deformity: validation of chin-brow vertical angle, slope of line of sight, and McGregor's slope with health-related quality of life. *Neurosurgery.* 2016;79(1):108–115.
55. Yan YZ, Shao ZX, Pan XX, et al. Acceptable chin-brow vertical angle for neutral position radiography: preliminary analyses based on parameters of the whole sagittal spine of an asymptomatic Chinese population. *World Neurosurg.* 2018;120:e488–e496.
56. Kim KT, Lee SH, Son ES, Kwack YH, Chun YS, Lee JH. Surgical treatment of "chin-on-pubis" deformity in a patient with ankylosing spondylitis: a case report of consecutive cervical, thoracic, and lumbar corrective osteotomies. *Spine (Phila Pa 1976).* 2012;37(16):E1017–E1021.
57. Deviren V, Scheer JK, Ames CP. Technique of cervicothoracic junction pedicle subtraction osteotomy for cervical sagittal imbalance: report of 11 cases. *J Neurosurg Spine.* 2011;15(2):174–181.
58. Gopalakrishnan KC, el Masri W. Prevertebral soft tissue shadow widening-an important sign of cervical spinal injury. *Injury.* 1986;17(2):125–128.
59. Penning L. Prevertebral hematoma in cervical spine injury: incidence and etiologic significance. *AJR Am J Roentgenol.* 1981;136(3):553–561.
60. Wholey MH, Bruwer AJ, Baker Jr HL. The lateral roentgenogram of the neck; with comments on the atlanto-odontoid-basion relationship. *Radiology.* 1958;71(3):350–356.
61. Haug RH, Wible RT, Lieberman J. Measurement standards for the prevertebral region in the lateral soft-tissue radiograph of the neck. *J Oral Maxillofac Surg.* 1991;49(11):1149–1151.
62. Oon CL. Some sagittal measurements of the neck in normal adults. *Br J Radiol.* 1964;37:674–677.
63. Chi LJ, Wang ADW, Chen LK. Prevertebral soft tissue measurements on lateral roentgenogram of cervical spine in Chinese. *Chin J Radiol.* 2002;27:151–155.
64. Jarraya M, Hayashi D, Roemer FW, et al. Radiographically occult and subtle fractures: a pictorial review. *Radiol Res Pract.* 2013;2013:370169.
65. Genant HK, Wu CY, van Kuijk C, Nevitt MC. Vertebral fracture assessment using a semiquantitative technique. *J Bone Miner Res.* 1993;8(9):1137–1148.
66. Mikula AL, Hetzel SJ, Binkley N, Anderson PA. Validity of height loss as a predictor for prevalent vertebral fractures, low bone mineral density, and vitamin D deficiency. *Osteoporos Int.* 2017;28(5):1659–1665.
67. Seo JY, Kwon YS, Kim KJ, Shin JY, Kim YH, Ha KY. Clinical importance of posterior vertebral height loss on plain radiography when conservatively treating osteoporotic vertebral fractures. *Injury.* 2017;48(7):1503–1509.
68. Kuhns LR, Strouse PJ. Facet coverage in children on flexion lateral cervical radiographs. *Spine (Phila Pa 1976).* 1999;24(4):339–341.
69. Oliveira ORGd, Martins SPR, Lima WGd, Gomes MM. The use of bone morphogenetic proteins (BMP) and pseudarthrosis, a literature review. *Rev Bras Ortop.* 2016;52(2):124–140.
70. Fraser JF, Hartl R. Anterior approaches to fusion of the cervical spine: a metaanalysis of fusion rates. *J Neurosurg Spine.* 2007;6(4):298–303.
71. Buser Z, Brodke DS, Youssef JA, et al. Synthetic bone graft versus autograft or allograft for spinal fusion: a systematic review. *J Neurosurg Spine.* 2016;25(4):509–516.
72. Ray CD. Threaded fusion cages for lumbar interbody fusions. An economic comparison with 360 degrees fusions. *Spine (Phila Pa 1976).* 1997;22(6):681–685.
73. Young PM, Berquist TH, Bancroft LW, Peterson JJ. Complications of spinal instrumentation. *Radiographics.* 2007;27(3):775–789.
74. Raizman NM, O'Brien JR, Poehling-Monaghan KL, Yu WD. Pseudarthrosis of the spine. *J Am Acad Orthop Surg.* 2009;17(8):494–503.

75. Hilibrand AS, Robbins M. Adjacent segment degeneration and adjacent segment disease: the consequences of spinal fusion? *Spine J.* 2004;4(6 suppl):190s–194s.

76. Zhang C, Berven SH, Fortin M, Weber MH. Adjacent segment degeneration versus disease after lumbar spine fusion for degenerative pathology: a systematic review with meta-analysis of the literature. *Clin Spine Surg.* 2016;29(1):21–29.

77. Kong L, Cao J, Wang L, Shen Y. Prevalence of adjacent segment disease following cervical spine surgery: a PRISMA-compliant systematic review and meta-analysis. *Medicine (Baltimore).* 2016;95(27), e4171.

78. Hashimoto K, Aizawa T, Kanno H, Itoi E. Adjacent segment degeneration after fusion spinal surgery-a systematic review. *Int Orthop.* 2019;43(4):987–993.

79. Alhashash M, Shousha M, Boehm H. Adjacent segment disease after cervical spine fusion: evaluation of a 70 patient long-term follow-up. *Spine (Phila Pa 1976).* 2018;43(9):605–609.

80. Samartzis D, Marco RA, Jenis LG, et al. Characterization of graft subsidence in anterior cervical discectomy and fusion with rigid anterior plate fixation. *Am J Orthop (Belle Mead, NJ).* 2007;36(8):421–427.

CHAPTER 7

Magnetic Resonance Imaging Techniques for the Evaluation of the Subaxial Cervical Spine

ASHLYN A. FITCH • SAMUEL S. RUDISILL • GARRETT K. HARADA • HOWARD S. AN
Department of Orthopaedic Surgery, Rush University Medical Center, Chicago, IL, United States

INTRODUCTION

The advancement of magnetic resonance imaging (MRI) has made high-quality visualization of the normal and pathologic spine, as well as associated neural tissue, readily available. Relative to plain radiography and computed tomography (CT), MRI boasts excellent visualization of soft tissues without exposing the patient to harmful radiation. Within the cervical spine specifically, MRI is routinely used for evaluation of neck pain and radicular symptoms.[1] Several pathologies including spinal stenosis, degenerative disc disease, and tumors can be identified on MRI. However, as with any imaging modality, MRI also has the potential to highlight clinically insignificant pathologies, thus correlation with clinical exam findings is critically important to confirm a diagnosis. Regardless, high-quality visualization of anatomic structures and their associated soft tissues makes MRI a highly valuable clinical and diagnostic tool.

MRI PRINCIPLES AND IMAGE SEQUENCES OF THE SUBAXIAL CERVICAL SPINE

When clinical pathology is suspected in the cervical spine, classic radiographs are often the first imaging study to be performed. However, the inability to visualize soft tissues in detail leaves potential for certain diseases to be overlooked. Conversely, MRI is a non-invasive technique offering excellent soft tissue resolution. Because it does not involve the use of harmful ionizing radiation, MRI has quickly become the imaging modality of choice for many patients. Several MRI sequences exist to image the cervical spine in multiple planes, including T1-weighted spin echo (SE), T2-weighted fast spin echo (FSE), axial gradient-recalled echo (GRE), and more[2,3] (Table 1). Each sequence is uniquely different to highlight different elements of cervical anatomy and physiology, therefore appropriate sequence selection is imperative to diagnostic evaluation.

With good image resolution and signal-to-noise ratios, T1-weighted SE sequences are best used to evaluate cervical anatomy, fracture lines, and osseous details.[4,5] Superior depiction of bone marrow intensity also makes T1-weighted imaging a useful tool in identifying processes of bone marrow replacement, such as metastatic disease.[2,6] However, T1-weighted imaging is less sensitive to many pathologies requiring clear differentiation of tissues. For example, poor distinction between intervertebral discs and the posterior longitudinal ligament or between muscle and nonfatty structures makes adequate assessment of these structures potentially difficult.[7]

T1-gadolinium contrast-enhanced (T1-Gd) sequences may be considered for detection of necrosis or inflammatory conditions. Increased blood vessel permeability secondary to disease permits accumulation of contrast agent which appears hyperintense to surrounding tissues.[8] However, the use of contrast makes these sequences relatively invasive, time-consuming, and costly to perform.

T2-weighted sequences are produced using longer echo time (TE) and repetition time (TR) to improve visualization of pathologic changes in soft tissues (i.e., intervertebral discs), evaluation of cellular processes altering local water content, and assessment of spinal cord parenchyma for lesions and edema.[3,5,9,10] In contrast to T1-weighted imaging, the spinal cord appears with intermediate signal intensity surrounded by high-intensity cerebrospinal fluid (CSF) on T2-weighted sequences, enabling clear identification of any areas of compromised central canal integrity.[2]

Atlas of Spinal Imaging. https://doi.org/10.1016/B978-0-323-76111-6.00011-0

TABLE 1
Summary of Clinically Relevant Magnetic Resonance Image (MRI) Sequences for Evaluation of the Cervical Spine

MRI Sequence	Clinical Context	Strengths	Weaknesses
T1-weighted spin echo	• Cervical anatomy • Fracture lines • Osseous detail • Bone marrow replacement	• Signal-to-noise ratio • Image resolution • Depiction of bone marrow intensity	• Tissue differentiation
T1-gadolinium contrast-enhanced	• Necrosis • Inflammatory conditions	• Contrast accumulation indicates blood vessel permeability	• Invasive • Time-consuming • Cost
T2-weighted fast spin echo	• Soft tissues • Local water content • Spinal cord parenchymal lesions • Edema	• Depiction of spinal canal • Fast acquisition • Image resolution • Signal-to-noise ratio • Decreased motion artifact	• Insensitivity to focal calcification • Insensitivity to focal hemorrhage • Hypersensitivity to fat and cerebrospinal fluid
Gradient-recalled echo	• Osteophytosis • Neural foraminal integrity • Traumatic injury/hemorrhage	• Fast acquisition • Decreased motion artifact • Extradural disease sensitivity	• Intradural disease sensitivity
Short tau inversion recovery	• Fat suppression • Orthopedic hardware • Traumatic injury/edema	• Fast acquisition • Low sensitivity to metal	• Cannot be used after gadolinium injection
Fluid-attenuated inversion recovery	• Motion artifact suppression • Orthopedic hardware • Degenerative disease • Demyelinating disease	• Fast acquisition • Low sensitivity to metal	
Metal artifact reduction sequences	• Orthopedic hardware	• Reduced metal artifact • Signal-to-noise ratio	
Kinetic MRI	• Motion-dependent pathology • Gravitational effects on alignment	• Visualizes effects of gravity and motion	
Susceptibility-weighted	• Calcified structures	• High sensitivity and specificity for osteophytes	

Specifically, T2-weighted FSE sequences have largely replaced SE sequences due to their faster imaging speed, improved resolution, superior signal-to-noise ratio, and decreased motion artifact. Disadvantages of T2-weighted FSE sequences include a decreased ability to detect small areas of calcification or hemorrhage, for which susceptibility-weighted MRI (SW-MRI) and T2-weighted GRE sequences provide better differentiation. Additionally, T2-weighted FSE may exhibit overly bright appearances of fat and CSF. Short tau inversion recovery (STIR) and fluid-attenuated inversion recovery (FLAIR) sequences are more appropriate for appreciating these tissues, respectively.[3]

Although both T1-weighted SE and T2-weighted FSE sequences are good at detecting degenerative changes,[4] each has its disadvantages. Neither clearly shows ossification of ligaments, so CT is the imaging study of choice should there be concern for this pathology. Further, fat can pose interference within these sequences, particularly in T1-weighted images. Fat-suppression sequences may therefore be necessary to achieve adequate contrast enhancement within the anatomic area of interest.[1]

Artifact, such as CSF pulsation on T2-weighted imaging or esophageal swallowing motions, may be present and should not be mistaken for pathology.[1] Lastly, as with all MRI techniques, it is important to recognize that significant disease may be harbored within the areas between imaging planes on sequences.[2] Gap size may need to be decreased in some cases to visualize tissues with more precise depth.

Should T1-weighted SE and T2-weighted FSE sequences produce inadequate images, axial GRE sequences can be ordered to supplement. Decreased imaging time and susceptibility to motion artifact establish GRE as superior in detecting many degenerative changes such as osteophyte formation and neural foraminal narrowing.[3] Additionally, this sequence is also useful in detecting the presence of blood following spinal cord hemorrhage in the context of trauma or vascular malformation.[1,3,11,12] While GRE demonstrates good sensitivity for extradural disease processes, its sensitivity for intradural pathology is less impressive.[1]

Increasing in popularity are inversion recovery sequences such as STIR and FLAIR. With their reduced scan time and low susceptibility to metal, these sequences are ideal for imaging patients with orthopedic hardware. As mentioned previously, STIR is a fat-suppression sequence that proves useful when adipose tissue is obstructing the images.[1] STIR can be added onto T1- or T2-weighted sequences, but it cannot be used after a gadolinium injection due to inadvertent nulling of certain tissues. Due to its superior sensitivity for detecting edema, STIR sequences are commonly ordered for the evaluation of traumatic injury.[11] FLAIR sequences may be added onto T2-weighted scans for suppression of motion artifact caused by water, making them a preferred sequence for pediatric patients or those who cannot remain supine for extended periods of time. By attenuating the high-intensity signal of CSF, these sequences can better distinguish the spinal cord, CSF, and intervertebral disc for evaluation of degenerative changes.[13] FLAIR further serves as a valuable tool in assessment of demyelinating disease, such as multiple sclerosis.[1]

Artifact reduction is also achievable using metal artifact reduction sequences (MARS). These sequences are particularly useful for imaging the cervical spine in patients with metal implants, as use of a low-powered magnet reduces the size and intensity of metal artifact produced by magnetic field distortion without sacrificing signal-to-noise ratio.

Kinetic MRIs, such as flexion/extension sequences, are newly emerging techniques used to assess the effects of movement and gravity on the cervical spine. Utilizing these methods may allow physicians to unveil motion-dependent pathologies not seen in more classic imaging orientations.[14,15] Several pathologies can be exacerbated with movement and should be evaluated using kinetic MRI, including central spinal stenosis, spondylolisthesis, and rheumatoid arthritis (RA). Furthermore, cervical alignment may also be better assessed with these techniques, as the effects of gravity contribute to a more accurate clinical evaluation of spinal curvature.

Susceptibility-weighted MRI (SW-MRI) is an emerging MR technique that has demonstrated improved visualization of calcified structures, such as osteophytes. SW-MRI has high sensitivity and specificity for identifying and locating osteophytes relative to classic T1- and T2- weighted images, which often fail to distinguish osteophytes from disc herniations. Whereas T1- and T2-weighted sequences show both as hypointense, SW-MRI depicts calcified structures with a hyperintense signal,[16] a useful benefit for preoperative planning not available with conventional 2D radiography.

ANATOMY
Vertebral Anatomy

The cervical spine consists of seven vertebrae arranged vertically from the base of the skull to the level of the shoulders. In coordination with associated muscles, tendons, and ligaments, these bony structures provide structure, support, and flexibility to the neck while serving to protect the spinal cord coursing within. Generally, the cervical spine shares characteristics with other spinal segments, including a vertebral body, vertebral arches, transverse processes, a spinous process, and facet joints. In midsagittal view, MRI of the healthy cervical spine shows small lips protruding from the anteroinferior border of the vertebral bodies,[17] facilitating a normal lordotic curvature from C2-T2 with the apex around C4-C5.[18] In contrast, the superior faces appear concave in the lateral direction and convex anteroposteriorly,[19] and the vertebral body walls are slightly concave in nature.[18] The fatty composition of the marrow within the healthy vertebral body conveys a bright signal intensity to T1-weighted images. Moving parasagittally brings the transverse processes into frame, which serve as significant points of attachment for various muscles and ligaments and provide conduits for neurovasculature. The vertebral artery and venous systems can be seen in the axial perspective passing vertically through the foramen transversarium of the transverse processes on each side of the vertebra.[17] Notably, the spinous processes of the typical cervical vertebrae demonstrate a classically bifid structure. Representative MRI images of the normal cervical spine are shown in Fig. 1.

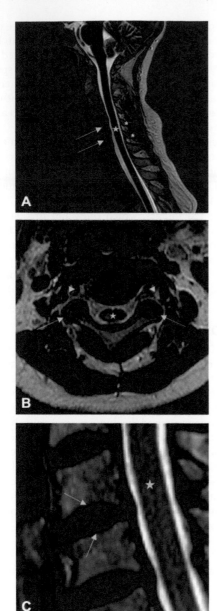

FIG. 1 T2-weighted MRI of the human cervical spine. The C1-C7 vertebral bodies *(arrows)*, spinous processes *(asterisks)*, and spinal cord *(star)* within the spinal canal is best appreciated in the midsagittal perspective (A). Axial view shows the facet joints *(arrows)*, transverse processes and foramina *(arrowheads)*, and a cross-section of the spinal cord *(star;* B). Higher magnification in the midsagittal frame allows enhanced visualization of the intervertebral discs *(star)* and vertebral endplates *(arrows;* C).

There are a few exceptions to these anatomic generalizations within the cervical spine. C1, often referred to as the atlas, is unique in its replacement of a vertebral body with the anterior tubercle. As the only vertebra without a vertebral body, the atlas assumes a ring-like shape and connects the occipital condyle above with the proper cervical spine below via the atlanto-occipital joint. Extensions of the anterior longitudinal ligament and ligamentum flavum comprise the atlanto-occipital membranes, which support the atlanto-occipital joint in conferring a majority of the flexion/extension motion to the head. Inferior to the atlas is the C2, or axis, so named due to the bony odontoid process protruding upward into the ring of C1 with which it forms the atlanto-axial joint. This synovial joint permits the atlas to rotate around the axis and accounts for nearly 50% of the rotational motion of the head.[17] Because they exhibit such unique morphologies, C1 and C2 are classified as atypical vertebrae. Additionally, the most inferior vertebra of the cervical spine, C7, has a number of distinguishing features. Known as vertebra prominens, C7 can be identified on midsagittal view by its particularly prominent spinous process, which is not bifid as in the rest of the cervical spine. This specialized projection ensures optimum fit with T1 in the cervicothoracic junction and provides attachment points for more muscles than any other cervical vertebra. Furthermore, the foramina in the transverse processes where the vertebral arteries normally pass are absent at this level and will not be seen on axial view.

Facet Joints

At each vertebral level except C1, the laminae and pedicles merge laterally into lateral masses before separating into the paired superior and inferior articular processes. The inferior processes from the vertebra above articulate with the superior processes of the vertebra below to form the facet joints. Formally termed zygapophyseal joints, these true synovial joints contain cartilage and menisci to permit small movements across the motion segment while restricting hyperflexion and hyperextension. Movement across each motion segment is quite limited; however, the cumulative effect across the entire spine enables significant rotation, flexion, extension, and lateral bending.[17] Notably, whereas these joints are oriented vertically within the lumbar spine, their 45-degree orientation within the cervical spine facilitates flexion and extension.[20] Paired with the abundance of proprioceptive and pain receptors innervating the area, the susceptibility of the facet joints to age- or trauma-related degeneration denotes a plausible role for the facet joints in chronic neck pain.[17] Visualization of the facet joints is best achieved with T2-weighted imaging, which shows a smooth homogenous signal of the hyaline cartilage overlying the low-signal cortical bone.[21] Despite the paucity of literature surrounding visualization of the normal facet joints with MRI, this imaging method becomes increasingly important in the context of pathology such as joint inflammation[22] and age-related cartilage degeneration.[2]

Intervertebral Discs

With the exception of the atlanto-occipital and atlanto-axial joints, intervertebral discs are interspersed between adjacent vertebral bodies throughout the cervical spine. These avascular structures provide support to vertebral bodies, permit flexibility throughout the full range of head and neck movements, and cushion the impact of various stresses and loads on the cervical spine. The anatomy of the intervertebral disc consists of two basic components. The nucleus pulposus is the soft inner core of mucoprotein gel that assists in providing cushioning and flexibility to the disc. Surrounding the nucleus pulposus is the annulus fibrosus, a durable external layer composed of concentric rings of alternating obliquely oriented collagen fibers functioning to distribute forces, protect the inner core, and stabilize the motion segment.[23] MRI is used to assess the integrity of the intervertebral discs through quantification of disc hydration primarily based on proton density and water content. Specifically, normal discs exhibit a bright signal within the nucleus pulposus on both T1- and T2-weighted images due to its high water and proteoglycan content, often with a horizontally oriented area of decreased intensity at the core's center in the adult. The more fibrous composition of the annulus fibrosus emits a darker signal, generating a marked distinction between the nucleus pulposus and annulus fibrosus in the healthy disc[24] (Fig. 1C). Coronal views show the superior face of the disc is concave, while the inferior face is convex.[19] In midsagittal view, one can determine that the six intervertebral discs of the cervical spine are thinner than the greater load-bearing discs of the lumbar spine but thicker than those of the less-mobile thoracic region.[23] The discs of the healthy cervical spine also demonstrate greater thickness anteriorly, which in conjunction with the lipped nature of the vertebral bodies facilitates a lordotic curvature.[17] Normally, an intervertebral disc will be entirely contained within the anterior and posterior margins of the vertebral bodies and will not vary in height by more than 25% compared to adjacent normal disc spaces.[25]

Vertebral endplates mark the transition between the intervertebral disc and the adjacent vertebral body.

Without a blood supply of its own, the intervertebral discs rely on the transport of nutrients and small amounts of blood from the subchondral bone through the hyaline cartilage and porous bone of the vertebral endplate for nourishment. These structures also function to buffer disc pressures on the vertebral bodies and limit protrusion, provide points of insertion for the inner fibers of the annulus, and serve as growth plates responsible for endochondral ossification. On T1-weighted MRI, normal endplates display uniform intensity with the vertebral body and a clear demarcation from the adjacent intervertebral disc, whereas alterations in signal intensity relative to the vertebral body indicate endplate abnormalities[26-28] (Fig. 1C).

Spinal Canal

One of the most critical functions of the vertebral column is to house and protect the spinal cord within a spinal canal created by stacked vertebral foramen. The spinal cord itself is immediately surrounded by the pia mater, subarachnoid space, arachnoid mater, and dura mater. At the level of each intervertebral disc, bilateral spinal nerves project off of the spinal cord to innervate their respective body segments. The entirety of the cervical spinal cord is best visualized in midsagittal view. On T1-weighted images, the spinal cord will appear with an intermediate signal due to abundance of lipids within the cord. However, due to low water content of the cord, this structure emits low-intensity on T2-weighted images.[1]

Despite the paucity of MR-based studies describing the normal configuration of the cervical canal, dural tube, and cord, a few generalizations can be made.[29-31] From the axial and sagittal perspectives of T2-weighted sequences, the healthy spinal cord will show a homogeneous signal without intrinsic abnormalities.[4] Typically measured on T2-weighted images, canal size varies by vertebral level, as well as by the sex and age of the patient.[32-35] Canal diameter normally tapers from the first vertebrae to the third vertebrae, where the spinal cord undergoes a slight enlargement before retaining a more uniform diameter throughout the remainder of the cervical spine.[4] Notably, cross-sectional area, sagittal diameter, and axial diameter of the spinal cord peak in the third decade of life and tends to decrease thereafter[29,33,36] (Table 2).

Vertebral Column Alignment

In sagittal view, the entirety of the vertebral column assumes a slightly S-shaped appearance to efficiently perform the necessary functions of each spinal region (Fig. 1A). Generally, the curves of the spinal column

TABLE 2
Average Spinal Canal Diameter for Men and Women in Their 20s and 70s Measured at the Level of the Intervertebral Disc[43]

Age	Men	Women
20–29	12.7–14.4 mm	12.6–14.3 mm
70–79	11.0–13.6 mm	10.8–13.5 mm

serve to absorb shock, provide balance, and permit motion. To aid in supporting the weight of the head, the cervical spine maintains a lordotic curvature that should be apparent in sagittal view of any radiograph or MRI sequence.[4,37–39] The extent of lordosis is best measured on upright/standing X-ray, as conventional MRI is performed in the supine position where gravity can alter the patient's typical alignment. However, if upright/standing films are not available, methods do exist to estimate the extent of lordosis on MRI (in supine position), such as Cobb angles.[38] However, the translation of these measurements to MRI sequences has been only scarcely reported in literature and their validity is yet to be established.[40]

Soft Tissues

The soft tissue of the cervical spine refers to the muscles, ligaments, fascia, blood vessels, nerves, and lymphatics that traverse and supply structures of the region.

Muscle

Musculature accounts for the majority of soft tissue volume and contributes to movement of the head, neck, upper back, and shoulders. At the dorsolateral aspect of the cervical spine from superficial to deep are the trapezius, splenius capitis, splenius cervicis, levator scapulae, rotatores, rectus capitis, obliquus capitis, and semispinalis muscles. Anterolaterally are the platysma, sternocleidomastoid, strap muscles of the larynx, hyoid muscles, scalenes, longus cervicis, and longus colli muscles. The bodies of these muscles are illustrated well on nonfat-saturated T1-weighted MRI, while T2-weighted imaging allows assessment of edema and fluid.[41]

Ligaments

Muscles are assisted in providing stability to the cervical spine by a network of ligaments, including the anterior longitudinal ligament (ALL), posterior longitudinal ligament (PLL), and posterior ligamentous complex (PLC). The ALL and PLL course along the anterior and posterior aspects of the subaxial vertebral bodies, respectively, demonstrating a narrow, thick morphology over the bodies but stretching wide and thin while coursing over the intervertebral discs. The PLC is located posterior to the neural arch, consisting of the ligamentum flavum (LF), interspinous ligaments, and ligamentum nuchae. Within the cervical spine, the interspinous ligaments are particularly thin and poorly developed.[17] Due to their fibrous composition, ligaments appear as dark bands on all MRI pulse sequences,[42,43] with discontinuities in signal void suggesting acute ligament rupture.[44]

Vasculature

Structures of the cervical spine are supplied by branches of the vertebral, ascending cervical, deep cervical, and occipital arteries. The vertebral arteries originate from the subclavian arteries, coursing between the longus colli and anterior scalene before entering the vertebral column at the level of C6 and ascending through the transverse foramina toward the foramen magnum.[41] Anterior and posterior vertebral veins accompany the vertebral arteries, surrounding them in a venous plexus at the lateral aspect of the spine.[45] Upon entering the spinal canal, the left and right vertebral arteries merge to form the basilar artery that supplies the brainstem.[17] Several segmental radicular arteries stem from the vertebral arteries, mostly directed toward the ALL, intervertebral disc, and vertebral body.[45] Others feed into the muscles of the neck, where they anastomose with branches of the ascending cervical artery traveling between the anterior scalene and longus capitis along the transverse processes.[41] The deep cervical artery arises from the costovertebral trunk and travels between the facet joints toward the posterior spinal muscles,[45] while the occipital artery stems from the external carotid artery on its way to supply the posterior scalp.[41] Conventional MRI can be used to evaluate vasculature in the cervical spine.[46] Because MRI cannot recognize flow, however, vasculature is illustrated as focal areas of absent signal, or "flow voids" (Fig. 1B). Normal vasculature should exhibit a single lumen and generally follow the course outlined above.[45,47] Administration of contrast dye in magnetic resonance angiography (MRA) enables enhanced visualization of these structures and is the preferred method for their assessment.[48,49]

Nerves

Assessment of the nerves and the foramina through which they pass is a critical component MR-based evaluation of the cervical spine. On midsagittal view, the spinal cord can be appreciated extending inferiorly from the medulla oblongata and pons. At each vertebral level, branches stem from the spinal cord to form the eight spinal nerves of the cervical spine, termed C1 through C8. These then travel along the costotransverse lamella and between the anterior and posterior tubercles of the transverse processes before exiting the vertebral column via the intervertebral foramina toward their respective dermatomes and myotomes. Parasagittal views depict normal spinal nerves with intermediate intensity surrounded by high-intensity fat on T1-weighted imaging.[42] Because of the 45-degree oblique orientation of the intervertebral foramina, however, oblique imaging offers optimal viewing to assess whether compression or irritation may be contributing to any pain or dysfunction.

PATHOLOGIES OF THE CERVICAL SPINE
Central Spinal Stenosis

Central spinal stenosis encompasses a spectrum of structural changes within the cervical spine causing narrowing of the canal.[2,38] This disease can result from several spinal abnormalities and often manifests clinically with neck pain and/or upper extremity radiculopathy.[2,50] Stenosis severe enough to cause impingement and injury to the spinal cord is referred to as myelopathy, a disease predominantly associated with aging populations and most commonly diagnosed in patients over 50.[51] With its clear depiction of the spinal cord and avoidance of the magnification errors that commonly affect radiographs, MRI is an essential tool for evaluating for spinal stenosis.[2,14,52] Furthermore, MRI offers superior visualization of the intervertebral discs, osteophytes, ligaments, and degree of stenosis for superior determination of potential causes and severity of disease.[2,14,52-55] Because cervical spinal stenosis can vary with dynamic change, often worsening upon extension, kinetic MRI sequences may be considered.[53,56] These sequences may prove useful when selecting a level for cervical decompression during preoperative planning. Generally, patients with suspected cervical myelopathy should undergo MRI to confirm the diagnosis before considering surgical intervention. If confirmed, treatment should be pursued promptly as prolonged spinal cord compression can permanently damage the structure, resulting in residual symptoms and functional disabilities. Studies have shown treatment initiated within 6 months of symptom onset confer the greatest chance of recovery.[51,57]

At the level of stenosis, intramedullary signal changes can be seen within the spinal cord on T1- and T2-weighted images.[38] T2-weighted MRIs will additionally show CSF as hyperintense signal both anterior and

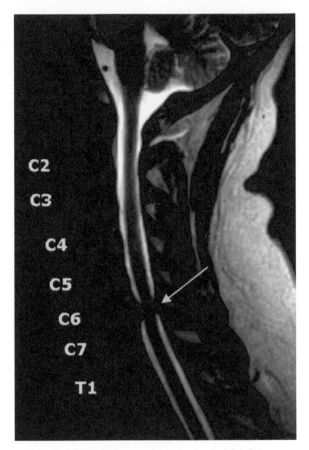

FIG. 2 Central spinal stenosis at the level of C6-C7 on a T2-weighted FSE sequence. There is notable disruption of hyperintense cerebral spinal fluid signal due to herniated disc protrusion *(arrow)*, potentially causing impingement of the spinal cord with associated clinical symptoms.

posterior to the cord on midsagittal images, as well as circumferentially around the cord on axial images, making physical compromise of the cord easily distinguishable regardless of compression mechanism[3] (Fig. 2). Disease progression may bring an increase in spinal cord edema, increasing T2-weighted and potentially decreasing T1-weighted signal intensity. Signal hyperintensity on T2-weighted sagittal images is often considered to be a diagnostic marker of myelopathy in the cervical spine, but the signal change is not pathognomonic for myelopathy.[38] Axial imaging is seldom used to assess for myelopathy as its validity remains uncertain. However, a "snake eye" appearance on T1-weighted axial scans has been noted in literature to be associated.[38,58] T1-Gd studies may be necessary to rule out vascular, inflammatory, infective, neoplastic, and demyelinating processes that may present similarly to myelopathy on conventional MRI sequences.[59]

C5-C6 is often the level most severely affected by myelopathy, followed by C4-C5[56] Central canal size varies among individuals; therefore, it is crucial to evaluate the affected level in reference to adjacent levels when assessing for stenosis and associated myelopathy.[32,35,38,60] Nevertheless, an inverse relationship between canal size and cord compression has been thoroughly described throughout the literature.[54,61–74] Reliable methods have been developed for quantification of central spinal stenosis severity, regardless of etiology. For example, Muhle et al. and Kang et al. have each suggested grading systems, as described later in this chapter.

Surgical intervention is commonly pursued in patients who exhibit clinical symptoms and display evidence of compression that could cause radiculopathy, myelopathy, or a combination of the two on MRI. For many, spinal cord decompression is an effective treatment for alleviation of symptoms and prevention of disease progression.[51,53] Specifically, patients with hyperintense intramedullary signal change on T2-weighted images are more likely to experience good surgical outcomes and reversal of MRI abnormality, while those with low intramedullary signal on T1-weighted scans may experience less favorable outcomes.[75] The limited regenerative capacity of the spinal cord should always be appreciated during spinal surgery, requiring adequate precautions and proper technique throughout the perioperative period to minimize risk of permanent injury.[51]

Certain risk factors for spinal stenosis should be discussed with patients if identified on imaging. For example, congenital narrowing of the cervical spinal canal less than 13 mm in diameter is associated with increased the risk of developing cervical spinal stenosis.[61–63,73,76,77] Specifically, a congenital canal diameter of less than 13 mm is diagnosed as relative stenosis, whereas a diameter of less than 10 mm is classified as absolute stenosis.[76] More recently, Nouri et al. suggested a SCOR measurement of greater than 70% is diagnostic for congenital spinal stenosis. These patients are more likely to develop myelopathy at a younger age with a greater degree of impairment and disability. However, these patients demonstrate comparable surgical outcomes to patients without congenital spinal stenosis.[78]

Degenerative Disc Disease

Degeneration within the cervical spine can affect many different structures, including the vertebral bodies, spinal ligaments, and facet joints.[68,79,80] However, initial stages of degenerative change typically present as a loss of structural integrity of the intervertebral discs, known as degenerative disc disease (DDD).[68] Symptoms

associated with DDD can present at any age, often with gradual-onset chronic pain. Progressive disc degeneration can lead to unequal exertion of forces on the adjacent vertebral bodies, resulting in bone restructuring and/or osteophyte formation characteristic of spondylosis.[79,80] On MRI, a healthy nucleus pulposus will appear hyperintense on T1- and T2-weighted images, but it loses intensity with age as water and proteoglycan content decreases.[81–86] This normal physiologic process predisposes the discs to further degradation, leading to diminished disc height, annular tears, disc herniation, and autofusion of adjacent vertebral bodies in the event of complete collapse.[37,38,87]

T1- and T2-weighted sequences are considered to be the most sensitive imaging methods for evaluating the intervertebral discs[88,89] (Fig. 3). However, MRI often fails to distinguish clinically relevant findings from incidental

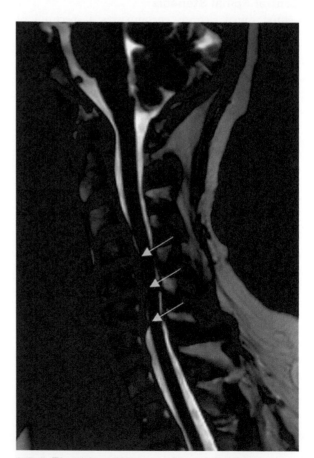

FIG. 3 T2-weighted FSE image of the cervical spine exhibiting signs of degenerative disc disease. Progressive disc degeneration is indicated by loss of signal intensity, signal void, and multilevel posterior disc bulging (see dark protrusions into the hyperintense cerebral spinal fluid; *arrows*).

ones. This can be disadvantageous in the context of DDD as signs apparent on imaging do not always correlate with symptoms.[25,90] Furthermore, it is important to recognize that decreased T2-weighted signal intensity in the nucleus pulposus due to loss of water and proteoglycan can be detected by as early as the second decade of life, as the core undergoes transitions to a more fibrocartilaginous structure and the distinct border between nucleus pulposus and annulus fibrosus becomes attenuated.[26,91,92] Loss of clear demarcation between these structures is not considered significant unless acute injury is suspected.[25,93] Several additional signs of DDD are apparent on MRI. Loss of disc height can be determined by comparison to normal values[94] or to normal adjacent disc heights, with decreases of greater than 25% serving as the diagnostic threshold for degeneration. More progressive degeneration characterized by accumulation of nitrogen within the disc results in the vacuum phenomenon, appearing as signal void on both T1- and T2-weighted imaging.[95] These degenerative changes can be more specifically diagnosed using any of the grading systems described below, such as Pfirrmann grades.[38,92,93]

Herniated Disc

A common and severe complication of degenerative disc disease is herniation of the intervertebral disc, a pathology in which a fragment of the nucleus pulposus extrudes through a tear or rupture in the annulus fibrosus. As DDD progresses, nucleus pulposus contents may be forced to migrate anteriorly, posteriorly, or laterally. Posterior herniations can project beyond the vertebral body margin to potentially cause cord compression, myelopathy, and radicular symptoms.[38] Disc herniations posterolaterally are particularly likely to impinge on spinal nerves exiting the vertebral column to produce clinically relevant symptoms, while anterior herniations have been reported to cause dysphagia by compressing the esophagus.[96]

MRI is considered the superior imaging method for evaluation of disc herniation. Herniated discs are most commonly found at the levels of C5-C6 and C6-C7, causing impingement of the C6 and C7 nerve roots, respectively. Conversely, impingement of the C3 nerve root by a herniated disc is rare.[19] On T2-weighted images, disc herniations are appreciable on sagittal and axial scans as hypointense protrusions of the disc into the vertebral foramen (Fig. 4). Cord compression is best visualized from the sagittal perspective as a hypointense herniation impinging on the hyperintense spinal cord. Disc herniation is also commonly associated with Modic changes within the vertebral endplates superior and inferior to the disc, described later in this chapter.[97] Clinically, it is not possible to determine the age of the disc herniation unless the disc appears well hydrated

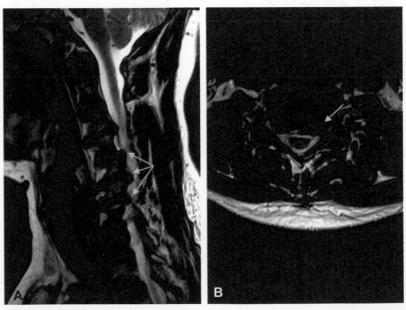

FIG. 4 T2-weighted FSE images demonstrating herniated discs in sagittal (A) and axial (B) views. Multiple herniated discs are visible as dark protrusions into hyperintense cerebral spinal fluid in the sagittal perspective *(arrows)*. On axial view, the C6-C7 disc herniation appears as a dark protrusion on the posterolateral edge of the intervertebral disc (B; *arrow*).

without any osseous ridging, suggesting the herniation is acute or subacute in nature.[2] Chronic herniations secondary to DDD are more common, however.[19]

Characteristic of all herniated intervertebral discs is the presence of high-intensity zones (HIZs) within the affected disc.[37] HIZs are focal areas of high intensity often within the posterior annulus fibrosus seen in sagittal view on T2-weighted imaging[37,98] (Fig. 5). Notably, HIZs do not result from normal aging, making them a reliable marker of DDD when differentiating from pathologically aging discs.[37,98-101] Appearing most commonly in the posterior aspect of the annulus fibrosus, HIZs are produced by a protrusion of the hyperintense nucleus pulposus through a tear in the annulus. These findings are highly correlated with significant lumbar discogenic pain, though their clinical relevance in the cervical spine remains to be elucidated.

Spondylolisthesis

Spondylolisthesis is a relatively common condition resulting from degeneration of the facet joints or hypermobility syndromes.[68,102-104] On imaging, spondylolisthesis will appear as a horizontal translation of one vertebral body out of alignment with adjacent vertebral bodies in sagittal view (Fig. 6). This disease is often associated with significant degeneration, disc herniation, and instability of the cervical spine.[38,102,104] With significant displacement, the diameter of the spinal canal can become compromised to produce spinal stenosis. Anterolisthesis, or forward slippage of the vertebral body, is commonly associated with more severe degeneration or trauma, though RA and other inflammatory arthropathies are known correlates of atraumatic spondylolisthesis.[102]

Since many spondylolistheses in the cervical spine are dependent upon normal upright positioning, diagnoses are commonly overlooked on conventional supine MRIs. Additionally, movement-dependent spondylolistheses may not be apparent on static

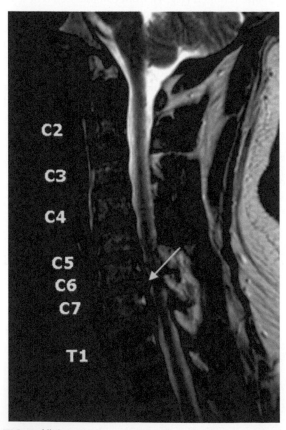

FIG. 5 High-intensity zone within the C2-C3 intervertebral disc on T2-weighted MRI *(arrow)*. High-intensity zones are seen within herniated discs as small areas of high intensity on T2-weighted sequences.

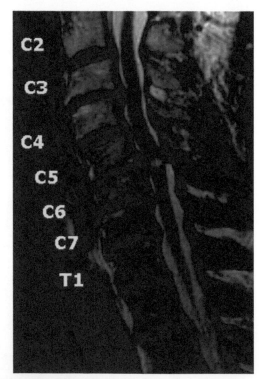

FIG. 6 T2-weighted FSE sequence showing spondylolisthesis at the level of C6. Posterior translation of the C6 vertebral body is seen impeding on the vertebral canal as illustrated by the loss of hyperintense cerebral spinal fluid signal.

MRI, requiring flexion/extension kinematic sequences.[103,105,106] The current gold standard method for evaluating spondylolisthesis is the Meyerding classification system using upright radiographs, though few studies have examined the validity of this system with MRI. More recently, however, Kawasaki et al. described a method for measuring severity of spondylolisthesis that is performed on upright kinetic MRI (see below).[103]

Osteoarthritis of the Facet Joints

Osteoarthritis of the facet joints may develop independently but most often occurs secondary to degeneration of the intervertebral disc with loss of disc space height.[107–109] As in any true synovial joint, degeneration of the facet joint is marked by fibrillation, fissuring, and ulceration of the hyaline articular cartilage advancing from superficial to deeper layers.[22] Although less accurate in visualizing bony pathology, T2-weighted MRI demonstrates moderate-to-good correlation with CT in identifying osteoarthritis and offers enhanced definition of nonbony structures in multiple planes, making it an acceptable substitute for assessing facet joint morphology[22,107,110] (Fig. 7). In early stages of the disease, cartilage degeneration causing narrowing of the joint space can be detected on axial view as decreased distance between the superior and inferior articulating facets. As the disease progresses, progressive decrease in joint space is accompanied by facet bone proliferation, forming osteophytes that appear isointense to adjacent bone.[111] Subchondral sclerosis may also develop, emitting hypointense signal on both T1- and T2-weighted images. In contrast, formation of cysts in the subchondral bone generates hyperintense T2-weighted signal if there is direct communication with the facet joint and hyperintense T1-weighted signal if there is a hemorrhagic or proteinaceous component, as seen from the axial or sagittal perspective.[109] Joint hypertrophy denotes later stages of facet joint osteoarthritis and is better appreciated on CT. With the potential to narrow the central canal, lateral recesses, and foramina,[26] facet joint osteoarthritis has significant implications in the etiology of neck and back pain.

Osteophytes

Osteophytes are projections of bone resulting from abnormal osteogenic proliferation commonly seen in the degenerative cervical spine at points experiencing chronic strain.[26,112] In the cervical spine specifically, osteophyte development is commonly a response to inhomogeneity in pressure on the vertebral endplate and facet joint secondary to intervertebral disc degeneration.[113] Three types of osteophytes have been described according to their shape and location[109,111] (Fig. 8). Traction osteophytes refer to 2–3-mm bony structures projecting horizontally from the vertebral endplate. Claw osteophytes also project from the endplate, arching over the disc toward the adjacent vertebral body to form a claw shape. The third type, known as wraparound bumper osteophytes, may be found along the capsular insertion of the facet joints and are commonly seen in progressive facet joint osteoarthritis.[108] MRI can be used to identify the presence of osteophytes; however, they can be difficult to distinguish from disc herniations as both will appear hypointense on T1- and T2-weighted imaging. SW-MRI can be used for improved differentiation of these structures, conveying a hyperintense signal to calcified structures such as osteophytes on inverse magnitude and phase-filtered images. Another benefit of SW-MRI is its ability to determine the dimensions and precise location of osteophytes, which is difficult to achieve on 2D radiography and useful in preoperative planning.[16]

Cervical Injury

Imaging of the cervical spine after trauma is essential for proper identification and classification of injury morphology. The development of the subaxial cervical spine injury classification system (SLIC) has sought to normalize assessment by dividing spinal injuries into three categories: compression, distraction, and translation/rotation[114] (Table 3). Compression injuries include those causing loss of height in part or all of the vertebral body and/or disruption of the vertebral endplate, including compression fractures, burst fractures, sagittal or coronal plane fractures, and flexion compression fractures. Trauma causing vertical dissociation of the vertebral column are labeled as distraction injuries and usually involve disruption of the ligaments at the level of the disc space or facet joints. Hyperextension injuries to the ALL resulting in either anterior disc expansion or posterior compression causing posterior element fracture or spinal cord compression are included in this category. Translational/rotational injuries refer to those demonstrating greater than 11 degrees of horizontal displacement of one vertebral segment relative to another. Trauma of this nature typically includes fracture or dislocation of the facet joints, lateral mass separation, or bilateral pedicle fractures.[114] The integrity of the discoligamentous complex (DLC), consisting of the intervertebral discs, ALL, PLL, ligamentum flavum, interspinous ligaments, supraspinous ligaments, and facet capsules, is another component of the SLIC as these structures directly contribute to stability of the cervical spine.[115] Widening of

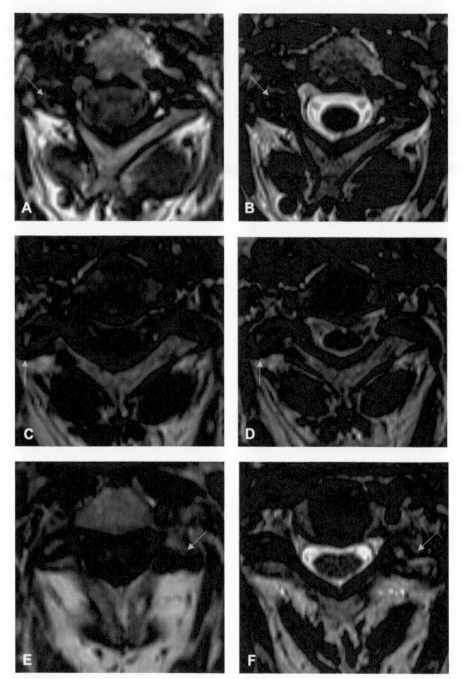

FIG. 7 Three cases of osteoarthritis of the facet joints depicted on T1-weighted (left) and T2-weighted (right) sequences. Joint space narrowing characterizes early stages of disease (A and B), while proliferation of isointense bone (C and D) and development of hyperintense subchondral sclerosis (D and E) indicate disease progression. A normal MRI of the facet joint is shown in Fig. 1B.

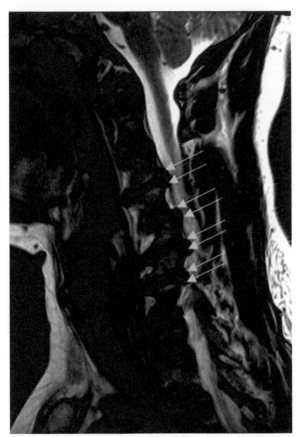

FIG. 8 T2-weighted MRI in midsagittal view with marked osteophyte formation surrounding at the posterior margins of vertebral levels C3-C7 *(arrows)*. Note: posterolateral disc herniations are also present within this segment as indicated in Fig. 4.

TABLE 3
Morphologic Classification of Injury to the Cervical Spine (Vaccaro)

Injury Type	Morphology
Compression	• Loss of vertebral body height • Endplate disruption
Distraction	• Anatomic dissociation of the vertebral column • Ligamentous disruption at level of disc space or facet joint
Translation/ rotation	• Horizontal displacement between adjacent vertebrae > 11 degrees • Disruption of anterior and posterior structures

the space between adjacent spinous processes, dislocation (< 50% articular apposition) or separation of the facet joints, subluxation of the vertebral bodies, and abnormal disc space widening are indicators of DLC compromise. The third and final component of SLIC is evaluation of neurologic status. As the spinal cord and nerve roots are normally protected within the spinal canal, neurologic impairment following traumatic injury is thus a logical indicator of severity of spinal cord injury.[114]

MRI is regarded as the preferred imaging modality for evaluating patients with traumatic injury and neurologic compromise as it provides optimal assessment of soft tissue injury.[116–119] Image acquisition performed within 72 h of injury prior to resorption of edema or extravasated blood is ideal, as the hypersensitivity of these fluids on T2-weighted imaging serves as an excellent natural contrast medium for ligament visualization. Comprehensive imaging should include T1-weighted, T2-FSE, gradient-echo, and FSE inversion recovery sequences in the sagittal plane as well as T2-weighted or gradient-echo sequences in the axial plane. Coronal T1-weighted or gradient-echo sequences may also be performed.[117] The presence of fracture on MRI is determined by altered configuration of the vertebra or a break in cortical continuity with or without changes in signal intensity on T1- or T2-weighted scans. Edema of the marrow emits low intensity on T1-weighted and high intensity on T2-weighted imaging, while spinal cord edema shows intramedullary foci of T2-weighted hyperintensity. Intramedullary hematoma is indicated by foci of high signal intensity on T1-weighted and low intensity on T2-weighted, spin-echo, and gradient-echo sequences. Traumatic disc herniation is identified by disc protrusion with increased T2-weighted signal intensity in the disc tissue and associated paraspinal soft tissue or spinal cord damage. Whereas normal intact ligaments appear as dark bands on T2-weighted scans, high signal intensity in the ligament itself or clear interruption of the dark band suggests ligament injury. Pre- and paravertebral hemorrhage or edema can present with or without soft tissue swelling and presents as T1-hypointense and T2-hyperintense.[120] Overall, MRI has been shown to be superior to CT in evaluation of traumatic and focal disc herniation, cord edema and compression, canal stenosis, ligament damage, and pre- and paravertebral hemorrhage and edema. However, appreciation of osseous injury such as degenerative subluxation, facet spondylosis, foraminal stenosis, and fracture is best achieved on CT.[120]

Tumors
Metastatic tumors
Although less common than metastases to the thoracic and lumbar spine, metastatic tumors in the cervical spine are more common than primary bone sarcomas.[121] The aggressiveness of the tumor, level within the spine location within the vertebra, and inclusion of associated anatomic structures each play a role in the clinical effects of the disease. Tumor growth requires the displacement or destruction of native bone tissue, compromising the integrity of the vertebrae and potentially leading to kyphotic deformities and compression of neurovasculature, causing neurologic dysfunction and ischemia.[122] Metastatic disease most often affects the mid-cervical region (C3-C6), where a narrower spinal canal increases the risk of myelopathy, sagittal imbalance, and pain. At the level of the vertebra, the tumor usually begins at the posterior aspect of the vertebral body and advances anteriorly, destroying cortical bone within the pedicles, lateral masses, and transverse processes along the way.[121] Diagnostic imaging of spinal neoplasia is best performed with MRI due to its superior visualization of soft tissue, assessment of edema, differentiation between normal and pathologic tissue, and identification of solid and cystic components. Although there are no specific features of metastatic disease on MRI, tumors and associated edema and syrinx generally emit intense signal on T2-weighted imaging.[123]

Primary spinal cord tumors
Approximately half of spinal cord tumors are primary tumors,[123] which are categorized into two types: intradural extramedullary spinal cord tumors (IESCTs) and intramedullary spinal cord tumors (ISCTs). IESCTs arise from within the spinal cord and account for 80% of primary spinal cord tumors.[124] These include nerve sheath tumors (NSTs), such as schwannomas and neurofibromas arising from the perineural cells, and meningiomas originating from arachnoidal cells along the neuraxis. While each of these tumors has characteristic findings on MRI, extramedullary tumors generally show displacement and compression of the spinal cord, expansion of the thecal sac, and a distinct interface with surrounding cerebrospinal fluid. Most IESCTs are depicted with high intensity on T2-weighted and intermediate intensity on T1-weighted imaging.[125] The remaining 20% of primary spinal cord tumors are the ISCTs, which originate from the dura and are located within the subarachnoid space.[124] ISCTs typically present with reactive cysts and extensive edema, causing mild expansion of the spinal cord. The most common

tumors in this category are ependymomas, astrocytomas, gangliomas, and hemangioblastomas,[123] most of which appear as well-circumscribed masses emitting iso- or hypointense signal on T1-weighted and hyperintense signal on T2-weighted MRI.[126]

Primary bony tumors
Tumors originating in bone may also develop within the cervical spine. Most primary bone tumors are benign, including aneurysmal bone cysts, giant cell tumors, osteoid osteomas, and osteoblastomas. These often mimic the general pattern of the spinal cord tumors on MRI: low to intermediate intensity on T1-weighted and high intensity on T2-weighted scans.[123] Although much more rare, metastatic primary bone tumors carry a very poor prognosis as they are difficult to excise with wide margins.[124] The most common primary metastatic bone tumors of the cervical spine are chordomas, osteosarcomas, chondrosarcomas, and Ewing sarcomas, each exhibiting a rather variable appearance on MRI based on subtype, progression, and extent of mineralization.[127]

Spinal Deformity
Spinal deformity, such as scoliosis, hyperlordosis, and kyphosis, can lead to a plethora of secondary conditions with a variety of clinical presentations. MRI is seldom the imaging method of choice to evaluate vertebral alignment but is required to assess for infantile or juvenile idiopathic scoliosis, congenital bony abnormalities, and scoliosis when associated with neurologic symptoms.[128] Should MRI be used or if upright radiographs are unavailable, vertebral alignment can be estimated by calculating the Cobb angle.[129-133] However, the reliability and validity of this measuring technique for MRI have yet to be adequately established. Many patients with spinal deformities choose to undergo surgical therapy with implantation of hardware, potentially making postoperative imaging of the spine difficult. Subsequent imaging studies should employ metal artifact reduction MRI sequences for optimal visualization of structures. An example of MRI representing loss of cervical lordosis is shown in Fig. 9.

Ligamentous Pathologies
There are several ligaments associated with the cervical spine. Hypertrophy, ossification, or calcification of these ligaments over time, particularly the PLL and LF, most commonly affects the cervical spine,[134] potentially leading to a reduction in cervical canal size and spinal cord compression.[68] MRI is not regarded as an ideal method for visualizing ligamentous pathologies,

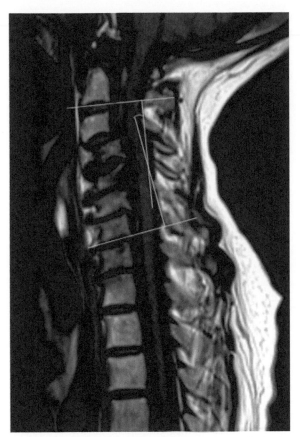

FIG. 9 Loss of natural lordotic curvature in the cervical spine demonstrated by a reduced Cobb angle on T1-weighted imaging.

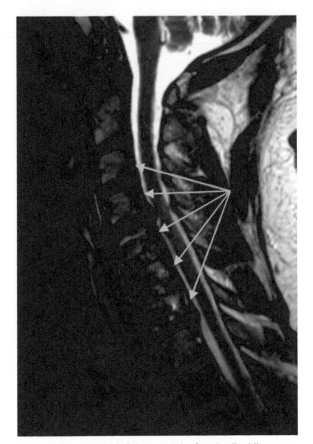

FIG. 10 Ossification of the posterior longitudinal ligament on T2-weighted MRI *(arrows)*. OPLL can appear as a hypo- or isointense signal immediately posterior to the vertebral bodies on T2-weighted sequences.

as ossification and hypertrophy, especially within the PLL, and disc material are difficult to differentiate on T1- and T2-weighted images.[38,135,136] However, effacement of CSF over multiple spinal levels is highly suggestive of ligamentous pathology on MRI.[38] Should there be concern for ligamentous pathology, CT is the preferred imaging modality for optimal visualization.

Both hypertrophy of the PLL (HPLL) and ossification of the PLL (OPLL) can lead to anterior compression of the spinal cord.[135] HPLL is typically secondary to herniated disc and often precedes ossification.[137] On T1-weighted imaging, HPLL appears isointense to paravertebral muscles.[137,138] OPLL can be seen in asymptomatic patients; thus, it is imperative to correlate findings with clinical signs and symptoms.[33] OPLL can be classified into four different categories, namely continuous, segmental, mixed, and nodular/circumscribed/bridged,[139,140] and demonstrates hypointense or absent signal on T1- and T2-weighted sequences

(Fig. 10). The LF tends to be thinnest at the midline; thus, it is best appreciated in parasagittal view as hypointense bands on T1- and T2-weighted imaging.[141] Hypertrophy, ossification, and rarely calcification of the LF can contribute to central and lateral canal stenosis, though it conveys little to no difference in signal intensity on MRI.[38,135] Notably, LF hypertrophy has the potential to lead to development of calcification, cysts, and fissures.[37] Ossification usually occurs secondary to degenerative changes of the spine.[142,143] While PLL pathology can contribute to anterior spinal cord stenosis, pathology of the LF has the potential to compress the spinal cord posteriorly.[68,144,145]

Inflammatory Conditions

Inflammatory conditions, such as RA, ankylosing spondylitis, Paget disease of bone, gout, and other spondylotic arthropathies, show a predilection for the cervical spine.[19,146] Significant abnormality identified on radiographs or apparent neurologic compromise in patients with these diseases necessitates further evaluation with MRI.[19,147] As the modality of choice for evaluating inflammatory conditions potentially involving the cervical spine, MRI demonstrates high sensitivity in detecting inflammatory changes of the joints and adjacent soft tissues (including the spinal cord and nerve roots). T2-weighted sequences are generally used to assess for spinal cord edema and demyelination commonly associated with chronic inflammatory conditions. Sensitivity to intramedullary disease processes can be increased by using STIR sequences.[1]

Rheumatoid arthritis

RA is a common chronic, systemic inflammatory disease with implications in the cervical spine, especially in patients with inadequate treatment or severe disease.[148–153] Cervical spine involvement is postulated to be a consequence of intense chronic synovitis leading to pannus formation within the joints.[151] Progressively worsening disease may entail bone erosion and consequent ligamentous laxity, compromising spinal stability.[149,154] After obtaining plain films in patients with RA, MRI should be performed to determine involvement of the cervical spine as it is sensitive to inflammatory changes within the joints even before symptoms arise.[5,155] Similarly, patients exhibiting signs of myelopathy or radiculopathy should undergo MRI for further investigation of their cause. It should be noted that patients may exhibit signs of myelopathy and cervical pain in the absence of radiographic evidence with neutral MRI sequences, necessitating kinematic sequences including flexion/extension studies to visualize any occult instabilities not apparent while supine.[148] Additionally, diffusion-weighted imaging (DWI) sequences offer superior depiction of disrupted water molecule flow to easily visualize spinal cord damage secondary to RA.[5] The use of MRI has also proven useful in determining prognosis, with T1-weighted spinal cord signal changes being associated with poorer clinical and final postoperative outcomes.[156,157]

Due to the inflammatory pannus formation, T2-hyperintense signals may appear within the synovial joints.[5] Formation of erosive pannus within the atlanto-axial joint is common in patients with RA and can lead to ligamentous laxity, resulting in atlanto-axial instability and potential subluxation.[154,158] Subluxation is typically in the anteriorly, though rarely posterior subluxation is seen secondary to fracture of the dens.[154] Extensive atlanto-axial subluxation may progress to cranial settling. If left untreated, this can cause pannus

development and subsequent brainstem compression, increasing the risk of cardiac arrest, stroke, or sudden death.[154,159] Subaxial subluxation is the second most common form of cervical instability seen in RA, and destruction of the facet joint and intervertebral disc secondary to pannus formation is commonly evident in MRI studies (Fig. 11). Clinically, this deformity may lead to symptoms of cervical stenosis, causing myelopathy and/or radiculopathy.[154,158] Notably, RA may manifest at a single level or affect multiple levels, resulting in a "staircase deformity" due to concurrent subluxations.

Seronegative spondyloarthropathies

Seronegative spondylitis is a term encompassing chronic inflammatory arthropathies that may manifest as disease within the cervical spine. Common seronegative spondyloarthropathies include ankylosing spondylitis (AS), enteropathic arthritis, psoriatic arthritis, and reactive arthritis, accounting for a significant portion of chronic low back pain cases.[160] The radiographic hallmark to these diseases is sacroiliitis. Rheumatoid factors are negative for these diseases but many are associated with the HLA-B27 antigen,[161] and many cases are accompanied by inflammatory bowel disorders. Cervical involvement typically occurs later in the course of disease, but symptoms can predominate. For example, psoriatic arthritis is known to manifest within the cervical spine before the appearance of characteristic skin lesions. On MRI, disc space narrowing and erosions of the vertebral endplates and spinous processes may also be seen.[76]

Ankylosing spondylitis is a seronegative spondyloarthropathy of particular importance primarily affecting synovial joints along the entirety of the spine. Bony fusion of these joints, along with OPLL, can result in significant immobility and chronic back pain.[160] Early stages of the disease are characterized by sacroiliitis on plain radiography in conjunction with inflammatory back pain, limited mobility in the lumbar spine, and/or restricted chest expansion.[160] However, inflammatory changes extend to all areas of the spine, including the cervical region, as the disease progresses.[160] The capability of MRI to show osseous and ligamentous inflammatory changes makes it the preferred imaging technique for diagnosis and monitoring of AS. T1-weighted sequences provide good differentiation of anatomic structures, while acute inflammatory changes can be visualized as hyperintense signal on T2-weighted FSE or STIR sequences. With its ability to detect abnormal free water content, STIR also offers the added benefit of highlighting hyperintense areas of bone marrow edema.[160] Andersson lesions are also

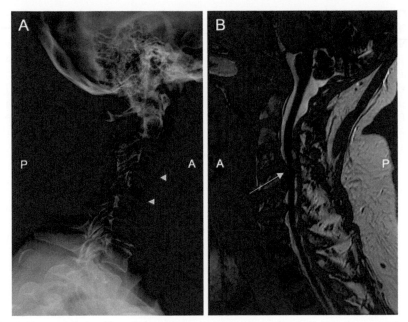

FIG. 11 Cervical spondylosis with radiculopathy and myelopathy in the setting of rheumatoid arthritis shown on radiograph (A) and T2-weighted MRI images (B). Subluxation is evident in radiograph at the C3-C4 and C4-C5 levels *(arrowheads)*, while MRI shows formation of pannus causing cervical stenosis and myelopathy *(arrow)*.

frequently found within the intervertebral spaces, appearing hypointense on T1-weighted and hyperintense on STIR sequences.[147] Early development of AS may be indicated on MRI by acute nondisplaced fractures of the ankylosed spine, an abnormality often missed on radiographic analysis. Patients with AS also often develop secondary osteoporosis, further increasing their risk of complications such as spinal fracture.[162,163] Consequently, these patients should undergo MR-based evaluation for spinal fractures and ligamentous injury even after trivial or minor trauma.[164] Apparent spinal deformity may require surgical stabilization to avoid worsening neurologic deficit.[162]

Paget's disease

Paget's disease of bone (PD) is a chronic metabolic bone disease characterized by increased formation of disorganized bone due to excessive osteoclast activity and compensatory osteoblast activity. Deposition of abnormal bone results in mechanically weaker, less compact, highly vascularized bone that is more susceptible to fracture. Although the cervical spine is rarely affected by PD, spinal stenosis-like symptoms may be still present in this region. MRI is therefore necessary to rule out metastasis that commonly presents with

similar symptoms. Particularly, T1, T2, and STIR sequences provide the best visualization of marrow infiltration, spinal stenosis, and facet joint hypertrophy when assessing for PD.[165]

Gout and pseudogout

Gout is a common metabolic disease involving deposition of monosodium urate crystals in joints. While not commonly affected by this disease, gout within the cervical spine can affect a multitude of structures including the facet joints, LF, and vertebral bodies. The clinical presentation of gout is largely nonspecific, and MRI and CT are of limited clinical value when differentiating the disease from infection and malignancy.[166] When MRI is used, gouty lesions range from hypo- to isointense on T1-weighted sequences and hypo- to hyperintense on T2-weighted sequences.[3,166]

Deposition of calcium pyrophosphate dihydrate crystals within articular cartilage, tendons, and ligaments causing arthropathy is known as pseudogout. Manifestation within the cervical spine is rare but can affect the intervertebral discs and ligaments.[167] LF calcification secondary to pseudogout is reflected as T1-isointense and T2-hyperintense signals with marked peripheral enhancement on T1-Gd sequences.[168,169]

MEASUREMENTS AND GRADING SCALES FOR MRI-BASED EVALUATION OF THE CERVICAL SPINE

MRI is a useful visualization tool for identification and quantification of several pathologies. Numerous measurements, hallmarks, and grading schemes have been developed to ensure effective and efficient diagnosis and monitoring of disease. Schemes that evaluate severity can also inform clinical decision-making regarding conservative and more invasive treatment options and assist in preoperative planning. More broadly, these measurement and grading scales offer clinicians and researchers a more formal and uniform method of evaluating and classifying the cervical spine.

As advancements continue to be made in functional MRI techniques such as T2/T2* mapping, T2 relaxation time, diffusion quantitative imaging, chemical exchange saturation transfer, delayed contrast-enhanced cartilage imaging, and MR spectroscopy, novel methods for evaluating the cervical spine are rapidly being developed.[170]

Intervertebral Disc Degeneration

Although radiographic techniques have long been used for the evaluation of intervertebral discs, MRI has been established as the most accurate method for assessing disc integrity in the clinical setting.[25,92,171–173] T2-weighted FSE has been widely used in spinal imaging since the 1990s due to its reduced scanning time, improved signal-to-noise ratio, and fewer motion artifacts.[174] Subsequently, several grading systems have been developed in efforts to normalize evaluation of cervical and/or lumbar disc integrity and degeneration in the clinical and research settings.[24,110,171,175–183] These systems each focus on quantifying various known markers of degenerative disease. Loss of disc height, decreased T2-weighted signal intensity of the intervertebral disc, and signal void on both T1- and T2-weighted imaging may be noted. Furthermore, the presence of annular tears, disc protrusion, osteophytes, and endplate sclerosis serve as additional indicators of progressive disc degeneration (Table 4).

Pfirrmann grades

Originally designed for use in the lumbar spine, the Pfirrmann grading system is a widely used tool for assessing macroscopic intervertebral disc degeneration that can be utilized in evaluation of the cervical spine.[92] Grades of 1–5 are assigned based on comprehensive appraisal of disc structure, signal intensity, distinction between nucleus and annulus, and height on T2-weighted FSE imaging. Specifically, grade 1 discs present with a homogenous structure, hyperintense signal, clear distinction between nucleus and annulus, and normal height. Discs demonstrating loss of homogenous structure but maintaining other parameters are designated as grade 2. Grade 3 discs appear inhomogeneous and gray with an unclear border between annulus and nucleus, intermediate signal intensity, and normal to slightly decreased disc height. Progression to grade 4 is characterized by conversion to black structure, loss of distinction between nucleus and annulus, intermediate/hypointense signal, and normal to slightly decreased disc height. Discs appearing inhomogeneous and

---

TABLE 4
Popular Grading Systems and Parameters for Evaluation of Intervertebral Disc Degeneration

Grading System	Spinal Region	Disc Height	Signal Intensity	Annular Tears	Disc Protrusion	Osteophytes	Endplate Sclerosis
Christe	Cervical	•		•	•	•	
Jacobs	Cervical	•	•		•	•	
Kolstad	Cervical	•	•		•		•
Lehto	Cervical	•	•		•	•	
Miyazaki	Cervical	•	•		•		
Suzuki	Cervical	•	•		•		
Walraevens	Cervical	•				•	•
Pfirrmann	Lumbar	•	•		•		
Benneker	Lumbar	•	•	•	•	•	•
Thompson	Lumbar	•	•		•	•	•

TABLE 5
Pfirrmann Grading System for Classification of Lumbar Intervertebral Disc Degeneration Using Midsagittal T2-Weighted MRI

Grade	Disc Height	Signal Intensity	Disc Structure	Distinction Between Annulus and Nucleus
I	Normal	Hyperintense	Homogeneous, bright white	Clear
II	Normal	Hyperintense	Inhomogeneous, with or without horizontal bands	Clear
III	Normal to slightly decreased	Intermediate	Inhomogeneous, gray	Unclear
IV	Normal to moderately decreased	Intermediate to hypointense	Inhomogeneous, gray to black	Lost
V	Collapsed disc space	Hypointense	Inhomogeneous, black	Lost

Although developed based on findings in the lumbar spine, the Pfirrmann grading system can be applied to evaluation of cervical discs (Pfirrmann).

black, lacking division between nucleus and annulus, emitting hypointense signal, and occupying a collapsed disc space represent the greatest extent of disc degeneration and are assigned a grade of 5 (Table 5). Although Pfirrmann grading system demonstrates high reliability in the evaluation of disc degeneration, related endplate integrity is not included in the assessment. Therefore, it is recommended Pfirrmann grading be supplemented with classification of Modic change.[27]

Endplate Abnormalities

MRI is commonly used to assess vertebral endplate integrity and identify changes associated with normal aging and pathological degeneration. Regardless of etiology, endplate thinning and depressurization of the intervertebral disc permit the nucleus pulposus to penetrate through the endplate into adjacent bone marrow.[184] Resulting inflammation and edema within the vertebral body are nonstructural changes represented on MRI as alterations in subchondral bone marrow intensity.[109,185] More extensive herniation into the bone

is associated with structural abnormalities including fractures, erosions, microtraumas, and vertebral rim lesions, collectively referred to as Schmorl's nodes on MRI.[179,186,187] Nonetheless, identification and evaluation of both nonstructural and structural changes in the endplate are important as they are a hallmark of degeneration in the spine.

Modic changes
Systematic quantification of nonstructural endplate degeneration was first performed by Modic et al.[27] who classified changes according to severity (Table 6). Healthy endplates emit a signal homogenous with surrounding vertebral body marrow and are labeled as Modic type 0. In Modic type 1, pathologic vascularization and edema within the endplate cause decreased T1-weighted signal intensity and increased T2-weighted signal intensity. Notably, this pattern of intensity is similar to that seen during infection. However, diffusion-weighted imaging can be used to distinguish the clearly marginated, linear hyperintensities at bone

TABLE 6
Modic Change Grading System for Classification of Nonstructural Vertebral Endplate Degeneration

Modic Type	T1 Signal	T2 Signal	Nonstructural Change
0	Normal	Normal	Healthy endplate
1	Hypointense	Hyperintense	Pathologic vascularization and edema
2	Hyperintense	Intermediate to hyperintense	Replacement of fatty marrow
3	Hypointense	Hypointense	Microfracture and sclerosis

marrow margins characteristic of degeneration from the more diffuse, poorly defined edematous borders of infectious etiology.[109] Reversion to Modic type 0 has been documented,[188] but classic progression of degeneration involves transition to Modic type 2.[27] At this stage, replacement of normal red marrow with yellow marrow appears as increased signal on T1-weighted imaging, while T2-weighted scans show intermediate or slightly elevated signal. The most advanced stage of degeneration is Modic type 3, characterized by the replacement of bone marrow with sclerosis and exhibiting decreased signal on both T1- and T2-weighted scans.[109,189]

Classification of Schmorl's nodes

Structural defects in the vertebral endplates known as Schmorl's nodes have been associated with the presence and severity of spinal degeneration.[190,191] Although no current grading schemes currently exist for classification of Schmorl's nodes in the cervical spine specifically, Samartzis et al. developed a classification system in the lumbar region that can readily be applied to cervical MRI analysis. Focusing on morphologic and topographic features, this system evaluates structural defects according to disc level, endplate involvement (rostral, caudal, or both), shape, size, location relative to endplate, and presence of associated marrow changes. Further, smaller defects exhibiting indented, sharp, or round shapes are classified as "typical" Schmorl's nodes, whereas larger rectangular or irregularly shaped defects are termed "atypical." Recognition and classification of Schmorl's nodes on MRI is of significant clinical relevance, as typical and atypical Schmorl's nodes

were found to carry a 2–4-fold and 5–13-fold greater risk of severe disc degeneration, respectively.[191]

Total endplate score

The total endplate scoring (TEPS) system serves as a more comprehensive method of analyzing the vertebral motion segment by combining evaluation of nonstructural (Modic changes) and structural (Schmorl's nodes) endplate integrity with assessment of physiological function.[184] The TEPS system classifies endplates into six types based on the extent of damage as assessed on T1-weighted MRI: (I) endplates exhibit no damage and appear as symmetric concave bands of hypointense signal without breaks or Modic changes, representing healthy discs; (II) endplates similarly lack breaks and Modic changes but demonstrate focal thinning either at the center or periphery, indicative of aging; (III) endplates show focal areas of disc-marrow contact commonly seen in the aging spine, though the contour of the endplate is maintained; (IV) endplate damage characterized by depression and a typical Schmorl's node occupying < 25% of the endplate, an indication of endplate degeneration; (V) endplates affected by a Schmorl's node covering < 50% of the endplate with associated subchondral change, also indicating degeneration; and (VI) completely damaged endplates with gross irregularity or sclerosis (Table 7). Grade I indicates normal endplate morphology, while grades II–III represent age-related changes and grades IV–VI suggest degeneration. The TEPS for a particular intervertebral disc is determined by adding the score of the superior and inferior endplates. Notably, increasing TEPS scores

---

TABLE 7
Total Endplate Scoring (TEPS) System for Quantification of Structural and Nonstructural Changes of the Vertebral Endplate

TEPS Score	Characteristic Endplate Changes	Modic Change	Schmorl's Nodes
1	• Symmetrically concave without breaks • Uniform hypointense signal	Absent	Absent
2	• Focal thinning without breaks	Absent	Absent
3	• Focal disc-marrow contact • Normal endplate contour	Absent	Absent
4	• Endplate depression	Usually present	≤ 25%
5	• Endplate depression • Subchondral changes	Usually present	≤ 50%
6	• Complete endplate damage • Irregularity and sclerosis	Usually present	≤ 100%

Grade 1 indicates a healthy endplate. Grades 2 and 3 describe age-associated change. Grades 4–6 signify pathologic degeneration.

correlated with decreased diffusion and increased disc degeneration. Particularly as endplate damage reaches a critical score of 6 or greater, the structural and diffusion status may be too compromised to permit biological treatment or regenerative therapy.

Facet Joints

Although MRI is useful for visualizing edema in the degenerated facet,[192] CT remains the imaging modality of choice due to its superior demonstration of bony details, joint space narrowing, and subchondral sclerosis.[111] Facet joint osteoarthritis is instead most commonly assessed using CT-based grading systems that classify degradation according to severity.[110] Compared to a healthy joint, a facet joint in the early stages of osteoarthritis will demonstrate joint space narrowing, cyst formation, and small osteophytes without joint hypertrophy. As the disease progresses, joint hypertrophy becomes apparent secondary to the formation of large osteophytes before the bone eventually fuses in late-stage disease.[22,108,183,193,194] Although no MR-based facet joint grading system currently exists in the cervical spine, schemes have been developed in the lumbar spine. Weishaupt et al. utilized MRI to assess joint space narrowing, osteophyte formation, articular process hypertrophy, and subarticular bone erosion with moderate-to-good agreement with CT-based analysis,[22] while Grogan et al. quantified cartilage loss and articular process sclerosis as markers of facet joint degeneration.[195] Assessment of facet joint osteoarthritis is of high clinical importance, as facet joint degradation accounts for over 55% of overall pain in the cervical spine.[196,197]

Spondylolisthesis

Measurement of spondylolisthesis on MRI is a less common practice, as most established methods are based on radiographs.[38] Estimating the magnitude of listhesis is possible on MRI using the Meyerding classification system, though the reliability and validity of this method is limited. The Meyerding classification depends on the percentage of slip compared to adjacent vertebral bodies rather than absolute magnitude of the slip. Specifically, grade I spondylolisthesis is categorized as a 0%–25% slip, grade II as 26%–50% slip, grade III as 51%–75% slip, grade IV as 76%–100% slip, and grade V as greater than 100% slip (Table 8). Another method developed by Kawasaki et al. measures the distance of slippage relative to adjacent normal vertebral bodies, with patients exhibiting more than 3–3.5 mm of horizontal translation being considered as having severe listhesis.[103]

TABLE 8
Meyerding Classification System for Evaluation of Spondylolisthesis on Magnetic Resonance Imaging

Meyerding Grade	Disc Displacement (%)
I	0–25
II	26–50
III	51–75
IV	76–100
V	> 100

Disc displacement is expressed as a percentage relative to adjacent vertebral bodies.

Spinal Stenosis

Regardless of the extrinsic cause of central spinal stenosis, severity of the disease can be classified in a few different ways. Muhle et al. described one method using kinematic T2-weighted MRIs to evaluate the spine based on static and dynamic factors and classify stenosis into one of four grades. Grade 0 stenosis is classified as normal; grade 1 as partial obliteration of the anterior or posterior subarachnoid space; grade 2 as complete obliteration of the anterior or posterior subarachnoid space; and grade 3 as spinal cord compression or displacement[54,198] (Table 9). Though commonly used, this method is limited by the subjective nature of the grade 1 classification and the lack of consideration of spinal cord signal change, a parameter reported in literature as a reliable marker of myelopathy.[54,199]

TABLE 9
Muhle Classification System for Evaluation of Spinal Stenosis on Kinematic Magnetic Resonance Imaging

Spinal Stenosis Grade	MRI Findings
0	• Normal spinal canal
1	• Partial obliteration of anterior or posterior subarachnoid space
2	• Complete obliteration of anterior or posterior subarachnoid space
3	• Complete obliteration of anterior or posterior subarachnoid space with spinal cord compression or displacement

TABLE 10
Kang Classification System for Evaluation of
Spinal Stenosis on T2-Weighted Magnetic
Resonance Imaging

Spinal Stenosis Grade	MRI Findings
0	• Absence of spinal canal stenosis
1	• > 50% obliteration of subarachnoid space
2	• Presence of spinal cord deformity
3	• Presence of spinal cord signal change

Kang et al. created a similar grading system performed on T2-weighted images to address these limitations, classifying grade 0 stenosis as absence of canal stenosis; grade 1 as greater than 50% obliteration of the subarachnoid space; grade 2 as spinal cord deformity; and grade 3 as spinal cord signal change[54] (Table 10).

Measuring techniques such as the Torg-Pavlov body-to-canal ratio and space available for the cord may also be considered when quantifying severity of spinal stenosis.[70] However, these measurements are classically performed on radiographs and their translation to MRI has yet to be adequately established. Spinal cord occupation ratio (SCOR) is an MR-based assessment method that has been correlated to Torg-Pavlov ratios and serves as an effective criterion for diagnosing congenital spinal stenosis.[78] SCOR is measured from the midsagittal perspective of T2-weighted images. Because the space occupied by soft tissues such as the LF is taken into account, SCOR is regarded as an effective method of assessment. Specifically, the width of the cord (demarcated by the low-intensity spinal cord) and the width of the canal (demarcated by the delineation of the high-intensity CSF and low-intensity adjacent soft tissues) are measured at the vertebral levels above and below the suspected level of stenosis and used to calculate SCOR using Formula (1). Patients with a SCOR of greater than 70% on MRI may be considered to have congenital spinal stenosis, a prevalent risk factor for developing cervical myelopathy later in life.[78]

$$SCOR = \left(\frac{Cord\ Above + Cord\ Below}{Canal\ Above + Canal\ Below} \right) \times 100 \qquad (1)$$

Cobb Angles

Cobb angles are a measurement tool used to assess vertebral column misalignments such as lordosis, kyphosis, and scoliosis. Although typically performed on anteroposterior radiographs, multiple studies have demonstrated translation to thoracolumbar MRI sequences. However, the reliability of this method has not yet been established for use in MRIs of the cervical spine.[129,130,132,133,200] Cobb angles are produced by drawing a horizontal line across the inferior endplate of the C2 vertebrae and another line across the inferior endplate of C7. Perpendicular lines are then extended outward from both horizontals. The angle formed by the intersection of these perpendicular lines is the Cobb angle[128,200,201] (Fig. 12). Since MRIs are commonly performed while the patient is supine, cervical lordotic

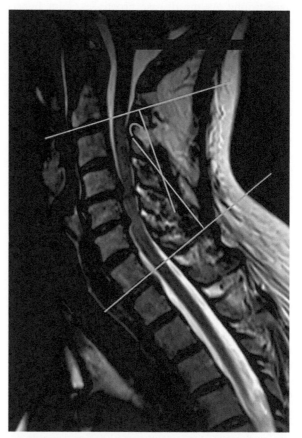

FIG. 12 Measurement of the Cobb angle. The Cobb angle is created by the intersection of the two lines drawn perpendicular to those parallel to the inferior vertebral endplates of C2 and C7. Although classically measured on standing radiographs, Cobb angles can be used on MRI in extreme circumstances.

curvature may be exaggerated and result in a slightly increased Cobb angle. However, results have been considered estimable compared to their radiographic counterparts.[38,200,202,203] Although normal Cobb angles will vary between patients, normal is considered between 20 and 35 degrees of lordosis.[204,205]

CONCLUSION

The rapid evolution of MRI has established this imaging technique as a valuable clinical and diagnostic tool for use in the cervical spine. Several unique imaging sequences exist to highlight various pathologies for optimal diagnosis, preoperative planning, treatment, and postoperative evaluation. Severity of disease can also be determined with the use of available grading schemes and measuring tools. However, it is important to correlate imaging abnormalities with symptomology to determine clinical significance and ensure implementation of the proper treatment regimen.

REFERENCES

1. Stone J. Imaging techniques in the adult spine. In: *Imaging of the Spine*; 2011:3–21. https://doi.org/10.1016/b978-1-4377-1551-4.50005-0.
2. Kaiser JA, Holland BA. Imaging of the cervical spine. *Spine*. 1998;23(24):2701–2712. https://doi.org/10.1097/00007632-199812150-00009.
3. Shen FH, Samartzis D, Fessler RG. *Textbook of the Cervical Spine E-Book*. Elsevier Health Sciences; 2014. https://play.google.com/store/books/details?id=4LeXBAAAQBAJ.
4. Khanna AJ, Carbone JJ, Kebaish KM, et al. Magnetic resonance imaging of the cervical spine. Current techniques and spectrum of disease. *J Bone Joint Surg Am Vol.* 2002;84-A(Suppl. 2):70–80. https://doi.org/10.2106/00004623-200200002-00009.
5. Mańczak M, Gasik R. Cervical spine instability in the course of rheumatoid arthritis—imaging methods. *Reumatologia/Rheumatology.* 2017;4:201–207. https://doi.org/10.5114/reum.2017.69782.
6. Engel G, Bender YY, Adams LC, et al. Evaluation of osseous cervical foraminal stenosis in spinal radiculopathy using susceptibility-weighted magnetic resonance imaging. *Eur Radiol.* 2019;29(4):1855–1862. https://doi.org/10.1007/s00330-018-5769-4.
7. Kaindl E. Clinical MR imaging: a practical approach. *Eur J Radiol.* 2004;51(1):97. https://doi.org/10.1016/s0720-048x(03)00176-1.
8. Baraliakos X. Assessment of acute spinal inflammation in patients with ankylosing spondylitis by magnetic resonance imaging: a comparison between contrast enhanced T1 and short tau inversion recovery (STIR) sequences. *Ann Rheum Dis.* 2005;64(8):1141–1144. https://doi.org/10.1136/ard.2004.031609.
9. Kim G, Khalid F, Oommen VV, et al. T1- vs. T2-based MRI measures of spinal cord volume in healthy subjects and patients with multiple sclerosis. *BMC Neurol.* 2015;15(1). https://doi.org/10.1186/s12883-015-0387-0.
10. Laiho K, Soini I, Kauppi M. Magnetic resonance imaging of the rheumatic cervical spine [Review of Magnetic resonance imaging of the rheumatic cervical spine]. *J Bone Joint Surg Am Vol.* 2003;85(12):2482. author reply 2483 https://doi.org/10.2106/00004623-200312000-00036.
11. Kumar Y, Hayashi D. Role of magnetic resonance imaging in acute spinal trauma: a pictorial review. *BMC Musculoskelet Disord.* 2016;17:310. https://doi.org/10.1186/s12891-016-1169-6.
12. Song S, Handwerker J. Spine MRI. In: *Basic Musculoskeletal Imaging*. US: McGraw-Hill Professional; 2013. 311.
13. Ganesan K, Bydder GM. A prospective comparison study of fast T1 weighted fluid attenuation inversion recovery and T1 weighted turbo spin echo sequence at 3 T in degenerative disease of the cervical spine. *Br J Radiol.* 2014;87(1041):20140091. https://doi.org/10.1259/bjr.20140091.
14. Gallucci M, Capoccia S, Colajacomo M. Spinal stenosis. In: Van Goethem JWM, van den Hauwe L, Parizel PM, eds. *Spinal Imaging: Diagnostic Imaging of the Spine and Spinal Cord.* Springer Berlin Heidelberg; 2007:185–209. https://doi.org/10.1007/978-3-540-68483-1_8.
15. Gallucci M, Puglielli E, Splendiani A, Pistoia F, Spacca G. Degenerative disorders of the spine. *Eur Radiol.* 2005;15(3):591–598. https://doi.org/10.1007/s00330-004-2618-4.
16. Bender YY-N, Diederichs G, Walter TC, et al. Differentiation of osteophytes and disc herniations in spinal radiculopathy using susceptibility-weighted magnetic resonance imaging. *Investig Radiol.* 2017;52(2):75–80. https://doi.org/10.1097/RLI.0000000000000314.
17. Dodwad S-NM, Khan SN, An HS. Cervical spine anatomy. In: Shen FH, Samartzis D, Fessler RIG, eds. *Cervical Spine Anatomy.* Elsevier/Saunders; 2015:3–21.
18. Rios JC, Naidich TP, Daniels DL, et al. The normal spinal column: overview and cervical spine. In: Naidich TP, Castillo M, Cha S, Raybaud C, Smirniotopoulos J, Kollias S, Kleinman G, eds. *Imaging of the Spine.* Elsevier/Saunders; 2011:45–74.
19. Malcolm GP. Surgical disorders of the cervical spine: presentation and management of common disorders. *J Neurol Neurosurg Psychiatry.* 2002;73(Suppl. 1):i34–i41. https://doi.org/10.1136/jnnp.73.suppl_1.i34.
20. Pal GP, Routal RV, Saggu SK. The orientation of the articular facets of the zygapophyseal joints at the cervical and upper thoracic region. *J Anat.* 2001;198(Pt 4):431–441. https://doi.org/10.1046/j.1469-7580.2001.19840431.x.
21. Hasegawa T, An HS, Haughton VM. Imaging anatomy of the lateral lumbar spinal canal. *Semin Ultrasound CT MR.* 1993;14(6):404–413. https://doi.org/10.1016/s0887-2171(05)80034-4.
22. Weishaupt D, Zanetti M, Boos N, Hodler J. MR imaging and CT in osteoarthritis of the lumbar facet joints. *Skelet*

Radiol. 1999;28(4):215–219. https://idp.springer.com/authorize/casa?redirect_uri=https://link.springer.com/article/10.1007/s002560050503&casa_token=oxgUOK-82kq4AAAAA:j7ghnQwlIV2YsBAAd_gq5vHXFI4MbX-N0CTzb9MRH63OhkeOVZ7KpHMLRoFaZGMFbVbZ-QUHeMbjLzG-Zxvw.

23. Newell N, Little JP, Christou A, Adams MA, Adam CJ, Masouros SD. Biomechanics of the human intervertebral disc: a review of testing techniques and results. *J Mech Behav Biomed Mater.* 2017;69:420–434. https://doi.org/10.1016/j.jmbbm.2017.01.037.

24. Jacobs LJ, Chen AF, Kang JD, Lee JY. Reliable magnetic resonance imaging based grading system for cervical intervertebral disc degeneration. *Asian Spine J.* 2016;10(1):70–74. https://doi.org/10.4184/asj.2016.10.1.70.

25. Matsumoto M, Fujimura Y, Suzuki N, et al. MRI of cervical intervertebral discs in asymptomatic subjects. *J Bone Joint Surg Br Vol.* 1998;80-B(1):19–24. https://doi.org/10.1302/0301-620x.80b1.0800019.

26. Modic MT, Masaryk TJ, Ross JS, Carter JR. Imaging of degenerative disk disease. *Radiology.* 1988;168(1):177–186. https://doi.org/10.1148/radiology.168.1.3289089.

27. Modic MT, Steinberg PM, Ross JS, Masaryk TJ, Carter JR. Degenerative disk disease: assessment of changes in vertebral body marrow with MR imaging. *Radiology.* 1988;166(1 Pt 1):193–199. https://doi.org/10.1148/radiology.166.1.3336678.

28. Rahme R, Moussa R. The Modic vertebral endplate and marrow changes: pathologic significance and relation to low back pain and segmental instability of the lumbar spine. *AJNR Am J Neuroradiol.* 2008;29(5):838–842. https://doi.org/10.3174/ajnr.A0925.

29. Ishikawa M, Matsumoto M, Fujimura Y, Chiba K, Toyama Y. Changes of cervical spinal cord and cervical spinal canal with age in asymptomatic subjects. *Spinal Cord.* 2003;41(3):159–163. https://doi.org/10.1038/sj.sc.3101375.

30. Okada E, Matsumoto M, Fujiwara H, Toyama Y. Disc degeneration of cervical spine on MRI in patients with lumbar disc herniation: comparison study with asymptomatic volunteers. *Eur Spine J: Official Publication of the European Spine Society, the European Spinal Deformity Society, and the European Section of the Cervical Spine Research Society.* 2011;20(4):585–591. https://doi.org/10.1007/s00586-010-1644-y.

31. Okada E, Matsumoto M, Ichihara D, et al. Does the sagittal alignment of the cervical spine have an impact on disk degeneration? Minimum 10-year follow-up of asymptomatic volunteers. *Eur Spine J: Official Publication of the European Spine Society, the European Spinal Deformity Society, and the European Section of the Cervical Spine Research Society.* 2009;18(11):1644–1651. https://doi.org/10.1007/s00586-009-1095-5.

32. Kameyama T, Hashizume Y, Ando T, Takahashi A. Morphometry of the normal cadaveric cervical spinal cord. *Spine.* 1994;19(18):2077–2081. https://doi.org/10.1097/00007632-199409150-00013.

33. Kato F, Yukawa Y, Suda K, Yamagata M, Ueta T. Normal morphology, age-related changes and abnormal findings of the cervical spine. Part II: magnetic resonance imaging of over 1,200 asymptomatic subjects. *Eur Spine J: Official Publication of the European Spine Society, the European Spinal Deformity Society, and the European Section of the Cervical Spine Research Society.* 2012;21(8):1499–1507. https://idp.springer.com/authorize/casa?redirect_uri=https://link.springer.com/article/10.1007/s00586-012-2176-4&casa_token=p6LBTPz64x-sAAAAA:USSr4j8vinMQ0yNrMJbwiNmkMs73h0XE2OU__CSOfd3rfU6cFX4dezW4e6L92bsmswueyjB2H3RYrPgg.

34. Nagata K, Yoshimura N, Hashizume H, et al. The prevalence of cervical myelopathy among subjects with narrow cervical spinal canal in a population-based magnetic resonance imaging study: the Wakayama Spine Study. *Spine J: Official Journal of the North American Spine Society.* 2014;14(12):2811–2817. https://doi.org/10.1016/j.spinee.2014.03.051.

35. Ros L, Mota J, Guedea A, Bidgood D. Quantitative measurements of the spinal cord and canal by MR imaging and myelography. *Eur Radiol.* 1998;8(6):966–970. https://doi.org/10.1007/s003300050497.

36. Sherman JL, Nassaux PY, Citrin CM. Measurements of the normal cervical spinal cord on MR imaging. *AJNR Am J Neuroradiol.* 1990;11(2):369–372. https://www.ncbi.nlm.nih.gov/pubmed/2107721.

37. Naidich TP, Castillo M, Cha S, Raybaud C, Smirniotopoulos JG, Kollias S. *Imaging of the Spine: Expert Radiology Series, Expert Consult-Online and Print.* Elsevier Health Sciences; 2010. https://play.google.com/store/books/details?id=NzyBq_wH1psC.

38. Nouri A, Martin AR, Mikulis D, Fehlings MG. Magnetic resonance imaging assessment of degenerative cervical myelopathy: a review of structural changes and measurement techniques. *Neurosurg Focus.* 2016;40(6):E5. https://doi.org/10.3171/2016.3.FOCUS1667.

39. Xing R, Liu W, Li X, Jiang L, Yishakea M, Dong J. Characteristics of cervical sagittal parameters in healthy cervical spine adults and patients with cervical disc degeneration. *BMC Musculoskelet Disord.* 2018;19(1):37. https://doi.org/10.1186/s12891-018-1951-8.

40. McAviney J, Schulz D, Bock R, Harrison DE, Holland B. Determining the relationship between cervical lordosis and neck complaints. *J Manip Physiol Ther.* 2005;28(3):187–193. https://doi.org/10.1016/j.jmpt.2005.02.015.

41. Tong CL. Paraspinal soft tissues. In: Naidich TP, Castillo M, Cha S, Raybaud C, Smirniotopoulos J, Kollias S, Kleinman GM, eds. *Imaging of the Spine.* Elsevier/Saunders; 2011:25–41.

42. Dewan AK, Malloy JP, Jay Khanna A. Magnetic resonance imaging of the cervical spine. In: Shen FH, Samartzis D, Fessler RG, eds. *Textbook of the Cervical Spine.* Elsevier/Saunders; 2015:86–104.

43. Saifuddin A, Green R, White J. Magnetic resonance imaging of the cervical ligaments in the absence of trauma.

Spine. 2003;28(15):1686–1691. discussion 1691–1692 https://doi.org/10.1097/01.BRS.0000083166.22254.BA.

44. Mirvis SE, Geisler FH, Jelinek JJ, Joslyn JN, Gellad F. Acute cervical spine trauma: evaluation with 1.5-T MR imaging. *Radiology.* 1988;166(3):807–816. https://doi.org/10.1148/radiology.166.3.3277249.

45. Arslan M, Acar HI, Comert A, Tubbs RS. The cervical arteries: an anatomical study with application to avoid the nerve root and spinal cord blood supply. *Turk Neurosurg.* 2018;28(2):234–240. https://doi.org/10.5137/1019-5149.JTN.19469-16.1.

46. Eskander MS, Drew JM, Aubin ME, et al. Vertebral artery anatomy: a review of two hundred fifty magnetic resonance imaging scans. *Spine.* 2010;35(23):2035–2040. https://doi.org/10.1097/BRS.0b013e31c9f3d4.

47. Jacobs A, Lanfermannb H, Neveling M, Szelies B, Schrijder R, Heissa W-D. MRI- and MRA-guided therapy of carotid and vertebral artery dissections. *Elsevier J Neurol Sci.* 1997;147:27–34.

48. Klufas RA, Hsu L, Barnes PD, Patel MR, Schwartz RB. Dissection of the carotid and vertebral arteries: imaging with MR angiography. *AJR Am J Roentgenol.* 1995;164(3):673–677. https://doi.org/10.2214/ajr.164.3.7863892.

49. Nguyen Bui L, Brant-Zawadzki M, Verghese P, Gillan G. Magnetic resonance angiography of cervicocranial dissection. *Stroke.* 1993;24(1):126–131. https://doi.org/10.1161/01.str.24.1.126.

50. Fox AJ, Lin JP, Pinto RS, Kricheff II. Myelographic cervical nerve root deformities. *Radiology.* 1975;116(02):355–361. https://doi.org/10.1148/116.2.355.

51. Davies BM, Mowforth OD, Smith EK, Kotter MR. Degenerative cervical myelopathy. *BMJ.* 2018;360:k186. https://doi.org/10.1136/bmj.k186.

52. Tierney RT, Maldjian C, Mattacola CG, Straub SJ, Sitler MR. Cervical spine stenosis measures in normal subjects. *J Athl Train.* 2002;37(2):190. https://www.ncbi.nlm.nih.gov/pmc/articles/pmc164344/.

53. Aikenmu K, Wubuli R, Wang Z, et al. Effect of surgical treatment on mild cervical spondylotic myelopathy with remarkable intramedullary magnetic resonance imaging signal changes. *Int J Clin Exp Med.* 2018;11(4):3289–3295. http://www.ijcem.com/files/ijcem0065310.pdf.

54. Kang Y, Lee JW, Koh YH, et al. New MRI grading system for the cervical canal stenosis. *AJR Am J Roentgenol.* 2011;197(1):W134–W140. https://doi.org/10.2214/AJR.10.5560.

55. Xu Y, Chen F, Wang Y, Zhang J, Hu J. Surgical approaches and outcomes for cervical myelopathy with increased signal intensity on T2-weighted MRI: a meta-analysis. *J Orthop Surg Res.* 2019;14(1):224. https://doi.org/10.1186/s13018-019-1265-z.

56. Lee Y, Kim SY, Kim K. A dynamic magnetic resonance imaging study of changes in severity of cervical spinal stenosis in flexion and extension. *Ann Rehabil Med.* 2018;42(4):584–590. https://doi.org/10.5535/arm.2018.42.4.584.

57. Tetreault LA, Côté P, Kopjar B, Arnold P, Fehlings MG. A clinical prediction model to assess surgical outcome in patients with cervical spondylotic myelopathy: internal and external validations using the prospective multicenter AOSpine North American and international datasets of 743 patients. *Spine J.* 2015;15(3):388–397. https://doi.org/10.1016/j.spinee.2014.12.145.

58. Al-Mefty O, Harkey LH, Middleton TH, Smith RR, Fox JL. Myelopathic cervical spondylotic lesions demonstrated by magnetic resonance imaging. *J Neurosurg.* 1988;68(2):217–222. https://doi.org/10.3171/jns.1988.68.2.0217.

59. Arvin B, Kalsi-Ryan S, Mercier D, Furlan JC, Massicotte EM, Fehlings MG. Preoperative magnetic resonance imaging is associated with baseline neurological status and can predict postoperative recovery in patients with cervical spondylotic myelopathy. *Spine.* 2013;38(14):1170–1176. https://doi.org/10.1097/brs.0b013e31828e23a8.

60. Fehlings MG, Rao SC, Tator CH, et al. The optimal radiologic method for assessing spinal canal compromise and cord compression in patients with cervical spinal cord injury. *Spine.* 1999;24(6):605–613. https://doi.org/10.1097/00007632-199903150-00023.

61. Edwards WC, LaRocca H. The developmental segmental sagittal diameter of the cervical spinal canal in patients with cervical spondylosis. *Spine.* 1983;8(1):20–27. https://doi.org/10.1097/00007632-198301000-00003.

62. Gore DR. Roentgenographic findings in the cervical spine in asymptomatic persons: a ten-year follow-up. *Spine.* 2001;26(22):2463–2466. https://doi.org/10.1097/00007632-200111150-00013.

63. Hayashi H, Okada K, Hamada M, Tada K, Ueno R. Etiologic factors of myelopathy. A radiographic evaluation of the aging changes in the cervical spine. *Clin Orthop Relat Res.* 1987;214:200–209. https://www.ncbi.nlm.nih.gov/pubmed/3791744.

64. Herzog RJ, Wiens JJ, Dillingham MF, Sontag MJ. Normal cervical spine morphometry and cervical spinal stenosis in asymptomatic professional football players. Plain film radiography, multiplanar computed tomography, and magnetic resonance imaging. *Spine.* 1991;16(6 Suppl):S178–S186. https://doi.org/10.1097/00007632-199106001-00001.

65. Kuwazawa Y, Bashir W, Pope MH, Takahashi K, Smith FW. Biomechanical aspects of the cervical cord: effects of postural changes in healthy volunteers using positional magnetic resonance imaging. *J Spinal Disord Tech.* 2006;19(5):348–352. https://doi.org/10.1097/01.bsd.0000203273.90004.eb.

66. Kuwazawa Y, Pope MH, Bashir W, Takahashi K, Smith FW. The length of the cervical cord: effects of postural changes in healthy volunteers using positional magnetic resonance imaging. *Spine.* 2006;31(17):E579–E583. https://doi.org/10.1097/01.brs.0000229228.62627.75.

67. Lee MJ, Cassinelli EH, Riew KD. Prevalence of cervical spine stenosis. Anatomic study in cadavers. *J Bone Joint Surg Am Vol.* 2007;89(2):376–380. https://doi.org/10.2106/JBJS.F.00437.

68. Nouri A, Tetreault L, Singh A, Karadimas SK, Fehlings MG. Degenerative cervical myelopathy: epidemiology, genetics, and pathogenesis. *Spine*. 2015;40(12):E675–E693. https://doi.org/10.1097/BRS.0000000000000913.

69. Okada Y, Ikata T, Katoh S, Yamada H. Morphologic analysis of the cervical spinal cord, dural tube, and spinal canal by magnetic resonance imaging in normal adults and patients with cervical spondylotic myelopathy. *Spine*. 1994;19(20):2331–2335. https://doi.org/10.1097/00007632-199410150-00014.

70. Pavlov H, Torg JS, Robie B, Jahre C. Cervical spinal stenosis: determination with vertebral body ratio method. *Radiology*. 1987;164(3):771–775. https://doi.org/10.1148/radiology.164.3.3615879.

71. Payne EE, Spillane JD. The cervical spine an anatomico-pathological study of 70 specimens (using a special technique) with particular reference to the problem of cervical spondylosis. *Brain*. 1957;80(4):571–596. https://doi.org/10.1093/brain/80.4.571.

72. Prasad SS, O'Malley M, Caplan M, Shackleford IM, Pydisetty RK. MRI measurements of the cervical spine and their correlation to Pavlov's ratio. *Spine*. 2003;28(12):1263–1268. https://doi.org/10.1097/01.BRS.0000065570.20888.AA.

73. Torg JS, Naranja Jr RJ, Pavlov H, Galinat BJ, Warren R, Stine RA. The relationship of developmental narrowing of the cervical spinal canal to reversible and irreversible injury of the cervical spinal cord in football players. An epidemiological study*. *JBJS*. 1996;78(9):1308. https://journals.lww.com/rca/00004623-199609000-00003.fulltext.

74. Torg JS, Pavlov H, Genuario SE, et al. Neurapraxia of the cervical spinal cord with transient quadriplegia. *J Bone Joint Surg Am Vol*. 1986;68(9):1354–1370. https://www.ncbi.nlm.nih.gov/pubmed/3782207.

75. Alafifi T, Kern R, Fehlings M. Clinical and MRI predictors of outcome after surgical intervention for cervical spondylotic myelopathy. *J Neuroimaging: Official Journal of the American Society of Neuroimaging*. 2007;17(4):315–322. https://doi.org/10.1111/j.1552-6569.2007.00119.x.

76. Khanna AJ. *MRI for Orthopaedic Surgeons*. Thieme; 2010.

77. Morishita Y, Naito M, Hymanson H, Miyazaki M, Wu G, Wang JC. The relationship between the cervical spinal canal diameter and the pathological changes in the cervical spine. *Eur Spine J: Official Publication of the European Spine Society, the European Spinal Deformity Society, and the European Section of the Cervical Spine Research Society*. 2009;18(6):877–883. https://doi.org/10.1007/s00586-009-0968-y.

78. Nouri A, Tetreault L, Nori S, Martin AR, Nater A, Fehlings MG. Congenital cervical spine stenosis in a multicenter global cohort of patients with degenerative cervical myelopathy: an ambispective report based on a magnetic resonance imaging diagnostic criterion. *Neurosurgery*. 2018;83(3):521–528. https://doi.org/10.1093/neuros/nyx521.

79. Baptiste DC, Fehlings MG. Pathophysiology of cervical myelopathy. *Spine J: Official Journal of the North American Spine Society*. 2006;6(6 Suppl):190S–197S. https://doi.org/10.1016/j.spinee.2006.04.024.

80. Galbusera F, van Rijsbergen M, Ito K, Huyghe JM, Brayda-Bruno M, Wilke H-J. Ageing and degenerative changes of the intervertebral disc and their impact on spinal flexibility. *Eur Spine J: Official Publication of the European Spine Society, the European Spinal Deformity Society, and the European Section of the Cervical Spine Research Society*. 2014;23(Suppl. 3):S324–S332. https://doi.org/10.1007/s00586-014-3203-4.

81. Aguila LA, Piraino DW, Modic MT, Dudley AW, Duchesneau PM, Weinstein MA. The intranuclear cleft of the intervertebral disk: magnetic resonance imaging. *Radiology*. 1985;155(1):155–158. https://doi.org/10.1148/radiology.155.1.3975396.

82 Boden S, Lee R, Herzog R. Magnetic resonance imaging of the spine. In: *The Adult Spine: Principles and Practice*. Philadelphia: Lippincott-Raven; 1997:563–629.

83. Boos N, Weissbach S, Rohrbach H, Weiler C, Spratt KF, Nerlich AG. Classification of age-related changes in lumbar intervertebral discs: 2002 Volvo Award in basic science. *Spine*. 2002;27(23):2631–2644. https://doi.org/10.1097/00007632-200212010-00002.

84. Mercer S, Bogduk N. The ligaments and anulus fibrosus of human adult cervical intervertebral discs. *Spine*. 1999;24(7):619. https://journals.lww.com/em-news/00007632-199904010-00002.fulltext.

85. Schiebler ML, Camerino VJ, Fallon MD, Zlatkin MB, Grenier N, Kressel HY. In vivo and ex vivo magnetic resonance imaging evaluation of early disc degeneration with histopathologic correlation. *Spine*. 1991;16(6):635–640. https://doi.org/10.1097/00007632-199106000-00007.

86. Sether LA, Yu S, Haughton VM, Fischer ME. Intervertebral disk: normal age-related changes in MR signal intensity. *Radiology*. 1990;177(2):385–388. https://doi.org/10.1148/radiology.177.2.2217773.

87. Van Goethem JWM, van den Hauwe L, Parizel PM, eds. *Spinal Imaging: Diagnostic Imaging of the Spine and Spinal Cord*. Berlin, Heidelberg: Springer; 2007. https://doi.org/10.1007/978-3-540-68483-1.

88. Albeck MJ, Hilden J, Kjaer L, et al. A controlled comparison of myelography, computed tomography, and magnetic resonance imaging in clinically suspected lumbar disc herniation. *Spine*. 1995;20(4):443–448. https://doi.org/10.1097/00007632-199502001-00006.

89. Parizel PM, Wilmink JT. Imaging of the spine: techniques and indications. In: *Diagnosis and Therapy of Spinal Tumors*; 1998:15–48. https://doi.org/10.1007/978-3-642-60254-2_2.

90. Haughton V. Medical imaging of intervertebral disc degeneration. *Spine*. 2004;29(23):2751–2756. https://doi.org/10.1097/01.brs.0000148475.04738.73.

91. Al-Hadidi MT, Badran DH, Al-Hadidi AM, Abu-Ghaida JH. Magnetic resonance imaging of normal lumbar intervertebral discs. *Saudi Med J*. 2001;22(11):1013–1018. https://www.ncbi.nlm.nih.gov/pubmed/11744977.

92. Pfirrmann CWA, Metzdorf A, Zanetti M, Hodler J, Boos N. Magnetic resonance classification of lumbar intervertebral disc degeneration. *Spine.* 2001;26(17):1873–1878. https://doi.org/10.1097/00007632-200109010-00011.

93. Nakashima H, Yukawa Y, Suda K, Yamagata M, Ueta T, Kato F. Cervical disc protrusion correlates with the severity of cervical disc degeneration. *Spine.* 2015;40(13):E774–E779. https://doi.org/10.1097/brs.0000000000000953.

94. Frobin W, Leivseth G, Biggemann M, Brinckmann P. Vertebral height, disc height, posteroanterior displacement and dens–atlas gap in the cervical spine: precision measurement protocol and normal data. *Clin Biomech.* 2002;17(6):423–431. https://doi.org/10.1016/S0268-0033(02)00044-X.

95. D'Anastasi M, Birkenmaier C, Schmidt GP, Wegener B, Reiser MF, Baur-Melnyk A. Correlation between vacuum phenomenon on CT and fluid on MRI in degenerative disks. *AJR Am J Roentgenol.* 2011;197(5):1182–1189. https://doi.org/10.2214/AJR.10.6359.

96. Ozdol C, Turk CC, Yildirim AE, Dalgic A. Anterior herniation of partially calcified and degenerated cervical disc causing dysphagia. *Asian Spine J.* 2015;9(4):612. https://doi.org/10.4184/asj.2015.9.4.612.

97. Kawaguchi K, Harimaya K, Matsumoto Y, et al. Effect of cartilaginous endplates on extruded disc resorption in lumbar disc herniation. *PLoS One.* 2018;13(4):e0195946. https://doi.org/10.1371/journal.pone.0195946.

98. Wang H, Li Z, Zhang C, et al. Correlation between high-intensity zone on MRI and discography in patients with low back pain. *Medicine.* 2017;96(30):e7222. https://doi.org/10.1097/MD.0000000000007222.

99. Khan I, Hargunani R, Saifuddin A. The lumbar high-intensity zone: 20 years on. *Clin Radiol.* 2014;69(6):551–558. https://doi.org/10.1016/j.crad.2013.12.012.

100. Peng B, Hou S, Wu W, Zhang C, Yang Y. The pathogenesis and clinical significance of a high-intensity zone (HIZ) of lumbar intervertebral disc on MR imaging in the patient with discogenic low back pain. *Eur Spine J.* 2006;15(5):583–587. https://doi.org/10.1007/s00586-005-0892-8.

101. Sugiura K, Tonogai I, Matsuura T, et al. Discoscopic findings of high signal intensity zones on magnetic resonance imaging of lumbar intervertebral discs. *Case Rep Orthop.* 2014;2014:1–5. https://doi.org/10.1155/2014/245952.

102. Dean CL, Gabriel JP, Cassinelli EH, Bolesta MJ, Bohlman HH. Degenerative spondylolisthesis of the cervical spine: analysis of 58 patients treated with anterior cervical decompression and fusion. *Spine J: Official Journal of the North American Spine Society.* 2009;9(6):439–446. https://doi.org/10.1016/j.spinee.2008.11.010.

103. Suzuki A, Daubs MD, Inoue H, et al. Prevalence and motion characteristics of degenerative cervical spondylolisthesis in the symptomatic adult. *Spine.* 2013;38(17):E1115–E1120. https://doi.org/10.1097/brs.0b013e31829b1487.

104. van den Hauwe L. Pathology of the posterior elements. In: *Spinal Imaging;* 2007:157–184. https://doi.org/10.1007/978-3-540-68483-1_7.

105. Hayashi T, Wang JC, Suzuki A, et al. Risk factors for missed dynamic canal stenosis in the cervical spine. *Spine.* 2014;39(10):812–819. https://doi.org/10.1097/brs.0000000000000289.

106. Ruangchainikom M, Daubs MD, Suzuki A, et al. Effect of cervical kyphotic deformity type on the motion characteristics and dynamic spinal cord compression. *Spine.* 2014;39(12):932–938. https://doi.org/10.1097/brs.0000000000000330.

107. Fujiwara A, Tamai K, Yamato M, et al. The relationship between facet joint osteoarthritis and disc degeneration of the lumbar spine: an MRI study. *Eur Spine J: Official Publication of the European Spine Society, the European Spinal Deformity Society, and the European Section of the Cervical Spine Research Society.* 1999;8(5):396–401. https://doi.org/10.1007/s005860050193.

108. Gellhorn AC, Katz JN, Suri P. Osteoarthritis of the spine: the facet joints. *Nat Rev Rheumatol.* 2013;9(4):216–224. https://doi.org/10.1038/nrrheum.2012.199.

109. Kushchayev SV, Glushko T, Jarraya M, et al. ABCs of the degenerative spine. *Insights Imaging.* 2018;9(2):253–274. https://doi.org/10.1007/s13244-017-0584-z.

110. Kettler A, Wilke H-J. Review of existing grading systems for cervical or lumbar disc and facet joint degeneration. *Eur Spine J: Official Publication of the European Spine Society, the European Spinal Deformity Society, and the European Section of the Cervical Spine Research Society.* 2006;15(6):705–718. https://doi.org/10.1007/s00586-005-0954-y.

111. Coste J, Judet O, Barre O, Siaud JR, Cohen de Lara A, Paolaggi JB. Inter- and intraobserver variability in the interpretation of computed tomography of the lumbar spine. *J Clin Epidemiol.* 1994;47(4):375–381. https://doi.org/10.1016/0895-4356(94)90158-9.

112. Bick EM. Vertebral osteophytosis: a clinical syndrome. *J Am Med Assoc.* 1956;160(10):828–829. https://doi.org/10.1001/jama.1956.02960450010002.

113. Butler D, Trafimow JH, Andersson GB, McNeill TW, Huckman MS. Discs degenerate before facets. *Spine.* 1990;15(2):111–113. https://doi.org/10.1097/00007632-199002000-00012.

114. Vaccaro AR, Hulbert RJ, Patel AA, et al. The subaxial cervical spine injury classification system: a novel approach to recognize the importance of morphology, neurology, and integrity of the disco-ligamentous complex. *Spine.* 2007;32(21):2365–2374. https://doi.org/10.1097/BRS.0b013e3181557b92.

115. White AA, Southwick WO, Panjabi MM. Clinical instability in the lower cervical spine a review of past and current concepts. *Spine.* 1976;1(1):15. https://journals.lww.com/spinejournal/Abstract/1976/03000/Clinical_Instability_in_the_Lower_Cervical_Spine_A.3.aspx.

116. Banagan K, Phillips FM. Subaxial cervical spine injuries. In: Shen FH, Samartzis D, Fessler RG, eds. *Textbook of the Cervical Spine.* Elsevier/Saunders; 2015:184–191.

117. Benedetti PF, Fahr LM, Kuhns LR, Hayman LA. MR imaging findings in spinal ligamentous injury. *AJR Am J Roentgenol.* 2000;175(3):661–665. https://doi.org/10.2214/ajr.175.3.1750661.

118. Dundamadappa SK, Cauley KA. MR imaging of acute cervical spinal ligamentous and soft tissue trauma. *Emerg Radiol.* 2012;19(4):277–286. https://doi.org/10.1007/s10140-012-1033-4.

119. Utz M, Khan S, O'Connor D, Meyers S. MDCT and MRI evaluation of cervical spine trauma. *Insights Imaging.* 2014;5(1):67–75. https://doi.org/10.1007/s13244-013-0304-2.

120. Katzberg RW, Benedetti PF, Drake CM, et al. Acute cervical spine injuries: prospective MR imaging assessment at a level 1 trauma center. *Radiology.* 1999;213(1):203–212. https://doi.org/10.1148/radiology.213.1.r99oc40203.

121. Bird JE, Marco RAW. Metastatic disease of the cervical spine. In: Shen FH, Samartzis D, Fessler RG, eds. *Textbook of the Cervical Spine.* Elsevier/Saunders; 2015:228–234.

122. Clohisy DR, Ramnaraine ML. Osteoclasts are required for bone tumors to grow and destroy bone. *J Orthop Res: Official Publication of the Orthopaedic Research Society.* 1998;16(6):660–666. https://doi.org/10.1002/jor.1100160606.

123. Kollias SS, Capper DM, Saupe N, Baráth K. Spinal tumors. In: Naidich TP, Castillo M, Cha S, Raybaud C, Smirniotopoulos J, Kollias S, Kleinman GM, eds. *Imaging of the Spine.* Elsevier; 2011:305–375.

124. Molina CA, (Jason) Yoon BM, Gokaslan ZL, Sciubba DM. Primary tumors of the spinal cord. In: Shen FH, Samartzis D, Fessler RG, eds. *Textbook of the Cervical Spine.* Elsevier/Saunders; 2015:213–218.

125. Beall DP, Googe DJ, Emery RL, et al. Extramedullary intradural spinal tumors: a pictorial review. *Curr Probl Diagn Radiol.* 2007;36(5):185–198. https://doi.org/10.1067/j.cpradiol.2006.12.002.

126. Abul-Kasim K, Thurnher MM, McKeever P, Sundgren PC. Intradural spinal tumors: current classification and MRI features. *Neuroradiology.* 2008;50(4):301–314. https://doi.org/10.1007/s00234-007-0345-7.

127. Drevelegas A, Chourmouzi D, Boulogianni G, Sofroniadis I. Imaging of primary bone tumors of the spine. *Eur Radiol.* 2003;13(8):1859–1871. https://doi.org/10.1007/s00330-002-1581-1.

128. Van Goethem J, Van Campenhout A, van den Hauwe L, Parizel PM. Scoliosis. *Neuroimaging Clin N Am.* 2007;17(1):105–115. https://doi.org/10.1016/j.nic.2006.12.001.

129. Bernstein P, Hentschel S, Platzek I, et al. The assessment of the postoperative spinal alignment: MRI adds up on accuracy. *Eur Spine J.* 2012;21(4):733–738. https://doi.org/10.1007/s00586-011-2115-9.

130. Schmitz A, Jaeger UE, Koenig R, et al. A new MRI technique for imaging scoliosis in the sagittal plane. *Eur Spine J.* 2001;10(2):114–117. https://doi.org/10.1007/s005860100250.

131. Smith JS, Lafage V, Ryan DJ, et al. Association of myelopathy scores with cervical sagittal balance and normalized spinal cord volume. *Spine.* 2013;38:S161–S170. https://doi.org/10.1097/brs.0b013e3182a7eb9e.

132. Street J, Lenehan B, Albietz J, Bishop P, Dvorak M, Fisher C. Intraobserver and interobserver reliabilty of measures of kyphosis in thoracolumbar fractures. *Spine J.* 2009;9(6):464–469. https://doi.org/10.1016/j.spinee.2009.02.007.

133. Wessberg P, Danielson BI, Willén J. Comparison of cobb angles in idiopathic scoliosis on standing radiographs and supine axially loaded MRI. *Spine.* 2006;31(26):3039–3044. https://doi.org/10.1097/01.brs.0000249513.91050.80.

134. Muthukumar N, Karuppaswamy U, Sankarasubbu B. Calcium pyrophosphate dihydrate deposition disease causing thoracic cord compression: case report. *Neurosurgery.* 2000;222. https://doi.org/10.1097/00006123-200001000-00047.

135. van Goethem JWM, van den Hauwe L, Parizel PM. *Spinal Imaging: Diagnostic Imaging of the Spine and Spinal Cord.* Springer Science & Business Media; 2007. https://play.google.com/store/books/details?id=gRhulSe79IAC.

136. Wong JJ, Leung OC, Yuen MK. Questionable adequacy of magnetic resonance for the detection of ossification of the posterior longitudinal ligament of the cervical spine. *Hong Kong J Radiol.* 2011;14:78–83. https://www.researchgate.net/profile/Ming_Keung_Yuen/publication/230629764_Questionable_Adequacy_of_Magnetic_Resonance_for_the_Detection_of_Ossification_of_the_Posterior_Longitudinal_Ligament_of_the_Cervical_Spine/links/553e3bbb0cf294deef6fcb92.pdf.

137. Mizuno J, Nakagawa H, Hashizume Y. Analysis of hypertrophy of the posterior longitudinal ligament of the cervical spine, on the basis of clinical and experimental studies. *Neurosurgery.* 2001;49(5):1091–1098. https://doi.org/10.1227/00006123-200111000-00013.

138. Inamasu J, Guiot BH, Sachs DC. Ossification of the posterior longitudinal ligament: an update on its biology, epidemiology, and natural history. *Neurosurgery.* 2006;58(6):1027–1039. https://doi.org/10.1227/01.neu.0000215867.87770.73.

139. Ono K, Yonenobu K, Miyamoto S, Okada K. Pathology of ossification of the posterior longitudinal ligament and ligamentum flavum. *Clin Orthop Relat Res.* 1999;359:18–26. https://doi.org/10.1097/00003086-199902000-00003.

140. Stapleton CJ, Pham MH, Attenello FJ, Hsieh PC. Ossification of the posterior longitudinal ligament: genetics and pathophysiology. *Neurosurg Focus.* 2011;30(3):E6. https://doi.org/10.3171/2010.12.focus10271.

141. Sugimura H, Kakitsubata Y, Suzuki Y, et al. MRI of ossification of ligamentum flavum. *J Comput Assist Tomogr.* 1992;16(1):73–76. https://doi.org/10.1097/00004728-199201000-00013.

142. Kishiya M, Sawada T, Kanemaru K, et al. A functional RNAi screen for Runx2-regulated genes associated with ectopic bone formation in human spinal ligaments.

J Pharmacol Sci. 2008;106(3):404–414. https://doi.org/10.1254/jphs.fp0072043.

143. Kong Q, Ma X, Li F, et al. COL6A1 polymorphisms associated with ossification of the ligamentum flavum and ossification of the posterior longitudinal ligament. *Spine.* 2007;32(25):2834–2838. https://doi.org/10.1097/brs.0b013e31815b761c.

144. Guo JJ, Luk KDK, Karppinen J, Yang H, Cheung KMC. Prevalence, distribution, and morphology of ossification of the ligamentum flavum. *Spine.* 2010;35(1):51–56. https://doi.org/10.1097/brs.0b013e31b3f779.

145. Miyasaka K, Isu T, Abe S, Takei H, Kaneda K, Tsuru M. Myelopathy due to ossification or calcification of the Ligamentum Flavum. *J Comput Assist Tomogr.* 1983;7(1):201. https://doi.org/10.1097/00004728-198302000-00181.

146. Bochkova AG, Levshakova AV, Bunchuk NV, Braun J. Spinal inflammation lesions as detected by magnetic resonance imaging in patients with early ankylosing spondylitis are more often observed in posterior structures of the spine. *Rheumatology.* 2010;49(4):749–755. https://doi.org/10.1093/rheumatology/kep419.

147. Jurik AG. Imaging the spine in arthritis—a pictorial review. *Insights Imaging.* 2011;2(2):177–191. https://doi.org/10.1007/s13244-010-0061-4.

148. Joaquim AF, Ghizoni E, Tedeschi H, Appenzeller S, Daniel Riew K. Radiological evaluation of cervical spine involvement in rheumatoid arthritis. *Neurosurg Focus.* 2015;38(4):E4. https://doi.org/10.3171/2015.1.focus14664.

149. Krauss WE, Bledsoe JM, Clarke MJ, Nottmeier EW, Pichelmann MA. Rheumatoid arthritis of the craniovertebral junction. *Neurosurgery.* 2010;66(Suppl. 3):A83–A95. https://doi.org/10.1227/01.neu.0000365854.13997.b0.

150. Matteson EL. Cervical spine disease in rheumatoid arthritis: how common a finding? How uncommon a problem? *Arthritis Rheum.* 2003;48(7):1775–1778. https://doi.org/10.1002/art.11085.

151. Meyer C, Bredow J, Heising E, Eysel P, Müller LP, Stein G. Rheumatoid arthritis affecting the upper cervical spine: biomechanical assessment of the stabilizing ligaments. *Biomed Res Int.* 2017;2017:1–7. https://doi.org/10.1155/2017/6131703.

152. Neva MH. High prevalence of asymptomatic cervical spine subluxation in patients with rheumatoid arthritis waiting for orthopaedic surgery. *Ann Rheum Dis.* 2005;65(7):884–888. https://doi.org/10.1136/ard.2005.042135.

153. Shen FH, Samartzis D, Jenis LG, An HS. Rheumatoid arthritis: evaluation and surgical management of the cervical spine. *Spine J: Official Journal of the North American Spine Society.* 2004;4(6):689–700. https://doi.org/10.1016/j.spinee.2004.05.001.

154. Joaquim AF, Appenzeller S. Cervical spine involvement in rheumatoid arthritis—a systematic review. *Autoimmun Rev.* 2014;13(12):1195–1202. https://doi.org/10.1016/j.autrev.2014.08.014.

155. Tehranzadeh J, Ashikyan O, Dascalos J. Magnetic resonance imaging in early detection of rheumatoid arthritis.

Semin Musculoskelet Radiol. 2003;7(2):79–94. https://doi.org/10.1055/s-2003-41342.

156. Bundschuh C, Modic MT, Kearney F, Morris R, Deal C. Rheumatoid arthritis of the cervical spine: surface-coil MR imaging. *Am J Roentgenol.* 1988;151(1):181–187. https://doi.org/10.2214/ajr.151.1.181.

157. Reijnierse M, Breedveld FC, Kroon HM, Hansen B, Pope TL, Bloem JL. Are magnetic resonance flexion views useful in evaluating the cervical spine of patients with rheumatoid arthritis? *Skelet Radiol.* 2000;29(2):85–89. https://doi.org/10.1007/s002560050015.

158. Glew D, Watt I, Dieppe PA, Goddard PR. MRI of the cervical spine: rheumatoid arthritis compared with cervical spondylosis. *Clin Radiol.* 1991;44(2):71–76. https://doi.org/10.1016/s0009-9260(05)80498-2.

159. Gurley JP, Bell GR. The surgical management of patients with rheumatoid cervical spine disease. *Rheum Dis Clin N Am.* 1997;23(2):317–332. https://doi.org/10.1016/s0889-857x(05)70332-x.

160. Taurog JD, Chhabra A, Colbert RA. Ankylosing spondylitis and axial spondyloarthritis. *N Engl J Med.* 2016;374(26):2563–2574. https://doi.org/10.1056/nejmra1406182.

161. Gran JT, Husby G. HLA-B27 and spondyloarthropathy: value for early diagnosis? *J Med Genet.* 1995;32(7):497–501. https://doi.org/10.1136/jmg.32.7.497.

162. Isla Guerrero A, Mansilla Fernández B, Hernández Garcia B, Gómez de la Riva Á, Gandía González ML, Isla Paredes E. Surgical outcomes of traumatic cervical fractures in patients with ankylosing spondylitis. *Neurocirugia.* 2018;29(3):116–121. https://doi.org/10.1016/j.neucir.2017.11.001.

163. Koivikko MP, Koskinen SK. MRI of cervical spine injuries complicating ankylosing spondylitis. *Skelet Radiol.* 2008;37(9):813–819. https://doi.org/10.1007/s00256-008-0484-x.

164. Rustagi T, Drazin D, Oner C, et al. Fractures in spinal ankylosing disorders: a narrative review of disease and injury types, treatment techniques, and outcomes. *J Orthop Trauma.* 2017;31(Suppl. 4):S57–S74. https://doi.org/10.1097/BOT.0000000000000953.

165. Lenehan B, Street J, Cassidy N. Paget's disease of the cervical spine: case report and review. *Ir J Med Sci.* 2012;181(3):369–372. https://doi.org/10.1007/s11845-010-0463-9.

166. Cheng CW, Nguyen QT, Zhou H. Tophaceous gout of the cervical and thoracic spine with concomitant epidural infection. In: *AME Case Reports.* vol. 2; 2018:35. https://doi.org/10.21037/acr.2018.07.01.

167. Turaga S, Thomas M, Savy L, Schreiber BE. Pseudogout or pseudolymphoma? Calcium pyrophosphate deposition disease of the cervical spine: a rare presentation and literature review. *BMJ Case Rep.* 2019;12(12). https://doi.org/10.1136/bcr-2019-231508.

168. Janssen H, Weissman BN, Aliabadi P, Zamani AA. MR imaging of arthritides of the cervical spine. *Magn Reson Imaging Clin N Am.* 2000;8(3):491–512. https://www.ncbi.nlm.nih.gov/pubmed/10947923.

169. Kobayashi T, Miyakoshi N, Abe T, et al. Acute neck pain caused by pseudogout attack of calcified cervical yellow ligament: a case report. *J Med Case Rep.* 2016;10(1). https://doi.org/10.1186/s13256-016-0928-1.

170. Lotz JC, Haughton V, Boden SD, et al. New treatments and imaging strategies in degenerative disease of the intervertebral disks. *Radiology.* 2012;264(1):6–19. https://doi.org/10.1148/radiol.12110339.

171. Benneker LM, Heini PF, Anderson SE, Alini M, Ito K. Correlation of radiographic and MRI parameters to morphological and biochemical assessment of intervertebral disc degeneration. *Eur Spine J: Official Publication of the European Spine Society, the European Spinal Deformity Society, and the European Section of the Cervical Spine Research Society.* 2005;14(1):27–35. https://doi.org/10.1007/s00586-004-0759-4.

172. Hong CH, Park JS, Jung KJ, Kim WJ. Measurement of the normal lumbar intervertebral disc space using magnetic resonance imaging. *Asian Spine J.* 2010;4(1):1–6. https://doi.org/10.4184/asj.2010.4.1.1.

173. Schneiderman G, Flannigan B, Kingston S, Thomas J, Dillin WH, Watkins RG. Magnetic resonance imaging in the diagnosis of disc degeneration: correlation with discography. *Spine.* 1987;12(3):276–281. https://doi.org/10.1097/00007632-198704000-00016.

174. Listerud J, Einstein S, Outwater E, Kressel HY. First principles of fast spin echo. *Magn Reson Q.* 1992;8(4):199–244. https://www.ncbi.nlm.nih.gov/pubmed/1489675.

175. Christe A, Läubli R, Guzman R, et al. Degeneration of the cervical disc: histology compared with radiography and magnetic resonance imaging. *Neuroradiology.* 2005;47(10):721–729. https://doi.org/10.1007/s00234-005-1412-6.

176. Kolstad F, Myhr G, Kvistad KA, Nygaard OP, Leivseth G. Degeneration and height of cervical discs classified from MRI compared with precise height measurements from radiographs. *Eur J Radiol.* 2005;55(3):415–420. https://doi.org/10.1016/j.ejrad.2005.02.005.

177. Lehto IJ, Tertti MO, Komu ME, Paajanen HE, Tuominen J, Kormano MJ. Age-related MRI changes at 0.1 T in cervical discs in asymptomatic subjects. *Neuroradiology.* 1994;36(1):49–53. https://doi.org/10.1007/bf00599196.

178. Miyazaki M, Hong SW, Yoon SH, Morishita Y, Wang JC. Reliability of a magnetic resonance imaging-based grading system for cervical intervertebral disc degeneration. *J Spinal Disord Tech.* 2008;21(4):288–292. https://doi.org/10.1097/BSD.0b013e31813c0e59.

179. Stäbler A, Bellan M, Weiss M, Gärtner C, Brossmann J, Reiser MF. MR imaging of enhancing intraosseous disk herniation (Schmorl's nodes). *AJR Am J Roentgenol.* 1997;168(4):933–938. https://doi.org/10.2214/ajr.168.4.9124143.

180. Suzuki A, Daubs MD, Hayashi T, et al. Patterns of cervical disc degeneration: analysis of magnetic resonance imaging of over 1000 symptomatic subjects. *Glob Spine J.* 2018;8(3):254–259. https://doi.org/10.1177/2192568217719436.

181. Thalgott JS, Albert TJ, Vaccaro AR, et al. A new classification system for degenerative disc disease of the lumbar spine based on magnetic resonance imaging, provocative discography, plain radiographs and anatomic considerations. *Spine J: Official Journal of the North American Spine Society.* 2004;4(6 Suppl):167S–172S. https://doi.org/10.1016/j.spinee.2004.07.001.

182. Thompson JP, Pearce RH, Schechter MT, Adams ME, Tsang IK, Bishop PB. Preliminary evaluation of a scheme for grading the gross morphology of the human intervertebral disc. *Spine.* 1990;15(5):411–415. https://doi.org/10.1097/00007632-199005000-00012.

183. Walraevens J, Liu B, Meersschaert J, et al. Qualitative and quantitative assessment of degeneration of cervical intervertebral discs and facet joints. *Eur Spine J: Official Publication of the European Spine Society, the European Spinal Deformity Society, and the European Section of the Cervical Spine Research Society.* 2009;18(3):358–369. https://doi.org/10.1007/s00586-008-0820-9.

184. Rajasekaran S, Venkatadass K, Naresh Babu J, Ganesh K, Shetty AP. Pharmacological enhancement of disc diffusion and differentiation of healthy, ageing and degenerated discs: results from in-vivo serial post-contrast MRI studies in 365 human lumbar discs. *Eur Spine J: Official Publication of the European Spine Society, the European Spinal Deformity Society, and the European Section of the Cervical Spine Research Society.* 2008;17(5):626–643. https://doi.org/10.1007/s00586-008-0645-6.

185. Zhang Y-H, Zhao C-Q, Jiang L-S, Chen X-D, Dai L-Y. Modic changes: a systematic review of the literature. *Eur Spine J: Official Publication of the European Spine Society, the European Spinal Deformity Society, and the European Section of the Cervical Spine Research Society.* 2008;17(10):1289–1299. https://doi.org/10.1007/s00586-008-0758-y.

186. Pfirrmann CW, Resnick D. Schmorl nodes of the thoracic and lumbar spine: radiographic-pathologic study of prevalence, characterization, and correlation with degenerative changes of 1,650 spinal levels in 100 cadavers. *Radiology.* 2001;219(2):368–374. https://doi.org/10.1148/radiology.219.2.r01ma21368.

187. Zehra U, Bow C, Lotz JC, et al. Structural vertebral endplate nomenclature and etiology: a study by the ISSLS Spinal Phenotype Focus Group. *Eur Spine J: Official Publication of the European Spine Society, the European Spinal Deformity Society, and the European Section of the Cervical Spine Research Society.* 2018;27(1):2–12. https://doi.org/10.1007/s00586-017-5292-3.

188. Marshman LAG, Trewhella M, Friesem T, Bhatia CK, Krishna M. Reverse transformation of Modic type 2 changes to Modic type 1 changes during sustained chronic low-back pain severity: report of two cases and review of the literature. *J Neurosurg Spine.* 2007;6(2):152–155. https://thejns.org/spine/view/journals/j-neurosurg-spine/6/2/article-p152.xml.

189. Mann E, Peterson CK, Hodler J, Pfirrmann CWA. The evolution of degenerative marrow (Modic) changes in the cervical spine in neck pain patients. *Eur Spine J: Official Publication of the European Spine Society, the European Spinal Deformity Society, and the European Section*

of the Cervical Spine Research Society. 2014;23(3):584–589. https://doi.org/10.1007/s00586-013-2882-6.

190 Wang Y, Videman T, Battié MC. ISSLS prize winner: lumbar vertebral endplate lesions: associations with disc degeneration and back pain history. *Spine (Phila Pa 1976).* 2012;37(17):1490–1496 [2013].

191. Samartzis D, Mok FPS, Karppinen J, Fong DYT, Luk KDK, Cheung KMC. Classification of Schmorl's nodes of the lumbar spine and association with disc degeneration: a large-scale population-based MRI study. *Osteoarthr Cartil/OARS, Osteoarthritis Research Society.* 2016;24(10):1753–1760. https://doi.org/10.1016/j.joca.2016.04.020.

192. Friedrich KM, Nemec S, Peloschek P, Pinker K, Weber M, Trattnig S. The prevalence of lumbar facet joint edema in patients with low back pain. *Skelet Radiol.* 2007;36(8):755–760. https://doi.org/10.1007/s00256-007-0293-7.

193. Park MS, Lee YB, Moon S-H, et al. Facet joint degeneration of the cervical spine: a computed tomographic analysis of 320 patients. *Spine.* 2014;39(12):E713–E718. https://doi.org/10.1097/BRS.0000000000000326.

194. Pathria M, Sartoris DJ, Resnick D. Osteoarthritis of the facet joints: accuracy of oblique radiographic assessment. *Radiology.* 1987;164(1):227–230. https://doi.org/10.1148/radiology.164.1.3588910.

195. Grogan J, Nowicki BH, Schmidt TA, Haughton VM. Lumbar facet joint tropism does not accelerate degeneration of the facet joints. *AJNR Am J Neuroradiol.* 1997;18(7):1325–1329. https://www.ncbi.nlm.nih.gov/pubmed/9282864.

196. Gellhorn AC. Cervical facet-mediated pain. *Phys Med Rehabil Clin N Am.* 2011;22(3):447–458. viii https://doi.org/10.1016/j.pmr.2011.02.006.

197. Manchikanti L, Boswell MV, Singh V, Pampati V, Damron KS, Beyer CD. Prevalence of facet joint pain in chronic spinal pain of cervical, thoracic, and lumbar regions. *BMC Musculoskelet Disord.* 2004;5:15. https://doi.org/10.1186/1471-2474-5-15.

198. Muhle C, Metzner J, Weinert D, et al. Kinematic MR imaging in surgical management of cervical disc disease, spondylosis and spondylotic myelopathy. *Acta Radiol.* 1999;40(2):146–153. https://doi.org/10.3109/02841859909177730.

199. Takahashi M, Yamashita Y, Sakamoto Y, Kojima R. Chronic cervical cord compression: clinical significance of increased signal intensity on MR images. *Radiology.* 1989;173(1):219–224. https://doi.org/10.1148/radiology.173.1.2781011.

200. Liu W, Fan J, Bai J, et al. Magnetic resonance imaging: a possible alternative to a standing lateral radiograph for evaluating cervical sagittal alignment in patients with cervical disc herniation? *Medicine.* 2017;96(39):e8194. https://doi.org/10.1097/MD.0000000000008194.

201. Mohanty C, Massicotte EM, Fehlings MG, Shamji MF. Association of preoperative cervical spine alignment with spinal cord magnetic resonance imaging hyperintensity and myelopathy severity: analysis of a series of 124 cases. *Spine.* 2015;40(1):11–16. https://doi.org/10.1097/BRS.0000000000000670.

202. Harrison DE, Harrison DD, Cailliet R, Troyanovich SJ, Janik TJ, Holland B. Cobb method or Harrison posterior tangent method: which to choose for lateral cervical radiographic analysis. *Spine.* 2000;25(16):2072–2078. https://doi.org/10.1097/00007632-200008150-00011.

203. Karabag H, Iplikcioglu AC. The assessment of upright cervical spinal alignment using supine MRI studies. *Clin Spine Surg.* 2017;30(7):E892–E895. https://doi.org/10.1097/bsd.0000000000000495.

204. Gore DR, Sepic SB, Gardner GM. Roentgenographic findings of the cervical spine in asymptomatic people. *Spine.* 1986;11(6):521–524. https://doi.org/10.1097/00007632-198607000-00003.

205 Katsuura Y, Lemons A, Lorenz E, Swafford R, Osborn J, Cason G. Radiographic analysis of cervical and spinal alignment in multilevel ACDF with lordotic interbody device. *Int J Spine Surg.* 2017;11(2):13. https://doi.org/10.14444/4013.

CHAPTER 8

Subaxial Cervical Spine CT

MICHAEL L. MARTINI[a] • SEAN N. NEIFERT[a] • JONATHAN J. RASOULI[b] •
THOMAS E. MROZ[b]
[a]Icahn School of Medicine at Mount Sinai, New York, NY, United States, [b]Cleveland Clinic, Cleveland, OH, United States

INTRODUCTION

Computed tomography (CT) scans have become the mainstay modality for screening patients in the setting of cervical trauma and identifying fractures in the subaxial cervical spine. High-resolution CT imaging, in particular, has become the primary radiologic means for screening patients at most trauma centers,[1] largely replacing radiographs given a superior sensitivity (90%–100%) in identifying traumatic bony injuries.[2–5] It is therefore critical for spine surgeons and neuroradiologists to understand: (1) normal subaxial cervical anatomy on CT imaging, including commonly used measures of spine relationships and CT-based landmarks for discs and joint spaces; (2) CT findings in the setting of subaxial cervical spine trauma; and (3) CT-based scoring systems for subaxial cervical spine injury.

SUBAXIAL CERVICAL SPINE MEASUREMENTS AND ANATOMICAL RELATIONSHIPS ON CT IMAGING
Coronal CT Imaging

In coronal CT imaging of the subaxial cervical spine, three of the most important measurements and anatomical relationships to understand include the uncovertebral joints (UVJs), the facet joints, and the disc heights.

The UVJs are articulations between the uncinate processes and the inferior vertebral bodies (Fig. 1). They are located between the five vertebral bodies of C2–7 (C2–3, C3–4, C4–5, C5–6, and C6–7) and form part of the anterior wall of the vertebral foramen. Functionally, the UVJs provide posterolateral reinforcement of the intervertebral disc, prevent posterior translation of the vertebral bodies, and provide stability to the cervical spine during movement. UVJ measurements can be obtained via CT imaging by measuring at the inferolateral corner of the vertebral body to the corresponding uncinate process of the vertebral body as discussed later. Previous studies have suggested that

the mean length of the UVJ on coronal CT imaging in normal anatomical subjects ranged from 1.27 to 1.87 mm, with expected variations between different cervical levels.[6]

The intervertebral disc height is another important measurement that may be examined in coronal CT imaging of the subaxial cervical spine. The height of the intervertebral discs may be measured on coronal imaging by taking the vertical length of the disc at the point halfway between the left and right UVJ measurements (Fig. 2). The average disc height in the subaxial cervical spine has been reported to a range from 4.62 to 5.03 mm in CT studies conducted on patients without cervical pathologies.[6]

The facet joints represent another important articulation that lends stability to the subaxial cervical spine by holding the adjacent vertebrae together via connections between the superior and inferior articulating facets. In the cervical spine, the superior facets face superiorly and medially, while the inferior facets are oriented inferiorly and laterally. Three different measurements can be taken of the cervical facet joint space on coronal CT imaging, including measurements of the lateral, medial, and midpoint of the joint space. The lateral and medial portions of the facet joint space are measured at the most lateral and most medial edges of the joint from a line drawn perpendicularly to the edges of the bones. The middle of the facet joint is measured as the midpoint between the lateral and medial facet measurements. The mean measurements for the medial, lateral, and midpoint portions of the subaxial cervical facet joints have been reported as 0.50–0.68 mm, 0.48–0.54 mm, and 1.04–1.37 mm, respectively, in normal anatomical subjects.[6]

Sagittal CT Imaging
There are several critical bone and joint measurements that one should examine on sagittal CT imaging of the subaxial cervical spine to reflect spinal articulation, alignment, and positioning. These measurements

Atlas of Spinal Imaging. https://doi.org/10.1016/B978-0-323-76111-6.00014-6

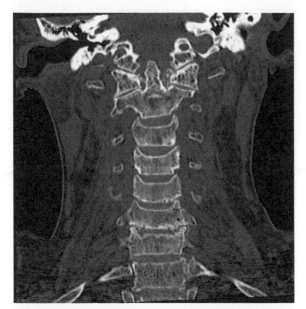

FIG. 1 Examples of UVJ joints on coronal imaging. Coronal CT demonstrating moderately spondylotic UVJ *(red circle)* and severely spondylotic UVJ *(green circle)*.

include the interspinous distances (ISDs); vertebral translations; anterior, posterior, and middle facet distances; and anterior, posterior, and middle disc heights.

The ISD represents the distance between the spinous processes of two adjacent spinal segments and may be altered following acute trauma or in degenerative processes in the spinal column. The ISD may be measured by taking the distance between the superior edges of the most posterior portion of adjacent spinous processes on sagittal CT imaging, as demonstrated in Fig. 3. Previous studies have reported mean ISD values ranging from 13.15 to 15.76 mm in the normal subaxial cervical spine depending on the segments involved.[6]

Vertebral body translation, reflecting shifts in the anterior/posterior positioning of a vertebral body relative to adjacent vertebral bodies, may also be assessed with sagittal CT imaging. This measurement may be obtained by drawing lines parallel to the anterior cortical surfaces of two adjacent vertebral bodies and measuring the distance between these two lines. The typical value for the anterior/posterior vertebral body translation in the sagittal axis of normal patients has

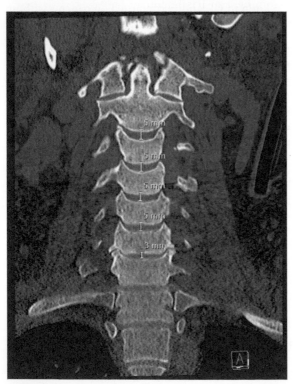

FIG. 2 Intervertebral disc height measurements on coronal imaging.

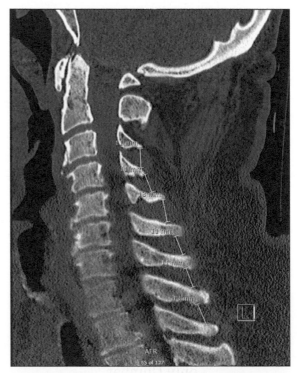

FIG. 3 ISD measurements on sagittal CT imaging.

been reported to be between 0.09 and 0.58 mm in the subaxial cervical spine.[6]

From sagittal CT imaging, the anterior and posterior portions of the cervical facet joint spaces can easily be visualized and measured using the most anterior and posterior edges of the facets. Similarly, the middle of the facet joint space can be measured at the midpoint of the facet joint between the anterior and posterior measurements. Similarly, one may also determine the percent of facet overlap. Changes or large deviations in the facet overlap may reflect certain pathological states in the facet joints. The percentage of facet overlap may be determined by taking the length of the superior and inferior facet that is covered by each other and dividing it by the total length from the most anterior aspect of the cranial facet to the most posterior aspect of the caudal facet. The mean value for the anterior facet measurement in healthy subjects has been reported to be between 0.83 and 0.92 mm in the subaxial cervical spine, while the posterior facet measurement ranges from 0.56 to 0.76 mm and the middle facet ranges from 0.97 to 1.27 mm.[6]

In a similar manner, the anterior, posterior, and middle portions of the intervertebral discs may be measured on sagittal CT imaging to comprehensively determine disc height in the subaxial cervical spine. The sagittal disc height may be obtained for the anterior and posterior portions of the intervertebral discs, using the anterior and posterior edges of the corresponding vertebral bodies, respectively. The line measuring the disc height is always drawn perpendicularly from the cortical edges of the vertebral bodies that interface with the intervertebral disc. A midpoint measurement of the intervertebral disc height may also be obtained halfway between the anterior and posterior measurements. Previous studies have reported that the mean anterior intervertebral disc height in the subaxial cervical region of healthy subjects has ranged from 2.70 to 3.46 mm. In comparison, the posterior and midpoint disc heights have ranged from 1.99 to 2.45 mm and from 4.66 to 5.24 mm, respectively.[6]

SUBAXIAL CERVICAL SPINE CT FINDINGS IN TRAUMA

Approximately 75% of cervical spine dislocations and 65% of cervical spine fractures occur in the subaxial region.[7] There are several types of subaxial cervical injuries that CT imaging is well-suited to assess. These include compression and burst fractures, distraction injuries, hyperflexion and hyperextension injuries, and translational or rotational injuries.

Compression and Burst Injuries

Compression and burst injuries present with a loss of height in the fractured vertebral body and do not show any signs of concomitant translational or distraction injury.[8] On CT scans, a fracture line or signs of endplate disruption are often observed in either sagittal or coronal sections (Fig. 4).[9, 10] Compression injuries also encompass fractures of the lateral mass, laminar, facet, and spinous processes that are only minimally displaced and lack any signs of distraction.[8]

Distraction Injuries

In contrast to compression and burst injuries, distraction injuries involve a dissociation in the vertical axis of the spine. Distraction often occurs in the posterior portion of the spine as a result of hyperflexion injuries and in the anterior portion of the spine following hyperextension injuries. Hyperflexion injuries often involve changes to the articulation at the facet joint and can range in severity from a mild facet subluxation to

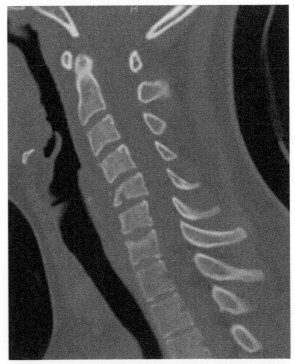

FIG. 4 Compression and burst injury in subaxial cervical spine on sagittal CT imaging.

a perched or jumped facet (Fig. 5), in which an inferior articulating process jumps on top of or over the ipsilateral superior articulating process of the more caudal vertebral level. A subluxation of a facet joint may be considered either when there is > 2 mm of diastasis between the articulating processes or when the overlap of the articulating surfaces drops below 50%.[7] Hyperflexion injuries are also often associated with widening of the posterior intervertebral disc space and are considered when the angulation in this space exceeds 11 degrees. Hyperextension injuries often involve injury or disruption to the anterior intervertebral disc and anterior longitudinal ligament, resulting in a widening of the anterior disc space (Fig. 6). On CT imaging, an avulsed fragment from the anteroinferior portion of the vertebral body, referred to as an "extension teardrop," is often observed.[11]

Translational and Rotational Injuries

A translational or rotational injury is characterized by a shift in vertebral positioning in the horizontal axis and may occur in the presence or absence of bony fracture (Fig. 7). Most translational injuries occur at the C5–6 and C6–7 levels. The translation is more likely to occur in the setting of bilateral disc oligamentous disruption, whereas rotation tends to occur with unilateral disruption, often with pivoting around an intact facet.[9, 12] In general, a distance of 3.5 mm between the posterior edges of two adjacent vertebral bodies is used to determine the presence of translational injury.[7, 10] Of note, traumatic anterior translation almost always occurs in the setting of a concurrent distraction injury, including a facet or fracture-dislocation.[8] For example, bilateral facet dislocations often result in 50% or more translation of the more cranial vertebral body.[13] Other injuries, including bilateral pedicle fractures or lateral mass fractures resulting in separation, can cause translation or rotation in the affected vertebral segments.[12] Rotational injuries can be observed on sagittal CT reconstructions of the spine as a misaligned midline sagittal plane at the affected level.[14]

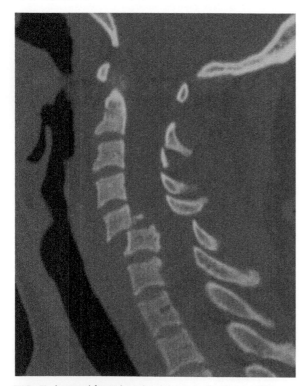

FIG. 5 Jumped facet in subaxial cervical spine on CT imaging.

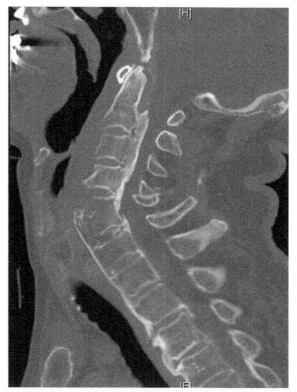

FIG. 6 C5 hyperextension fracture in patients with ankylosing spondylitis.

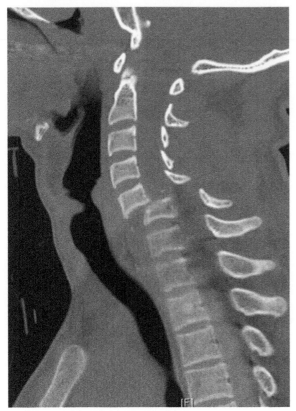

FIG. 7 Translational or rotational injury in subaxial cervical spine on CT imaging.

CT-BASED SCORING SYSTEMS FOR SUBAXIAL CERVICAL INJURY

Two primary scoring systems have been developed to classify subaxial cervical injury using multidetector CT imaging: the Cervical Spine Injury Severity Score[15] and the Subaxial Injury Classification and Scoring (SLIC) system.[7] Both of these scales draw heavily from the assessment of the morphological structure of the bony elements of the cervical spine and have been reported to have improved inter-rater reliability compared to previous radiography-based classification systems.[7, 16]

Cervical Spine Injury Severity Score

The Cervical Spine Injury Severity Score was originally introduced by Moore et al. and involves conceptually dividing the spine into four columns: anterior, posterior, and two lateral columns.[17] Each column is then assessed for evidence of displacement and ligamentous injury and is assigned a corresponding score ranging from 0 to 5 points. Injuries in each column are

characterized as either simple or complex depending on the type and extent of the injury. An injury is considered simple if it involves a bony element of the spine and only affects one column. Conversely, an injury is considered complex if it involves both ligamentous and bony injury in one column, or if an injury involves multiple columns. The final score is tallied by summing the individual scores from each of the four spinal columns, for a maximum possible score of 20 points. A score of $\geq$ 7 suggests that surgical fixation is indicated to correct the injury and stabilize the spine. Of note, this scoring system does not consider the patient's neurological status or findings from other imaging modalities.

Subaxial Injury Classification and Scoring (SLIC) System

The SLIC system was developed by Vacarro et al. in 2007[7] and is becoming increasingly favored in traumatic settings as a means of classifying traumatic injuries as surgical or nonsurgical. The SLIC system is comprised of three distinct grading components, each of which involves assessing an independent predictor of injury outcome. The SLIC components include morphological findings of bony injury, disc oligamentous complex structural integrity, and neurological status.[12] Each component is assessed and scored individually before being added to obtain a cumulative score. Cumulative scores of 3 or less are considered nonsurgical injuries, while a score of 4 is considered indeterminate and 5 or more is surgical.

The SLIC morphology score considers the remaining structural integrity and preserved bony relationships between vertebral segments at the site of injury. The morphology score is assessed using findings from CT imaging and ranges from 0 to 4, with more severe injuries receiving a higher numerical score. A score of 0 reflects no abnormality, while a score of 1 and 2 reflects a compression fracture and a burst fracture, respectively. Distraction injuries receive a score of 3, and translational or rotational injuries receive a score of 4. In cases featuring multiple injuries at a single spinal level, the most severe injury is considered for the SLIC morphology score. In addition, if multiple spinal levels are involved in a traumatic injury, a SLIC score is determined for each injured level. As an illustrative example, a patient with a distraction injury at C4–5 and both a distraction and a translational injury at C5–6 would receive a C4–5 morphology score of 3 and a C5–6 score of 4.

The SLIC disc oligamentous complex score considers the structural integrity of anterior spinal structures, including the anterior longitudinal ligament, the intervertebral disc, and the posterior longitudinal ligament, as well as posterior structures, including the facet joints, ligamentum flavum, supraspinous ligament, and the interspinous ligament. A score of 0 is given if the disc oligamentous complex is found to be intact, whereas a score of 1 is assigned if the integrity is indeterminate or 2 if it is disrupted. Given that the integrity of these structures is highly reflective of overall spinal stability at an injured segment, injury to the disc oligamentous complex is considered an independent predictor of injury outcome. It is important to note that disc oligamentous complex injuries are often initially appreciated by observing abnormal relationships between bony elements of the spine on CT imaging. There is also some degree of overlap in the scoring of the disc oligamentous complex and the bone morphology given that both scores are influenced by abnormal bony relationships secondary to traumatic injury. For example, an isolated distraction injury without neurological deficit would be given a morphology score of 3 and a disc oligamentous complex score of 2, resulting in a total score of 5 with recommended surgical intervention.

The SLIC neurologic status score considers the presence of neurological injury and whether or not the injury is reversible with surgical intervention. Accordingly, a score of 1 is assigned in cases involving only root injuries. A score of 2 is assigned in cases of complete cord injury, whereas a score of 3 is assigned if the cord injury is incomplete and a score of 4 is assigned if there is incomplete cord injury with continued cord compression. Again, this scoring reflects the surgical priority of these injuries, as a surgical intervention may be able to significantly improve patient outcomes in the setting of incomplete cord injuries compared to complete cord injuries. Despite its recognized importance in predicting patient outcomes, care must be taken when considering the presence of neurologic injury as it may be difficult to detect in polytraumatic settings or in obtunded patients.

LIMITATIONS OF CT IMAGING IN THE SUBAXIAL CERVICAL SPINE

Despite the significant clinical utility of CT imaging in the rapid detection and evaluation of bony and ligamentous injuries which plays a fundamental role in the decision-making process of whether or not surgical intervention is indicated, there are important limitations to this imaging modality with regard to other critical determinants that impact patient management. For example, CT imaging is not well suited to assess spinal

cord swelling, spinal cord contusion, or hemorrhage, intervertebral disc herniations, or epidural hematomas, whereas magnetic resonance imaging is able to clearly identify these pathologies. Similarly, for these reasons, magnetic resonance imaging also plays a central role in operative planning, particularly in deciding preferred surgical approaches for cases involving traumatic disc herniation or cord hemorrhage.

CONCLUSIONS

High-resolution CT imaging has become the imaging modality of choice for rapidly assessing traumatic injuries involving the subaxial cervical spine. Becoming familiar with the most common spine measurements and the normal spinal anatomical relationships on CT imaging is critical for understanding the structural and functional changes that may occur in the setting of traumatic cervical injuries. CT-based scoring systems are becoming increasingly used in clinical settings to assess cervical spine stability and injury severity based on changes in bone morphology and anatomic relationships around the site of injury. These scoring systems are useful tools for triaging traumatic cervical injuries and in guiding the appropriate delivery of surgical or nonsurgical treatments.

REFERENCES

1. Como JJ, Diaz JJ, Dunham CM, et al. Practice management guidelines for identification of cervical spine injuries following trauma: update from the eastern association for the surgery of trauma practice management guidelines committee. *J Trauma.* 2009;67(3):651–659.
2. Berne JD, Velmahos GC, El-Tawil Q, et al. Value of complete cervical helical computed tomographic scanning in identifying cervical spine injury in the unevaluable blunt trauma patient with multiple injuries: a prospective study. *J Trauma.* 1999;47(5):896–902. discussion 902–893.
3. Brohi K, Healy M, Fotheringham T, et al. Helical computed tomographic scanning for the evaluation of the cervical spine in the unconscious, intubated trauma patient. *J Trauma.* 2005;58(5):897–901.
4. Holmes JF, Akkinepalli R. Computed tomography versus plain radiography to screen for cervical spine injury: a meta-analysis. *J Trauma.* 2005;58(5):902–905.
5. Mathen R, Inaba K, Munera F, et al. Prospective evaluation of multislice computed tomography versus plain radiographic cervical spine clearance in trauma patients. *J Trauma.* 2007;62(6):1427–1431.
6. Cahill CW, Radcliff KE, Reitman CA. Enhancing evaluation of cervical spine: thresholds for normal CT relationships in the subaxial cervical spine. *Int J Spine Surg.* 2018;12(4):510–519.

7. Vaccaro AR, Hulbert RJ, Patel AA, et al. The subaxial cervical spine injury classification system: a novel approach to recognize the importance of morphology, neurology, and integrity of the disco-ligamentous complex. *Spine (Phila Pa 1976)*. 2007;32(21):2365–2374.

8. Dreizin D, Letzing M, Sliker CW, et al. Multidetector CT of blunt cervical spine trauma in adults. *Radiographics*. 2014;34(7):1842–1865.

9. Aarabi B, Walters BC, Dhall SS, et al. Subaxial cervical spine injury classification systems. *Neurosurgery*. 2013;72(Suppl 2):170–186.

10. Patel AA, Dailey A, Brodke DS, et al. Subaxial cervical spine trauma classification: the subaxial injury classification system and case examples. *Neurosurg Focus*. 2008;25(5):E8.

11. Edeiken-Monroe B, Wagner LK, Harris Jr JH. Hyperextension dislocation of the cervical spine. *AJR Am J Roentgenol*. 1986;146(4):803–808.

12. Dvorak MF, Fisher CG, Fehlings MG, et al. The surgical approach to subaxial cervical spine injuries: an evidence-based algorithm based on the SLIC classification system. *Spine (Phila Pa 1976)*. 2007;32(23):2620–2629.

13. Braakman R, Vinken PJ. Unilateral facet interlocking in the lower cervical spine. *J Bone Joint Surg (Br)*. 1967;49(2):249–257.

14. Vaccaro AR, Lehman Jr RA, Hurlbert RJ, et al. A new classification of thoracolumbar injuries: the importance of injury morphology, the integrity of the posterior ligamentous complex, and neurologic status. *Spine (Phila Pa 1976)*. 2005;30(20):2325–2333.

15. Anderson PA, Moore TA, Davis KW, et al. Cervical spine injury severity score. Assessment of reliability. *J Bone Joint Surg Am*. 2007;89(5):1057–1065.

16. Stone AT, Bransford RJ, Lee MJ, et al. Reliability of classification systems for subaxial cervical injuries. *Evid Based Spine Care J*. 2010;1(3):19–26.

17. Moore TA, Vaccaro AR, Anderson PA. Classification of lower cervical spine injuries. *Spine (Phila Pa 1976)*. 2006;31(11 Suppl):S37–S43. discussion S61.

CHAPTER 9

Clinical Correlations to Specific Phenotypes and Measurements With Classification Systems

WYLIE Y. LOPEZ • THOMAS D. CHA
Department of Orthopedic Surgery, Massachusetts General Hospital, Harvard Medical School, Boston, MA, United States

INTRODUCTION

Classification systems provide a common language through which physicians and researchers can communicate. They can help create a framework for standardized treatment algorithms through which surgeons can directly and reproducibly contribute to improvements in patient outcomes. In order for these algorithms to be generalized to the population, they must be clinically relevant, reliable, and validated.[1,2] If measurements are involved as part of the tool for outcome prediction, there must be a standardized way to obtain such data in an accurate way: whether that be through specific language to determine landmarks, image acquisition, imaging modalities, etc. This chapter will explore some of the more commonly used classification systems used in the subaxial cervical spine, specifically, within the domains of the traumatic, degenerative, and stenotic spine. It will also examine the literature for assessment of their reliability, validation and, if present, their clinical impact with focus on standard health-related quality of life (HRQOL) measures and surgeon expert opinion parameters thought to be relevant for evaluating and predicting outcomes.

THE TRAUMATIC SUBAXIAL CERVICAL SPINE

Classification systems in the traumatic subaxial cervical spine encompass a broad spectrum of pathology. They can assist the provider in making a quick assessment of initial stability for emergency triage and ultimately, in working out a finalized treatment plan. This becomes critical for the patient when assessing initial neurologic injury, recovery potential, and surgical timing. Sadiqi et al.[3] launched an international web-based survey to ascertain what parameters were thought to influence outcomes in patients with subaxial cervical spine trauma. They polled 279 AO Spine International and International Spinal Cord Society members and concluded that neurological status, implant failure within 3 months, and patient's satisfaction were the most relevant parameters in the short and long term: bony fusion was the most relevant in the long term, and surgical site infection, spinal canal encroachment on advanced imaging, facet or lateral mass fracture on radiographs, and age were the most relevant in the short term. These parameters, along with HRQOL scores, will be the basis for examining clinical correlates for three of the most widely used classification systems for subaxial cervical spine trauma, the Allen and Ferguson Classification, the Subaxial Injury Classification and Severity Scale (SLICS), and the AO Spine Subaxial Cervical Spine Injury Classification System.

Allen and Ferguson Classification of Subaxial Cervical Spine Injury
Overview
The Allen and Ferguson Classification, proposed in 1982, is regarded as one of the first broadly used classification systems for subaxial cervical spine trauma. It is based on the biomechanical concepts that allow the mechanism of injury to be deduced from radiographic patterns via "injury vectors." The following injury mechanisms make up the schema and are derived from the major injury vector involved: vertical compression, compressive flexion, compressive extension, lateral flexion, distractive flexion, and distractive extension. These injury vectors have a magnitude and produce a spectrum of injury, which the authors have termed, a phylogeny. Each phylogeny is made up of stages that

denote a specific type and degree of injury to a cervical motion segment, and it was noted by the authors that these stages correlated well with neurologic status.[4] An important point to this system is that it assumes an indirect injury mechanism; the assumption is that a direct injury mechanism (i.e., blow to the neck, and penetrating projectile) is biomechanically different and often causes a much less predictable pattern of injury that cannot readily be deduced.[4] The classification system is simplified in the following:

- **Vertical compression (VC):** compressive loading of the entire vertebral centrum—as the severity of the vertebral body fracture increases, the incidence of vertebral arch fractures increases (16%, 25%, and 40% in stages 1, 2, and 3, respectively)
  - VC Stage 1: fracture of a superior or inferior endplate with a cupping deformity
  - VC Stage 2: fracture of both endplates with cupping. Sometimes associated with a nondisplaced or minimally displaced fracture through the centrum
  - VC Stage 3: fracture of both endplates with a fragmented centrum
    - Fragments are displaced peripherally and sometimes, into the neural canal
- **Compressive flexion (CF):** anterior compression and burst fracture variants—the occurrence of multiple contiguous CF lesions suggests a greater magnitude of force imparted to the anterior elements
  - CF Stage 1: blunting of the anterior-superior vertebral margin to a rounded contour
  - CF Stage 2: CF 1 changes and obliquity of the anterior vertebral body with loss of height at the centrum. May see a fracture through the centrum
    - Resulting appearance is a "beaking" of the anterior-inferior vertebral body
  - CF Stage 3: CF 2 changes and a fracture line passing obliquely from the anterior surface of the vertebral body through the centrum and extending through the inferior subchondral plate
    - The "beak" in CF 2 is fractured
  - CF Stage 4: CF 3 changes and less than 3 mm of displacement of the inferior-posterior vertebral margin into the neural canal
  - CF Stage 5: CF 3 and gross displacement of the posterior portion of the vertebral body into the canal with signs of ligamentous failure
    - Separation of the articular facets and increased distance between the spinous processes at the injury level indicating failure of at least the posterior portion of the anterior ligamentous complex and entirety of the posterior ligamentous complex

- **Compressive extension (CE):** posterior compression/vertebral arch injuries—the severity of anatomic damage does not correlate well with the severity of the spinal cord lesion
  - CE Stage 1: unilateral vertebral arch fracture with or without anterorotary vertebral body displacement
    - Linear fracture through the articular process, compression of the articular process, pedicle or lamina fracture, or a combination of the two
    - Rotary listhesis of the centrum may occur
  - CE Stage 2: Bilaminar fractures
    - Typically, at contiguous multiple levels
  - CE Stage 3: Bilateral vertebral arch fractures without displacement of the vertebral body
  - CE Stage 4: CE Stage 3 with partial vertebral body displacement anteriorly
    - CE Stage 3 and 4 are theoretical and were actually not encountered in this study
  - CE Stage 5: CE stage 3 with full vertebral body width displacement anteriorly
    - Ligamentous failure occurs posteriorly between the above and fractured vertebra and anteriorly between the fractured and lower vertebra
    - The anterior-superior portion of the centrum is characteristically sheared off by the anteriorly displaced centrum
- **Lateral flexion (LF):** asymmetric lateral compression injury of the centrum and ipsilateral vertebral arch with distraction of the contralateral vertebral arch—sometimes associated with occult "kissing compressive lesions" of the uncovertebral joint
  - LF Stage 1: compression fracture on the centrum plus vertebral arch fracture on the ipsilateral side without displacement of the arch on the AP view
  - LF Stage 2: LF Stage 1 with displacement of the arch on the AP view or ligamentous failure on the contralateral side with separation of the articular processes
    - Both can occur simultaneously
- **Distractive flexion (DF):** spectrum of facet-displacing injury patterns—the degree of ligamentous failure is sequentially greater in each subsequent stage and this correlates well with neurologic status
  - DF Stage 1: failure of the PLC as evidenced by subluxation of the facet in flexion with abnormally great divergence of the spinous processes at the injury level
    - Can see blunting of the anterior-superior margin of the vertebra similar to CF 1

- DF Stage 2: unilateral facet dislocation
  - The range of ligamentous injury is variable and may require dynamic studies for full assessment
  - Facet subluxation on the opposite side of the dislocation would suggest severe ligamentous injury
- DF Stage 3: Bilateral facet dislocation with approximately 50% anterior displacement of the vertebral body
- DF Stage 4: DF Stage 3 with full vertebral body width displacement anteriorly or grossly unstable motion segment
- **Distractive extension (DE):** anterior ligamentous failure with posterior vertebral displacement—frequently resulting from a fall and occurred more commonly in older age groups as compared to the other fractures and dislocations
  - DE Stage 1: failure of the anterior ligamentous complex or a transverse nondeforming fracture of the centrum
    - Abnormal widening of the disc space is a radiographic hint
  - DE Stage 2: DE Stage 1 with failure of the posterior ligamentous complex with displacement of the upper vertebral body posteriorly into the canal
    - This type of displacement tends to reduce when the head is in neutral so radiographic hints may be subtle (often less than 3 mm).

Reliability and validation

Reliability of the classification system was not discussed in the initial manuscript by Allen and Ferguson but was explored separately in the literature. In the landmark manuscript by Vaccaro et al.,[5] reliability was assessed, along with the SLICS and Harris Scores, via surveys after 2 rounds of case presentations given to 20 members of the Spine Trauma Study Group (STSG). Because the Allen and Ferguson Classification system is nonordinal, it could not be assessed with intraclass correlation coefficient (ICC)—instead, it was assessed with Cohen's kappa coefficient (compares qualitative items). As compared to the SLICS and Harris classification systems, the interrater and intrarater reliability scores were highest in the Allen and Ferguson system (Intrarater reliability: AF [0.63], SLICS [0.60], and Harris [0.53]; Interrater reliability: AF [0.53], SLICS [0.51], and Harris [0.41]). Validation efforts were also made in the SLICS manuscript whereby the SLIC score and its recommendation to the participant's management recommendation were compared; raters agreed

with the SLIC score algorithm in 91.8% of cases. They also compared the SLIC morphology domain and the Ferguson and Allen description of morphology with 71.5% agreement between the two systems.

Stone et al.[6] assessed the reliability of the Cervical Spine Injury Severity Score (CSISS), SLICS, and Allen and Ferguson Classifications and found mixed results compared to some of the previous literature. Their team found that ICC values for CSISS and SLICS suggested excellent interobserver reliability. The kappa coefficient for Allen-Ferguson, however, suggested moderate to poor reliability, particularly when assessing the 6 main groups and all 21 groups, respectively. Urrutia et al.[7] showed similarly poor interobserver reliability but substantial intraobserver reliability.

Clinical correlates

There are no studies in the literature prospectively implementing the Allen and Ferguson Classification to assess patient outcomes. Instead, these concepts served as a steppingstone for the generation of subsequent subaxial cervical spine classification systems. Harris et al.[8] would expand on these ideas to produce their own classification system in 1986 that was followed by the Magerl[9] classification in 1994. These classification systems, while providing significant contributions to the language associated with classifying spine fractures, were unable to be reliably used or clinically validated in the literature.[5,7,10,11]

Subaxial Injury Classification and Severity Scale
Overview
The Subaxial Injury Classification Scale (SLICS, Fig. 1) is one of the most readily used classification systems in the traumatic subaxial cervical spine. Its development consisted of expert opinions of a subgroup within the Spine Trauma Study Group (STSG) and the amalgamation of a thorough literature review for cervical trauma with previously obtained surveys used to establish what was believed to be the most important characteristics for defining these injuries.[5,10] These surveys, previously used for thoracolumbar injuries, were thus adapted based on the literature search and developed into the current subaxial classification system. It was developed for the purpose of categorizing injuries in a standardized way and, at the time of its development, was the only classification attempting to predict treatment.[5]

This system uses three previously generated critical characteristics for clinical decision making that were also found to be appropriate for the subaxial cervical

SLIC system component	Points
morphology	
No abnormality	0
Compression	1
Burst	+ 1 = 2
Distraction (hyperflexion/extension without out dislocation [perched facet])	3
Translation/rotation (includes dislocations)	4
DLC injury	
Intact	0
Equivocal (e.g., MRI signal change only)	1
Injured	2
Neurological status	
Intact	0
Root injury	1
Complete cord injury	2
Incomplete cord injury	3
Continuous cord compression in setting of neuro deficit (neuro modifier)	+ 1

FIG. 1 SLIC scale.

spine—injury morphology (based on column disruption), integrity of the disco-ligamentous complex (DLC), and patient's neurologic status.[5,10] These characteristics can all be determined by traditional radiographic studies such as X-ray, CT, and MRI imaging. Each component within the three domains is given a numerical value (with 0 being normal) in an ascending manner based on presumed severity of outcome and/or necessity for requiring surgery. The point totals in the three domains are added such that higher point totals assume a more severe injury. A score of less than 4 would recommend for nonoperative treatment while a score greater than 4 would recommend for surgical intervention. The classification system is simplified in the following:

- **Injury morphology**
  - Compression (1 point): includes compression, burst, flexion/compression (teardrop), and non-displaced/minimally displaced lateral mass and facet fractures. The latter two only included if there is no visible translation between vertebral levels noted
    - Burst patterns (2 points) are considered higher energy and therefore scored higher than traditional compression fractures

- Distraction (3 points): includes anatomic dissociations in the vertical axis; hyperextension/hyperflexion injuries
  - Signifies a more severe injury pattern due to the force required to overcome the protective forces (i.e., facet capsule in flexion, anterior longitudinal ligament in extension)
  - Commonly involves ligamentous disruption traversing the disc space and facet joints, and therefore, MRI is useful for assessment
- Translation/rotation (4 points): includes anatomic dissociations in the horizontal axis; unilateral/bilateral facet fracture-dislocations, fracture separation of the lateral mass, and bilateral pedicle fractures
  - A relative angulation of $\geq$ 11 degrees implies displacement exceeding physiologic ranges
- **DLC integrity**
  - Components include the intervertebral disc, anterior/posterior longitudinal ligaments, ligamentum flavum, interspinous/supraspinous ligaments, and facet capsules
  - Indeterminant (1 point)
    - T2 MRI imaging showing only hyperintense signal

- Isolated interspinous ligament widening
- Indications of instability (2 points)
  - Abnormal facet alignment (articular apposition < 50% or diastasis > 2 mm through facet joint)
  - Abnormal widening of the disc space on either neutral or extension radiographs
  - Horizontal signal intensity on T2 sagittal MRI through a disc involving the nucleus and annulus
  - Subluxation of the vertebral bodies (i.e., translational/rotational abnormalities)
- **Neurologic status**
  - Root (1 point) injury: implies lower energy mechanism and less likelihood for catastrophic neurologic disability
  - Incomplete (3 points) vs complete (2 points): thought to warrant surgical intervention in the setting of ongoing compressive phenomenon in order to provide the patient's highest likelihood of improvement and therefore receives the highest score

Reliability and validation

Reliability was assessed via surveys after 2 rounds of case presentations given to 20 members of the STSG. Interrater and intrarater agreement were assessed by ICC scores of the morphology, DLC, and neurologic status, and compared with the same cases using the Allen and Ferguson and the Harris classifications. The interrater and intrarater reliability were variables among the three domains of the classification system; however, the overall reliability of the SLIC score was substantial with an interrater ICC of 0.71 and an intrarater ICC of 0.83.[4] The interrater and intrarater reliability ICC for the SLIC management recommendations were moderate and substantial, respectively (ICC of 0.58 and 0.77). As compared to the other two aforementioned systems, the SLIC interrater and intrarater reliability scores were higher than the Harris system, but lower than the Ferguson and Allen system.

Validation of the system was determined by testing the assumption that SLICS would be able to morphologically characterize injuries and predict treatments and that the expert panel would gain consensus on treatment. This was done via internal testing by comparing the SLIC score and its recommendation to the participant's management recommendation for the aforementioned cases. Raters agreed with the SLIC score management in 91.8% of cases. A comparison was also made between the SLIC morphology domain and the Ferguson and Allen description of morphology

with 71.5% agreement between the two systems. The authors describe the reliability of this system as moderate and the validity as sufficient.

Separate external validation studies in the literature confer mostly positive results; however, there have been disagreements on the morphology domain of the system. Urrutia et al.[7] published a study independently evaluating the reliability of the SLIC scale. They observed that the interobserver agreement was substantial when considering the main types and moderate when considering subtypes and the intraobserver agreement was substantial for both main and subtypes. Stone et al.[6] and Lee et al.,[12] in separate studies, observed excellent and significant reliability, respectively. More recently, in a study published by van Middendorp et al.,[13] poor agreement on morphologic injury characteristics and no improvement in agreement among surgeons with the SLICS treatment algorithm were seen.

Clinical correlates

There is a paucity of literature attempting to ascertain outcomes based on the prospective application of the SLICS system. The first and only to do so was Joaquim et al.[14]—in their study, they assessed neurologic status as the primary outcome of successful treatment; 48 patients were included. In the 23 patients treated nonoperatively (SLIC < 4), there was no neurological deterioration. There were 25 treated surgically (SLIC > 4); of those with incomplete deficits, 72% showed improvement in their American Spinal Injury Association (ASIA) score and no patient showed neurological worsening. As previously mentioned, neurologic status is one of the more relevant parameters in regard to short- and long-term outcome estimations.[3] With these data in mind, the authors concluded that SLICS was both safe and efficacious in guiding surgical treatment for the parameter of neurologic status.

The information generated from the SLICS study was the spark for a plethora of new manuscripts with important clinical correlates. In one such study, Dvorak et al.,[15] using the SLICS scale as their basis, undertook a systematic review of the literature to create an evidence-based algorithm for subaxial cervical spine injury surgical approach; their approach algorithm was based on the three morphological domains of the SLICS study. The systematic review verified that for the burst morphology, an anterior approach w/ vertebral body resection and stabilization provides mechanical reconstitution of the motion segment, optimal decompression of the neural elements, and ample bone graft to reinforce the fusion.[16,17] For distraction injuries, the surgical approach tends to be denoted by the pattern of DLC disruption—hyperextension injuries tend to be anterior and thus will require an anterior approach, hyperflexion injuries tend to be posterior, along with cases of severe spondylosis, DISH, or ankylosing spondylitis (these entities create long lever arms) and are thus best approached posteriorly.[15-17] The exception to this rule is for facet subluxation, where the approach is determined based on disc herniation—posteriorly displaced disc herniation is preferentially treated anteriorly, if there is no disc herniation, the case can be approached via surgeon preference.[15,18-20] Translational/rotational injuries are further subcategorized based on the presence of vertebral body fracture along with the presence and severity of neural compression. Facet-fracture dislocations associated with endplate fractures necessitate posterior fusion; if there is a concern for progressive kyphosis, significant discoligamentous injury on MRI, or severe comminuted fracture, then a combined approach is warranted. If there is no vertebral body fracture, the approach is determined by the presence of disc herniation, similarly to cases of facet subluxation (after attempted reduction).

AO Spine Subaxial Cervical Spine Injury Classification System
Overview
The AO Spine Subaxial Cervical Spine Injury Classification System (Fig. 2) is a morphology-based system that was constructed in response to the lack of wide acceptance for any one subaxial cervical spine classification system. While SLICS, both internally and externally, showed good reliability and validity, other studies in the literature showed disagreement in the domain of morphology—this was the basis for the creation of the AO system.[5,13,21] Its development stemmed from multiple assessments and revisions of concepts from the aforementioned thoracolumbar system and SLICS in conjunction with a database of AO spinal trauma cases and was considered complete once unanimous consensus was achieved in all domains.[5,10,21]

The components of the system include injury morphology and neurologic status—carried over from the thoracolumbar system and SLICS—with the inclusion of two new domains, facet integrity and case-specific modifiers. The inclusion of facet integrity arises from previous literature attesting to its role in stability and, when injured, the implied high-energy mechanism and the worse patient outcomes that are associated.[22-24] Injuries are described by their level, then morphologic type (the primary injury) with secondary injuries and modifiers placed in parentheses. The classification system is simplified in the following:

- **Injury morphology**
  - Type A: fractures that result in compression of the vertebra with intact tension band
    - A0: no bony or minor injury such as an isolated lamina or spinous process fracture
      - Includes patients with central cord syndrome and no fracture
    - A1: compression fractures involving a single endplate without the involvement of the posterior wall of the vertebral body
    - A2: coronal split or pincer fractures involving both endplates without the involvement of the posterior aspect of the vertebral wall
    - A3: burst fractures involving a single endplate
    - A4: burst fracture or sagittal split involving both endplates
  - Type B: failure of the posterior or anterior tension band through distraction with physical separation of the subaxial spinal elements while maintaining continuity of the alignment of the spinal axis without translation or dislocation
    - B1: posterior tension band injury of bony structures only with extension into the vertebral body
      - ⇒ Anterior structures such as disc or annulus may also be involved
    - B2: posterior tension band injury of the posterior capsuloligamentous or bony capsuloligamentous structures
      - ⇒ Anterior structures such as vertebral body or disc may also be involved and should be specified separately
    - B3: anterior tension band injury with tethering of the posterior elements
  - Type C: injuries with displacement or translation of one vertebral body relative to another in any direction; anterior, posterior, lateral translation, or vertical distraction
    - Because type C involves vertebra relative to one another, any associated injury should be specified as a subtype with a designation of Type A or B after the initial type C designation
- **Facet injury**
  - If there are multiple injuries to the same facet, the highest level injury gets classified
  - If both facets at the same level are injured, the right side is designated first
  - F1: nondisplaced facet fracture
    - < 1 cm fragment, < 40% of the lateral mass
  - F2: facet fracture with instability potential
    - > 1 cm fragment, > 40% of the lateral mass, or displacement

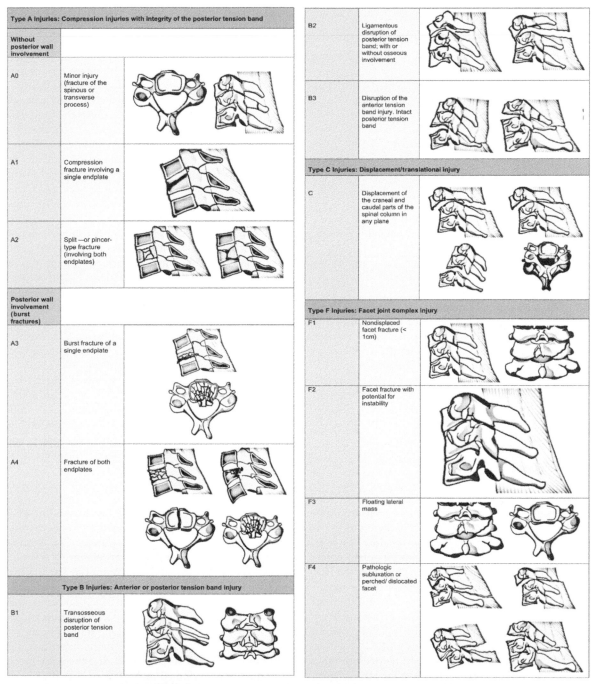

FIG. 2 AO Spine Subaxial Cervical Spine Injury Classification System.(From Urrutia J, Zamora T, Campos M, et al. A comparative agreement evaluation of two subaxial cervical spine injury classification systems: the AO Spine and the Allen and Ferguson schemes. Eur Spine J. 2016:25;2186–2187.)

- F3: floating lateral mass—pedicle and lamina disruption resulting in disconnection of the superior and inferior articular facets at a level
- F4: pathologic subluxation or perched/dislocated facet
- BL: The bilateral (BL) modifier is used if both facets have the same injury at the same level
- **Neurologic status**
  - N0: neurologically intact
  - N1: transient neurological deficit
  - N2: radiculopathy
  - N3: incomplete spinal cord injury
    - "+" is designated for ongoing cord compression
  - N4: complete spinal cord injury
  - NX: undetermined due to unexaminable patient
- **Case-specific modifiers**
  - M1: posterior capsuloligamentous complex injury without complete disruption
    - often identified on MRI
  - M2: critical disc herniation—evidence of nucleus pulposus protruding posteriorly to a vertical line drawn along the posterior border of the inferior vertebral body at the injured level
  - M3: Stiffening/metabolic bone disease
    - Diffuse skeletal hyperostosis (DISH), ossification of the posterior longitudinal ligament (OPLL), ankylosing spondylitis (AS), ossification of the ligamentum flavum (OLF)
  - M4: signs of vertebral artery injury

Reliability and validation

The authors assessed the interrater and intrarater reliability and validity of their system via an internal assessment of their data. They had 10 reviewers—beforehand, all received a paper with background information and purpose of the system—grade 10 cases to prove their competency against a gold standard determined by two of the senior authors. Once they felt that the authors had a correct understanding of the system (no incorrect grades given), they sent out 30 additional cases to be a review on two separate occasions. They found substantial overall interrater reliability when comparing levels of fracture severity (A/B/C/F) with k values of 0.64 and 0.65, respectively, between the two sessions. For intraobserver reliability, for all subtypes, they obtained a k value of 0.75, indicating substantial reliability. As for validation, for the first round of assessments, they found the range of correctness compared to the predetermined gold standard to be 20–29 cases. In the second round, the range was between 16 and 29 cases noting a decrease from the first round.

Several external studies agreed that this system has high reliability, validity, and repeatability.[7,25,26]

Clinical correlates

The young age of this classification system has resulted in a few available studies assessing its applicability in regard to HRQOL measures. One such study assessed the injury morphology and how it affects the long-term neurologic outcome. Mushlin et al.[27] determined the AO Spine Subaxial Cervical Spine Injury Classification System's morphology in a sample of 82 patients reviewed retrospectively and recorded the admission and 6-month follow-up ASIA Impairment Scale (AIS) and ASIA motor score (AMS). The A0 subtype was the most common and was found to have no complete injuries on admission or follow-up. They also showed significant improvement in AMS on follow-up from 70 to 90. Groups A3, A4, and C had the worst neurologic injuries and the highest percentage of patients with complete injuries; A3/A4 had the highest percentage at 55.6%, was the only subtype to have patients with complete injuries on follow-up, and also had the lowest AMS scores on follow-up. The authors hypothesized that this difference between A3/4 and C subtypes on follow-up was possibly due to the amenability of type C fractures to be decompressed by reduction maneuvers, which theoretically reduces time to decompression and ultimately improves long-term outcomes. This study successfully associates specific subtypes with ASIA designation and AMS score and can potentially influence timing to surgery and the risk/benefits discussion with patients in regard to long-term prognosis.

Du et al.[28] prospectively assessed the effects of early vs delayed decompression on AIS and the Spinal Cord Independence Measure III (SCIM version 3) at 12-month follow-up. They included 402 patients who were divided into early decompression (< 72 hours after injury) and delayed decompression (≥ 72 hours after injury) groups. After intervention, each group was subsequently broken down into five morphology subtypes (A0, A1–4, B, C/F4, or F1–3) and outcomes were measured. 100 patients in the early group and 76 patients in the late group showed AIS improvement ≥ 1 grade, with only B and C/F4 types being statistically significant. SCIM version 3 showed that the early group also showed better functional recovery, with B subtypes being statistically significant. The authors concluded that early decompression led to better neurologic and functional recovery for the B and C/F4 subtypes and that type A and F1–3 subtypes failed to show significant clinical advantages to undergoing aggressive early decompression.

THE DEGENERATIVE SUBAXIAL CERVICAL SPINE

The development of a classification system for spinal deformity, as seen in the Scoliosis Research Society-Schwab Classification, has proven clinically valuable by demonstrating correlation with standardized HRQOL measures.[29–31] The literature points to a correlation between the simultaneous occurrence of deformities of the thoracolumbar and cervical spine and to correlations between cervical spine sagittal imbalance and HRQOL measures, Neck Disability Index (NDI), and myelopathy (modified Japanese Orthopedic Association [mJOA] score).[31,32] As the spinal deformity literature matures, it is becoming increasingly clear that cervical deformity should be addressed in the context of global spinal alignment, as compensatory efforts are often made by the body to maintain horizontal gaze.[33,34] These correlations created the basis for the development of a cervical spine deformity classification. As of the publication of this chapter, the Ames Classification stands alone as the most comprehensive and widely studied classification system for subaxial cervical spine deformity.

The Ames Classification

Overview

The overall goal of the Ames Classification (Fig. 3) is to assess cervical spine deformity (CSD) in the context of global spinopelvic alignment and to address clinically relevant parameters.[29] This system is an adaptation of the SRS-Schwab classification for adult thoracolumbar deformity and uses a deformity descriptor and five modifiers that include sagittal, regional, and global spinopelvic alignment and neurologic status. According to the authors, in order to utilize the classification system in practice, the following requirements must be obtained: (1) full-length standing posteroanterior (PA) and lateral spine radiographs that include the cervical spine and femoral heads; (2) standing PA and lateral cervical spine radiographs; (3) completed and scored mJOA questionnaire; (4) a clinical photograph or radiograph that includes the skull for measurement of the chin-brow vertical angle (CBVA).

The deformity descriptors attempt to categorize the cervical spine alignment into basic groupings. The first three groupings are sagittal deformities that are distinguished based on the location of the apex of deformity—group C being in the cervical spine, CT in the cervicothoracic junction, and T being in the thoracic spine. The fourth grouping are coronal plane deformities in which the C2–C7 Cobb angle is greater than 15 degrees and the fifth are deformities of the craniovertebral junction.

The five modifiers, outlined in the following, were chosen based on extensive literature review and expert

Deformity descriptor	5 Modifiers
C: Primary sagittal deformity with apex in cervical spine	**C2-C7 Sagittal vertical axis (SVA)** **0:** C2–C7 SVA <4 cm **1:** C2–C7 SVA between 4 and 8 cm **2:** C2–C7 SVA >8 cm
CT: Primary sagittal deformity with apex at cervico -thoracic junction	**Horizontal gaze** **0:** CBVA between 1°–10° **1:** CBVA between −10°– 0° or 11°–25° **2:** CBVA <−10° or > 25°
T: Primary sagittal deformity with apex in thoracic spine	**Cervical lordosis minus T1 slope** **0:** TS-CL < 15° **1:** TS-CL between 15°–20° **2:** TS-CL > 20°
S: Primary coronal deformity (C2–C7 Cobb angle ≥ 15°)	**Myelopathy** **0:** mJOA = 18 (none) **1:** mJOA between 15–17 (mild) **2:** mJOA between 12–14 (moderate) **3:** mJOA < 12 (severe)
CVJ: Primary cranio -vertebral junction deformity	**SRS-Schwab Classification** **T, L, D, or N:** curve type **0, +, or ++:** PI-LL **0, +, or ++:** Pelvic Tilt **0, +, or ++:** C7-S1 SVA

FIG. 3 Ames classification.

opinion in regard to the most likely contributors to HRQOL measures. Higher number scores are associated with the worse deformity. The first three modifiers can all be measured on sagittal radiographs.

- **C2–C7 sagittal vertical axis (cSVA)** defines the sagittal balance of the cervical spine
  - corresponds to the distance from a plumb line drawn down the centrum of C2 to the posterosuperior corner of C7 (Fig. 4)
  - Normal C2–C7 SVA reported to be 16.8 ± 11.2 mm[35]
  - Correlated with multiple measures of HRQOL, negatively correlated with SF-36 physical component scores, positively correlated with NDI, significantly correlated with mJOA score[31–33]
  - Ames score:
    - 0: C2–C7 SVA < 4 cm
    - 1: C2–C7 SVA between 4 and 8 cm
    - 2: C2–C7 SVA > 8 cm
- **Horizontal gaze** is an estimate of the patient's direct line of vision with the head and neck at rest and the knees and hips extended
  - It is calculated via the CBVA (Fig. 5)
  - As discussed in Chapter 6, CBVA is defined as the angle between a line drawn from the patient's chin to brow and a vertical line
  - Can be measured on radiographs that include the skull or from a clinical photograph with the head/neck in neutral and hips/knees extended
  - No optimal target exists in the literature but CBVA between − 5 and 17 degrees considered

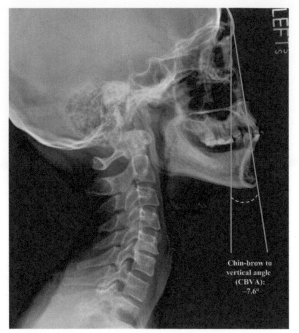

FIG. 5 Chin-brow to vertical angle.

optimal and associated with favorable outcomes when correcting spinal deformity including improved gaze and ambulation[31,36–38]

- Ames score:
  - 0: CBVA between 1 and 10 degrees
  - 1: CBVA between − 10 and 0 degrees or between 11 and 25 degrees
  - 2: CBVA <−10 degrees or > 25 degrees
- **Cervical lordosis minus T1 slope** is an equation analogous to the relationship between pelvic morphology and lumbar lordosis proposed by Schwab et al. (LL = PI ± 10 degrees). A greater magnitude of TS requires a greater magnitude of CL to balance the head over the trunk, similar to how a greater pelvic incidence requires a greater lumbar lordosis.[33,39]
  - CL (Fig. 6) is measured by drawing Cobb angles between C2 and C7
  - T1 slope (T1S, Fig. 7) is the angle created by drawing a horizontal axis through the posterosuperior corner of the T1 vertebral body and a line tangent to the superior endplate of T1
  - These measurements included as modifiers due to the literature suggesting that cervical kyphosis, an indicator of CL, is the most common CSD and associated with increased neck pain and less postoperative neurological improvement in patients with myelopathy[40–43]

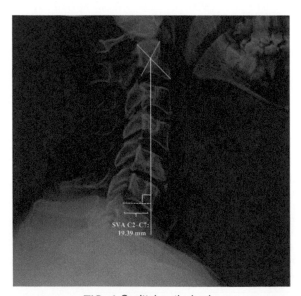

FIG. 4 Sagittal vertical axis.

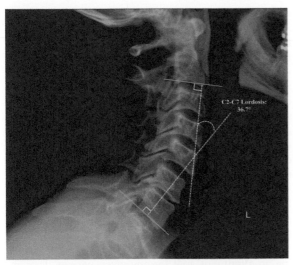

FIG. 6 C2–C7 cervical lordosis.

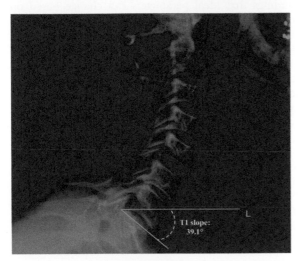

FIG. 7 T1 slope.

- Optimal target about 25 ± 5 degrees[44]
- Ames score:
  - 0: TS-CL < 15 degrees
  - 1: TS-CL between 15 and 20 degrees
  - 2: TS-CL > 20 degrees
- **Myelopathy** is a condition associated with progressive cervical kyphosis via the draping effect of the cord on structures anterior to it
  - Myelopathy is directly related to CSD and can often profoundly impact patient's function[33,45,46]
  - Scoring is based on the widely recognized and accepted mJOA score that provides a quantitative assessment of the severity of myelopathy[45]

- Ames score:
  - 0: mJOA = 18 (none)
  - 1: mJOA between 15 and 17 (mild)
  - 2: mJOA between 12 and 14 (moderate)
  - 3: mJOA < 12 (severe)
- **SRS-Schwab Classification** is a classification system used to provide a common language for adult thoracolumbar spinal deformity. It includes five thoracolumbar coronal curve types and three sagittal modifiers. These parameters were chosen by Schwab and colleagues because they have been shown to be highly correlated with pain and disability when abnormal.[47] As mentioned previously, it has proven clinically valuable by demonstrating correlation with standardized HRQOL measures. A more extensive description of this classification will be provided in a later chapter.

Reliability and validation

Reliability was assessed internally via a separate study, whereby 10 clinical cases were graded by 20 CSD experts. The cases were chosen as representative examples of the classification system's descriptors and modifiers. Sufficient patient history and appropriate imaging were provided, and image quality was controlled for. The experts graded the cases, then after a minimum of 1 week, the case order was randomized and resent for grading. Interrater and intrarater reliability were calculated based on the Fleiss K coefficient values. K values classified as: 0.00–0.20 (slight agreement), 0.21–0.40 (fair agreement), 0.41–0.60 (moderate agreement), 0.61–0.80 (substantial agreement), and 0.81–1.00 (almost perfect agreement). Interrater reliability for the deformity descriptor in rounds 1 and 2 was 0.489 (moderate agreement) and 0.280 (fair agreement), respectively, while mean intrarater reliability was 0.584 (moderate agreement). For the modifiers, interrater and intrarater reliabilities were C2–7 SVA 0.338/0.412 (fair/moderate) and 0.584 (moderate), horizontal gaze 0.779/0.430 (substantial/moderate) and 0.768 (substantial), TS-CL 0.721/0.567 (substantial/moderate) and 0.720 (substantial), myelopathy 0.602/0.477 (moderate/moderate) and 0.746 (substantial), SRS-Schwab classification curve type 0.590/0.433 (moderate/moderate) and 0.564 (moderate), PI-LL 0.554/0.386 (moderate/fair) and 0.826 (almost perfect), PT 0.714/0.627 (substantial/substantial) and 0.633 (substantial), and C7–S1 SVA 0.071/0.064 (slight/slight) and 0.233 (fair), respectively. Most of the K coefficients for interrater and intrarater reliability would be classified as moderate to substantial agreement. Validation of this system is a work in progress, as will be shown by the external studies cited in Clinical Correlates section.

Clinical correlates

In 2017, Passias et al.[48] published a retrospective review of a prospective cervical deformity database that attempted to characterize the deformity type and malalignment of their cohort with the Ames-ACD and the Schwab-ASD Classifications. Within this study, they also explored the relation between HRQOL measures and Ames-ACD descriptors before and after corrective surgery. They found that the Ames Classification was effective in describing the cervical deformity type in their cohort of 84 patients. Patients who showed improvements by either 1 or 2 modifier grades in cSVA, horizontal gaze, and TS-CL modifiers at 3 months postoperatively had reduced scores in NRS Neck (all 3 modifiers) and EQ5D scores (cSVA and horizontal gaze modifiers). In this cohort, 33.9% of the patients improved in cSVA, 27.4% in TS-CL, and 43.4% in horizontal gaze. While these results are encouraging, long-term follow-up would be important to determine whether they have a lasting effect. There was also no discussion on the minimal clinically important difference (MCID) needed to impart clinical relevance.

Passias et al.[49] revisited the topic in 2018 with a strikingly different conclusion. This time, in another retrospective study of 63 patients who underwent deformity correction, they explored the idea that the standard HRQOL measures are not cervical deformity-specific and therefore cannot capture the entire spectrum of a patient's deformity and outcomes. Their results showed that, at 1 year, 46% of the patients improved in mJOA, 71.4% in NDI scores, and 65.1% in EQ5D of which MCID was met in 19% of mJOA, 44.4% in NDI, and 19% in EQ5D. Despite the data suggesting clinical improvement in this cohort, they found no correlation between improvement in Ames radiographic modifier grades and HRQOL improvement. They did find, however, that improvement in Schwab SVA correlated with 1-year mJOA MCID and that Schwab PT and PI-LL improvements correlated with 1-year EQ5D MCID. Passias concluded that either radiographic parameters are being weighed too heavily or HRQOL measures were not specific enough to the CD population.

There is evidence in the literature that the Patient-Reported Outcomes Measurement Information System (PROMIS) metrics have outperformed the standard HRQOL measures.[50,51] With this idea in mind, Pierce and Passias attempted to evaluate the association of the Ames cervical alignment components with PROMIS metrics, specifically, Pain Intensity (PI), Physical Function (PF), and Pain Interference. Their retrospective cohort study assessed the cSVA and TS-CL modifiers in 208 patients. Their results indicated that there was no strong correlation between PROMIS scores and Ames deformity severity groups for cSVA and TS-CL; however, both trended toward lower PF and higher Pain Interference scores with increasing deformity severity.[52] Where they did see significance was in their ability to use conditional tree analysis to develop cutoff PROMIS metrics in relation to cSVA and TS-CL severity categories. Most parameters were significant or approached significance and showed that the cSVA modifier demonstrated more drastic cutoffs for moderate deformity that more closely mimicked the TS-CL modifier for severe deformity—PI: > 96, PF: < 14, Pain Intensity: > 57.4 versus PI: > 87, PF: ≤ 14, and Pain Intensity: > 56.5. These data suggest that, while not statistically significant, there is a relation between PROMIS scores and Ames Classification severity.

Paramount to the correction of CSD is determining an alignment goal for any given patient. This endeavor has been fraught with difficulty due to the findings that ideal parameters can change based on the mobility of the cervical spine and a patient's natural cervical curvature, which in some cases, can be kyphotic. Staub et al.[53] determined the T1S-CL in an asymptomatic population based on normal gaze and a mobile cervical spine and used that information to develop a formula to predict ideal cervical lordosis for a given patient: $CL = T1S - 16.5 \pm 2$ degrees. CL has been shown to directly correlate with HRQOL measures; Cho et al.[35] outlined the findings of multiple authors with respect to surgical correction of lordosis and their effect on HRQOL measures and found improvements in NDI, visual analog scale (VAS), mJOA, and Nurick Scale scores.[53-61] These findings underscore the potential strength of this formula as a predictor of improved HRQOL scores.

THE STENOTIC SUBAXIAL CERVICAL SPINE

The stenotic subaxial cervical spine can present with a constellation of symptoms including radiculopathy, myelopathy, or spinal cord injury (i.e., central cord syndrome) from even a minor traumatic event. Cervical stenosis can be congenital or acquired (degenerative, traumatic). Lee et al.[62] used calipers to measure the cervical canal diameter of 469 cadaveric specimens and extrapolated that, with the threshold for stenosis being a canal diameter < 12 mm, cervical stenosis was present in 4.9% of the adult population; 6.8% of the population greater than 50 years of age or older, and 9% of the population 70 years of age or older. Given the prevalence of this disease state and the potential for neurologic compromise associated with it, methods for accurate measurement and classification for the subaxial cervical spine are essential.

The Torg-Pavlov Ratio
Overview
Helene Pavlov and Joseph Torg were aware that the traditional method for measuring the canal diameter of the cervical spine could be influenced by technical factors involved with acquiring the image; this idea leads to the development of their ratio. They determined that their method, The Torg-Pavlov Ratio (also known as the ratio method) is independent of magnification factors caused by differences in target distance, object-to-film distance, or body type, because the spinal canal and vertebral body are in the same anatomic plane and are similarly affected by magnification.[63] The traditional method requires a sagittal spine X-ray and measures the cephalocaudal midpoint of the vertebral body to the nearest point of the corresponding spinal laminar line; < 13 mm is considered stenotic.

- **The Torg-Pavlov ratio** (Fig. 8) = a/b
  - $a/b < 0.80$ considered stenotic
  - a: the sagittal diameter of the spinal canal
    - measurement from the posterior surface of the vertebral body to the nearest point of the corresponding spinal laminar line
  - b: the sagittal diameter of the vertebral body
    - measurement from the midpoint of the anterior surface of the vertebral body to the midpoint of the posterior surface of the vertebral body.

Reliability and validation
This study used a control group of healthy patients (ages 15–38) who had cervical spine X-rays taken during an emergency room visit and compared them to a symptomatic group of athletes who developed transient cervical spinal neuropraxia (all male, ages 15–32, mostly football players). They found that when measuring with the conventional and the ratio method, there was statistically significant cervical stenosis in the entire symptomatic patient group vs the male control group. Sensitivity and specificity of the Torg-Pavlov ratio were assessed internally using receiver operating characteristic (ROC) curve analysis to compare the conventional method to the ratio method. When using an operating point of sagittal canal diameter less than 14 mm to indicate stenosis (i.e., the conventional method), there was a hit rate of 0.35 and a false-alarm rate of 0.01—this translates to 65% of stenotic canals being called normal. When using an operating point of spinal canal/vertebral body ratio of less than 0.82 to indicate stenosis, there was a hit rate of 0.92 and a false-alarm rate of 0.06—8% of stenotic canals being called normal and 6% of normal canals being called stenotic. The cumulative data showed that a ratio value of less than 0.80 represented a stenotic canal 96.3% of the time.

Several studies have assessed the reliability of the ratio method externally. Aebli et al.[64] noted excellent interobserver and intraobserver reliability when using the ratio method. Suk et al.[65] compared the ratio method to ratios obtained on CT and MRI and found

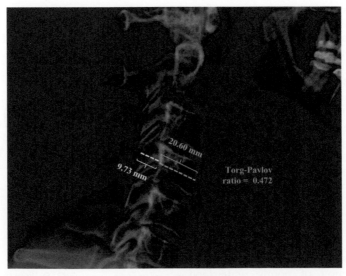

FIG. 8 Torg-Pavlov ratio.

positive correlations to both in patients who underwent laminoplasty for myelopathy.

Clinical correlates

There have been no studies published showing a relationship between the Torg-Pavlov ratio and quality of life metrics. When it comes to the stenotic cervical spine, the literature suggests clinical parameters (i.e., the severity of myelopathy and duration of symptoms) are much better predictors of outcome following surgery than radiographic parameters.[66,67] Irrespective of the lack of outcomes data, this ratio has still lead to the development of clinically applicable findings.

One of the more frightening aspects of CSM is how even a minor trauma can lead to a significant spinal cord injury. In 2012, Aebli et al.[68] showed how the Torg-Pavlov ratio can be used to predict this potentially catastrophic event. They compared Torg-Pavlov ratios of 45 patients suffering from tetraplegia or tetraparesis after minor trauma to 68 patients with no neurological injury after similar minor trauma; exclusion criteria were fractures (other than isolated spinous process fracture), discoligamentous injury on MRI, gunshots, stab injuries, high-voltage injuries, or patients younger than 20. Their data suggest that patients who sustained SCI after minor trauma had statistically significantly smaller Torg-Pavlov ratios than patients who did not have neurologic involvement with their injury. Using ROC curve analysis, they determined that a ratio value of less than 0.7 yielded the greatest positive likelihood ratio for predicting the occurrence of spinal cord injury. They concluded that patients at risk of acute SCI after minor trauma can be identified by applying a Torg-Pavlov cutoff value of 0.7.

Other studies have shown how the ratio can be used to predict postoperative neurologic dysfunction for patients with CSM. Sieh et al.[69] showed that a Torg-Pavlov ratio < 0.65 is a reliable predictor for the development of upper limb palsy after posterior cervical decompression. Similarly, Wang et al.[70] showed that a ratio of < 0.65 at the C5 level is a reliable predictor of C5 palsy after cervical laminoplasty for patients with myelopathy. These studies can be helpful in discussing risks of surgery and postoperative expectations for patients with CSM that will undergo decompression.

The K-line
Overview
Ossification of the posterior longitudinal ligament (OPLL) is a phenomenon of poorly understood pathogenesis whereby the PLL becomes hyperostotic secondary to ectopic calcification. A subset of patients with OPLL will progress to myelopathy due to the stenosing nature of this entity—an occupancy ratio between 30% and 60% is predictive of the development of myelopathy and some studies noted 100% of the patients with a ratio > 60% developed myelopathy.[71,72] A high surgical complication rate is associated with OPLL, particularly with respect to CSF leaks. This rate was noted to be even higher with an anterior approach, especially in patients with kyphotic spinal alignment and larger OPLL size.[73–75] Fujiyoshi et al. developed a novel radiographic marker, the Kyphosing Line (K-line), to evaluate the cervical alignment and OPLL size with 1 parameter and showed how this marker could be used as an index to determine surgical approach. Adequate posterior decompression is reliant on posterior shift of the cord and the amount of contact with the ventral OPLL mass, with the "noncontact" type being the most desirable.[76] K-line (+) patients were more likely to be noncontact types after posterior decompression during intraoperative ultrasound assessment and, therefore, were more likely to achieve sufficient posterior shift. The authors extrapolated that K-line (+) patients can be approached posteriorly while K-line (−) patients would not be expected to have appropriate posterior shift and should therefore be approached anteriorly. The K-line is acquired from the lateral view of the cervical radiograph with the patient in neutral. If C7 is excluded due to shoulder shadows, MRI could be evaluated as a surrogate (modified K-line).

- **The K-line** (Fig. 9): Find the midpoints of the spinal canal at C2 and C7 and connect them with a line.
  - K-line (+): OPLL stays ventral to the K-line and does not exceed it
  - K-line (−): OPLL exceeds the K-line and passes posterior to it

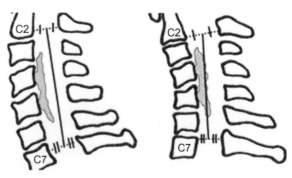

FIG. 9 View of K-line.

Reliability and validation

There are no studies published discussing the reliability or validation of the K-line proper. As a surrogate for the K-line, Marques et al.[77] assessed the reliability of various cervical spine radiographic parameters that included the K-line tilt, a variation of the K-line. The K-line tilt is the angle subtended by the K-line and a line drawn perpendicular to the horizon; this parameter was found to correlate with postoperative kyphosis after laminoplasty and showed a significant correlation with the C2–C7 SVA in predicting postoperative pain and disability.[78] In the aforementioned radiographic assessment, 758 lateral cervical radiographs were analyzed for Cobb angles, T1S, occipitocervical inclination, K-line tilt, and cSVA. Of all these parameters, K-line tilt was found to be the most reliable with an intraobserver ICC of 0.988 and interobserver ICC of 0.961. These numbers can attest to the simplicity of applying the K-line concept.

Clinical correlates

The original K-line study by Fujiyoshi et al. investigated the JOA score and % neurologic recovery for patients before and after posterior decompression. The authors discovered that patients in the K-line (+) group achieved a statistically significant improvement in the JOA score (K-line [+]: $8.9\pm0.7 \rightarrow 13.8\pm0.6$, K-line [−]: $7.3\pm0.7 \rightarrow 8.9\pm0.8$) and overall neurologic percent recovery (K-line [+]: $66.1\%\pm5.2\%$, K-line [−]: $13.9\%\pm12.2\%$) with a posterior decompressive surgery. These findings lead to the conclusion that a posterior decompression for K-line (−) patients would lead to inferior neurologic recovery and overall clinical picture.

Subsequent studies sought to understand if there was a difference between the types of posterior surgeries implemented in K-line (−) patients. Koda et al.[79] suggested that anterior decompression and instrumented fusion (ADF) obtained significantly higher postoperative JOA scores than both posterior decompression and instrumented fusion (PDF) and laminoplasty (LMP) but, PDF had significantly higher JOA scores than LMP. At 1-year follow-up, the JOA score continued to improve and was found to be significantly higher in the ADF and PDF groups when compared to laminoplasty, suggesting that PDF was a viable option for this group if ADF is unable to be performed. Similar findings were seen in multiple studies, with the general consensus that LMP performs the worst of the three, while ADF was the superior procedure and PDF filled an intermediary, yet clinically acceptable role, in K-line (−) patients.[80–82]

C5 Lateral Mass Divided by Canal Diameter Ratio
Overview

Developmental cervical stenosis poses additional problems, in that it can often be asymptomatic until there is an acute injury or until abnormal degenerative tissue causes neural compression sufficient for symptoms to develop. Several studies in the literature have analyzed that Torg-Pavlov ratio and found it to provide high sensitivity for cervical stenosis but low specificity for identifying developmental cervical stenosis and high variability among the sexes and between ethnicities.[83–85] Horne et al.[86] identified this void and synthesized the C5 Lateral Mass Divided By Canal Diameter Ratio (C5 LM/CD Ratio) in an attempt to develop an objective radiographic measurement to screen for developmental cervical stenosis. They used true lateral cervical spine projections (overlapping single projection of the facet joints) to obtain the ratios and compared these measurements to those made on CT midline sagittal cuts. These measurements were made at the mid-height level of the vertebral body between the closest points of the cortical margins at the C5 level. The C5 level was chosen via ROC curve analysis at each cervical level that showed C5 to have the best statistical profile. Their ratio predicted developmental cervical stenosis at any level between C3 and C6 and, an LM/CD ratio of > 0.735 at C5 demonstrated 76% sensitivity, 80% specificity, and a negative predictive value of 0.88. The ratio was not impacted by sex or ethnicity, unlike the Torg-Pavlov ratio.

- C5 LM/CD ratio (Fig. 10) = LM/CD
  - LM/CD ratio $\geq$ 0.735 indicates a canal diameter < 12 mm (developmental cervical stenosis)
  - LM = lateral mass-to-posterior vertebral body distance
  - CD = the spinolaminar line-to-vertebral body distance (spinal canal diameter).

Reliability and validation

Reliability of the C5 LM/CD ratio was tested internally using 22 of the 150 patient radiographs and having them measured by several of their authors—the primary investigator, spine surgery and anesthesia attending, and 2 spine fellows—in triplicate. They found excellent intra- and interobserver reliability with ICC > 0.96. Also measured were the correlation between C5 LM/CD and Torg-Pavlov ratios to the true canal diameter found on CT scan, which both correlated significantly. Sensitivity and specificity of the ratio were determined using ROC curve analysis. Curves were assessed for the LM/CD ratio at each spinal level and

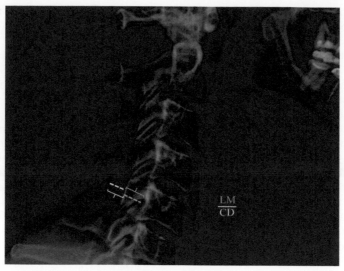

FIG. 10 C5 LM/CD ratio.

showed that C5 held the best statistical profile; an LM/CD ratio ≥ 0.735 indicated a canal diameter at the C5 level of $< 12\,$mm with a sensitivity of 83% and a false-positive rate of 25%. The ratio was also found to be able to predict cervical stenosis at any cervical level with a sensitivity of 75% and a false-positive rate of 20%. These findings were compared to the previous gold-standard Torg-Pavlov ratio that showed a statistical profile similar to the reference line of the ROC curve. The negative predictive value of 0.88 also suggests that a ratio below 0.735 is a strong indicator of the absence of developmental cervical stenosis between C3 and C6. There have been no other studies published exploring the reliability and/or validation of the C5 LM/CD ratio.

Clinical correlates
There have been no studies published showing a relationship between the LM/CD ratio and quality of life metrics.

CONCLUSION
Classification systems and measurements provide a common language through which Orthopedists and researchers can communicate information and create treatment algorithms. The topics described in this section are but a few available in the literature; however, these have generated considerable clinical correlates that prove their usefulness in clinical practice. Through the continued application and analysis of these systems, the clinical outcomes associated with the treatment of subaxial cervical spine pathology will continue to evolve and improve with time and patience.

REFERENCES
1. Garbuz DS, Masri B, Esdaile J, et al. Classification systems in orthopedics. *J Am Acad Orthop Surg.* 2002;10:290–297.
2. Middendorp JJ, Audigé L, Hanson B, et al. What should an ideal spinal injury classification system consist of? A methodological review and conceptual proposal for future classifications. *Eur Spine J.* 2010;19:1238–1249.
3. Sadiqi S, Verlaan J, Lehr M, et al. Surgeon reported outcome measure for spine trauma. *Spine.* 2016;41(24):E1453–E1459.
4. Allen Jr BL, Ferguson RL, Lehmann T. A mechanistic classification of closed, indirect fractures and dislocations of the lower cervical spine. *Spine.* 1982;7:1–27.
5. Vaccaro AR, Hulbert RJ, Patel AA, et al. The subaxial cervical spine injury classification system: a novel approach to recognize the importance of morphology, neurology, and integrity of the disco-ligamentous complex. *Spine.* 2007;32:2365–2374.
6. Stone AT, Bransford RJ, Lee MJ, et al. Reliability of classification systems for subaxial cervical injuries. *Evid Based Spine Care J.* 2010;1:19–26.
7. Urrutia J, Zamora T, Yurac R, et al. An independent inter- and intra-observer agreement evaluation of the AO Spine subaxial cervical spine injury classification system. *Spine.* 2017;42(5):298–303.
8. Harris JHJ, Edeiken-Monroe B, Kopaniky DR. A practical classification of acute cervical spine injuries. *Orthop Clin North Am.* 1986;17(1):15–30.
9. Magerl F, Aebi M, Gertzbein SD, et al. A comprehensive classification of thoracic and lumbar injuries. *Eur Spine J.* 1994;3(4):184–201.

10. Vaccaro AR, Lehman Jr RA, Hurlbert RJ, et al. A new classification of thoracolumbar injuries: the importance of injury morphology, the integrity of the posterior ligamentous complex, and neurologic status. *Spine*. 2005;30:2325–2333.

11. Oner FC, Ramos LMP, Simmermacher RKJ, et al. Classification of thoracic and lumbar spine fractures: problems of reproducibility. A study of 53 patients using CT and MRI. *Eur Spine J*. 2002;11(3):235–245.

12. Lee WJ, Yoon SH, Kim YJ, et al. Interobserver and intraobserver reliability of sub-axial injury classification and severity scale between radiologist, resident, and spine surgeon. *J Korean Neurol Assoc*. 2012;52:200–203.

13. van Middendorp JJ, Audigé L, Bartels RH, et al. The subaxial cervical spine injury classification system: an external agreement validation study. *Spine J*. 2013;13(9):1055–1063.

14. Joaquim AF, Ghizoni E, Tedeschi H, et al. Clinical results of patients with subaxial cervical spine trauma treated according to the SLIC score. *J Spinal Cord Med*. 2014;37(4):420–424.

15. Dvorak MF, Fisher CG, Fehlings MG, et al. The surgical approach to subaxial cervical spine injuries: an evidence-based algorithm based on the SLIC classification system. *Spine*. 2007;32:2620–2629.

16. Goffin J, Plets C, Van den Bergh R. Anterior cervical fusion and osteosynthetic stabilization according to Caspar: a prospective study of 41 patients with fractures and/or dislocations of the cervical spine. *Neurosurgery*. 1989;25:865–871.

17. Brodke DS, Anderson PA, Newell DW, et al. Comparison of anterior and posterior approaches in cervical spinal cord injuries. *J Spinal Disord Tech*. 2003;16:229–235.

18. Ianuzzi A, Zambrano I, Tataria J, et al. Biomechanical evaluation of surgical constructs for stabilization of cervical teardrop fractures. *Spine J*. 2006;6:514–523.

19. Dvorak MF, Pitzen T, Zhu Q, et al. Anterior cervical plate fixation: a biomechanical study to evaluate the effects of plate design, endplate preparation, and bone mineral density. *Spine*. 2005;30:294–301.

20. Ludwig SC, Vaccaro AR, Balderston RA, et al. Immediate quadriparesis after manipulation for bilateral cervical facet subluxation. A case report. *J Bone Joint Surg Am*. 1997;79:587–590.

21. Vaccaro AR, Koerner JD, Radcliff KE, et al. AOSpine subaxial cervical spine injury classification system. *Eur Spine J*. 2016;25:2173–2184.

22. Wilson JR, Vaccaro AR, Harrop JS, et al. The impact of facet dislocation on clinical outcomes after cervical spinal cord injury: results of a multicenter North American prospective cohort study. *Spine*. 2013;38:97–103.

23. Nadeau M, McLachlin SD, Bailey SI, et al. A biomechanical assessment of soft-tissue damage in the cervical spine following a unilateral facet injury. *J Bone Joint Surg Am*. 2012;94, e156.

24. Rasoulinejad P, McLachlin SD, Bailey SI, et al. The importance of the posterior osteoligamentous complex to subaxial cervical spine stability in relation to a unilateral facet injury. *Spine J Off J North Am Spine Soc*. 2012;12:590–595.

25. Vaněk P. New AOSpine subaxial cervical spine injury classification and its clinical usage. *Perspect Surg*. 2018;97(6):273–278.

26. Silva OT, Sabba MF, Lira HI, et al. Evaluation of the reliability and validity of the newer AOSpine subaxial cervical injury classification (C-3 to C-7). *J Neurosurg Spine*. 2016;25(3):303–308.

27. Mushlin H, Kole MJ, Chryssikos T, et al. AOSpine subaxial cervical spine injury classification system: the relationship between injury morphology, admission injury severity, and long-term neurologic outcome. *World Neurosurg*. 2019;130:e368–e374.

28. Du J, Fan Y, Zhang J, et al. Early versus delayed decompression for traumatic cervical spinal cord injury: application of the AOSpine subaxial cervical spine injury classification system to guide surgical timing. *Eur Spine J*. 2019;28:1855–1863.

29. Ames CP, Smith JS, Eastlack R, et al. Reliability assessment of a novel cervical spine deformity classification system. *J Neurosurg*. 2015;23(6):673–683.

30. Schwab F, Ungar B, Blondel B, et al. Scoliosis Research Society—Schwab adult spinal deformity classification: a validation study. *Spine*. 2012;37:1077–1082.

31. Smith JS, Klineberg E, Schwab F, et al. Change in classification grade by the SRS-Schwab Adult Spinal Deformity Classification predicts impact on health-related quality of life measures: prospective analysis of operative and nonoperative treatment. *Spine*. 2013;38:1663–1671.

32. Tang JA, Scheer JK, Smith JS, et al. Positive cervical sagittal alignment negatively impacts outcomes following adult posterior cervical fusion procedures. *Neurosurgery*. 2012;71:662–669.

33. Cho SK, Safir S, Lombardi JM, et al. Surgical spine deformity: indications, considerations, and surgical outcomes. *J Am Acad Orthop Surg*. 2019;27(12):e555–e567.

34. Diebo BG, Challier V, Henry JK, et al. Predicting cervical alignment required to maintain horizontal gaze based on global spinal alignment. *Spine*. 2016;41(23):1795–1800.

35. Cho SK, Safir S, Lombardi JM, et al. Cervical spine deformity: indications, considerations, and surgical outcomes. *J Am Acad Orthop Surg*. 2019;27:e555–e567.

36. Hardacker JW, Shuford RF, Capicotto PN, et al. Radiographic standing cervical segmental alignment in adult volunteers without neck symptoms. *Spine*. 1997;22:1472–1480.

37. Scheer JK, Tang JA, Smith JS, et al. Cervical spine alignment, sagittal deformity, and clinical implications: a review. *J Neurosurg Spine*. 2013;19:141–159.

38. Lee SH, Kim KT, Seo EM, et al. The influence of thoracic inlet alignment on the craniocervical sagittal balance in asymptomatic adults. *J Spinal Disord Tech*. 2012;25:E41–E47.

39. Ha Y, Schwab F, Lafage V, et al. Reciprocal changes in cervical spine alignment after corrective thoracolumbar deformity surgery. *Eur Spine J*. 2014;23:552–559.

40. Oshima Y, Takeshita K, Taniguchi Y, et al. Effect of preoperative sagittal balance on cervical laminoplasty outcomes. *Spine*. 2016;41:E1265–E1270.

41. Naderi S, Ozgen S, Pamir MN, et al. Cervical spondylotic myelopathy: surgical results and factors affecting prognosis. *Neurosurgery.* 1998;43:43–50.

42. Jenkins LA, Capen DA, Zigler JE, et al. Cervical spine fusions for trauma. A long-term radiographic and clinical evaluation. *Orthop Rev.* 1994;(suppl):13–19.

43. Suk KS, Kim KT, Lee SH, et al. Significance of chin-brow vertical angle in correction of kyphotic deformity of ankylosing spondylitis patients. *Spine.* 2003;28:2001–2005.

44. Xing R, Liu W, Li X, et al. Characteristics of cervical sagittal parameters in healthy cervical spine adults and patients with cervical disc degeneration. *BMC Musculoskelet Disord.* 2018;19(1):37.

45. Smith JS, Lafage V, Ryan DJ, et al. Association of myelopathy scores with cervical sagittal balance and normalized spinal cord volume: analysis of 56 preoperative cases from the AOSpine North America Myelopathy study. *Spine.* 2013;38(2.1):S161–S170.

46. Ames CP, Blondel B, Scheer JK, et al. Cervical radiographical alignment: comprehensive assessment techniques and potential importance in cervical myelopathy. *Spine.* 2013;38(22):S149–S160.

47. Lafage V, Schwab F, Patel A, et al. Pelvic tilt and truncal inclination: two key radiographic parameters in the setting of adults with spinal deformity. *Spine.* 2009;34:e599–e606.

48. Passias PG, Jalai CM, Smith JS, et al. Characterizing adult cervical deformity and disability based on existing cervical and adult deformity classification schemes at presentation and following correction. *Neurosurgery.* 2017;82(2):192–201.

49. Passias PG, Horn SR, Oh C, et al. Evaluating cervical deformity corrective surgery outcomes at 1-year using current patient-derived and functional measures: are they adequate? *J Spine Surg.* 2018;4:295–303.

50. Brodke DJ, Saltzman CL, Brodke DS. PROMIS for orthopaedic outcomes measurement. *J Am Acad Orthop Surg.* 2016;24:744–749.

51. Hung M, Clegg DO, Greene T, et al. Evaluation of the PROMIS physical function item bank in orthopaedic patients. *J Orthop Res.* 2011;29:947–953.

52. Pierce KE, Alas H, Brown AE, et al. PROMIS physical health domain scores are related to cervical deformity severity. *J Craniovertebr Junction Spine.* 2019;10(3):179–183.

53. Staub BN, Lafage R, Kim HJ, et al. Cervical mismatch: the normative value of T1 slope minus cervical lordosis and its ability to predict ideal cervical lordosis. *J Neurosurg Spine.* 2019;30:31–37.

54. Grosso MJ, Hwang R, Krishnaney AA, et al. Complications and outcomes for surgical approaches to cervical kyphosis. *J Spinal Disord Tech.* 2015;28:E385–E393.

55. Kim HJ, Piyaskulkaew C, Riew KD. Anterior cervical osteotomy for fixed cervical deformities. *Spine.* 2014;39:1751–1757.

56. Du W, Zhang P, Shen Y, et al. Enlarged laminectomy and lateral mass screw fixation for multilevel cervical degenerative myelopathy associated with kyphosis. *Spine J.* 2014;14:57–64.

57. Yeh KT, Lee RP, Chen IH, et al. Laminoplasty instead of laminectomy as a decompression method in posterior instrumented fusion for degenerative cervical kyphosis with stenosis. *J Orthop Surg Res.* 2015;10:138.

58. Lau D, Ziewacz JE, Le H, et al. A controlled anterior sequential interbody dilation technique for correction of cervical kyphosis. *J Neurosurg Spine.* 2015;23:263–273.

59. Kim HJ, Nemani VM, Riew DK. Cervical osteotomies for neurological deformities. *Eur Spine J.* 2015;24(1):S16–S22.

60. Kim HJ, Piyaskulkaew C, Riew DK. Comparison of Smith-Petersen osteotomy versus pedicle subtraction osteotomy versus anterior-posterior osteotomy types for the correction of cervical spine deformities. *Spine.* 2015;40:143–146.

61. Mahesh B, Upendra B, Vijay S, et al. Addressing stretch myelopathy in multilevel cervical kyphosis with posterior surgery using cervical pedicle screws. *Asian Spine J.* 2016;10:1007–1017.

62. Lee MJ, Cassinelli EH, Riew DK. Prevalence of cervical spinal stenosis: anatomic study in cadavers. *J Bone Joint Surg Am.* 2007;89(2):376–380.

63. Pavlov H, Torg JS, Robie B, Jahre C. Cervical spinal stenosis: determination with vertebral body ratio method. *Radiology.* 1987;164(3):771–775.

64. Aebli N, Wicki AG, Rüegg TB, et al. The Torg-Pavlov ratio for the prediction of acute spinal cord injury after a minor trauma to the cervical spine. *Spine J.* 2013;13(6):605–612.

65. Suk K, Kim K, Lee J, et al. Reevaluation of the Pavlov ratio in patients with cervical myelopathy. *Clin Orthop Surg.* 2009;1(1):6–10.

66. Aggarwal RA, Srivastava SK, Bhosale SK, et al. Prediction of surgical outcome in compressive myelopathy: a novel clinicoradiological prognostic score. *J Craniovertebr Junction Spine.* 2016;7(2):82–86.

67. Karpova A, Ranganathan A, Davis AM, et al. Predictors of surgical outcome in cervical spondylotic myelopathy. *Spine.* 2013;38(5):392–400.

68. Aebli N, Ruegg TB, Wicki AG, et al. Predicting the risk and severity of acute spinal cord injury after a minor trauma to the cervical spine. *Spine J.* 2013;13(6):597–604.

69. Sieh K, Leung S, Lam JSY, et al. The use of average Pavlov ratio to predict the risk of postoperative upper limb palsy after posterior cervical decompression. *J Orthop Surg Res.* 2009;24(4):1–9.

70. Wang B, Liu W, Shao Z, et al. The use of preoperative and intraoperative Pavlov ratio to predict the risk of postoperative C5 palsy after expansive open-door laminoplasty for cervical myelopathy. *Indian J Orthop.* 2019;53(2):309–314.

71. Matsunaga S, Nakamura K, Seichi A, et al. Radiographic predictors for the development of myelopathy in patients with ossification of the posterior longitudinal ligament: a multicenter cohort study. *Spine.* 2008;33(24):2648–2650.

72. Matsunaga S, Kukita M, Hayashi K, et al. Pathogenesis of myelopathy in patients with ossification of the posterior longitudinal ligament. *J Neurosurg.* 2002;96(2, suppl):168–172.

73. Chiba K, Ogawa Y, Ishii K, et al. Long-term results of expansive open-door laminoplasty for cervical myelopathy-average 14-year follow-up study. *Spine*. 2006;31:2998–3005.

74. Iwasaki M, Okuda S, Miyauchi A, et al. Surgical strategy for cervical myelopathy due to ossification of the posterior longitudinal ligament: part 1: clinical results and limitations of laminoplasty. *Spine*. 2007;32:647–653.

75. Yamazaki A, Homma T, Uchiyama S, et al. Morphologic limitations of posterior decompression by midsagittal splitting method for myelopathy caused by ossification of the posterior longitudinal ligament in the cervical spine. *Spine*. 1999;24:32–34.

76. Fujiyoshi T, Yamazaki M, Kawabe J, et al. A new concept for making decisions regarding the surgical approach for cervical ossification of the posterior longitudinal ligament: the K-line. *Spine*. 2008;33(26):E990–E993.

77. Marques C, Granstrom E, MacDowall A, et al. Accuracy and reliability of X-ray measurements in the cervical spine. *Asian Spine J*. 2020;14(2):169–176.

78. Kim H, Kim T, Park M, et al. K-line tilt as a novel radiographic parameter in cervical sagittal alignment. *Eur Spine J*. 2018;27:2023–2028.

79. Koda M, Mochizuki M, Konishi H, et al. Comparison of clinical outcomes between laminoplasty, posterior decompression with instrumented fusion, and anterior decompression with fusion for K-line (−) cervical ossification of the posterior longitudinal ligament. *Eur Spine J*. 2016;25:2294–2301.

80. Saito J, Maki S, Kamiya K, et al. Outcome of posterior decompression with instrumented fusion surgery for K-line (−) cervical ossification of the longitudinal ligament. *J Clin Neurosci*. 2016;32:57–60.

81. Chen Y, Guo Y, Lu X, et al. Surgical strategy for multilevel severe ossification of the posterior longitudinal ligament in the cervical spine. *J Spinal Disord Tech*. 2011;24:24–30.

82. Fujimori T, Iwasaki M, Okuda S, et al. Long-term results of cervical myelopathy due to ossification of the posterior longitudinal ligament with an occupying ratio of 60% or more. *Spine*. 2014;39:58–67.

83. Blackley HR, Plank LD, Robertson PA. Determining the sagittal dimensions of the canal of the cervical spine. The reliability of ratios of anatomical measurements. *J Bone Joint Surg Br*. 1999;81(1):110–112.

84. Kang Y, Lee JW, Koh YH, et al. New MRI grading system for the cervical canal stenosis. *AJR Am J Roentgenol*. 2011;197(1):134–140.

85. Lim JK, Wong HK. Variation of the cervical spinal Torg ratio with gender and ethnicity. *Spine J*. 2004;4(4):396–401.

86. Horne PH, Lampe LP, Nguyen JT, et al. A novel radiographic Indicator of developmental cervical stenosis. *J Bone Joint Surg Am*. 2016;98:1206–1214.

CHAPTER 10

Full-Length Spine—Plain Radiographs

STEFAN PARENT[a,b]
[a]Department of surgery, Université de Montréal, Montréal, QC, Canada
[b]Centre Hospitalier Universitaire Sainte-Justine, Montréal, QC, Canada

INTRODUCTION

The evaluation of spinal pathologies is dependent upon careful history, clinical examination, and appropriate full-length spine radiographs. Appropriate full-length spine radiographs should be obtained when evaluating a patient for suspected coronal, sagittal, or combined imbalance. Full-length spine should ideally include C7 and both femoral heads. This ensures that important landmarks used for parameter calculations are readily available. Plain radiographs can be obtained either through a standardized method using long-film acquisitions with a radiographic source located 72 inches away from the subject or, more recently, through the use of an EOS™ system. The EOS™ system is a slot-scanning device that allows simultaneous acquisition of full-length spine radiographs both in the PA (or AP) and in the lateral position with a significant dose reduction when compared with traditional digital radiography acquisitions.[1]

The thoracic spine is typically composed of 12 thoracic vertebrae each bearing a pair of ribs. The lumbar spine is typically composed of 5 lumbar vertebrae. Normal variations include 11 or 13 thoracic vertebrae and 4 or 6 lumbar vertebrae, and can be seen in as much as 10% of the population. The spine is normally straight in the coronal plane with an accepted variation up to 10° before being considered a scoliosis. In the sagittal plane, the thoracic spine is normally in kyphosis (normal range 20–50°) and the lumbar spine is in lordosis. Lumbar lordosis is usually well correlated with pelvic incidence.

Radiographic imaging of the spine is a static representation of the patient's everyday posture. It doesn't take into consideration gait compensatory mechanisms or one's functional limitations such as spasticity or limited range of motion. A careful evaluation of the patient's gait is of critical importance to better understand the subtle variations in the patient's sagittal and coronal profiles. Postural control is also highly dependent on integration at the central nervous system level of external stimuli, including proprioception, vestibular information, and visual information. This information is processed centrally, and posture derives from this complex and intricate process. Horizontal gaze (vision) is a central part of posture and plays an important role in the patient's ability to stand with a normal posture. The other determinant of sagittal alignment is pelvic morphology, which dictates how the lumbar spine and, to some extent, how the thoracic spine will be aligned.

IMAGE ACQUISITION

Radiographs should be acquired with the patient standing in a natural physiological load-bearing position. Hips and knees should be in their natural position for the patient but don't need to be fully extended. These compensation mechanisms should, however, be noted during physical examination. If possible, head-to-toe image acquisition (as is possible with the EOS™ system) will give an insight into these compensation mechanisms. The arms should be positioned in a way allowing a good assessment of the thoracic spine. Classically, this is done either through a hands-on-clavicle (or hands-on-cheek) position or with the arms holding a support. More recently, a hands-on-wall in the EOS™ system has been advocated with the added benefit of being able to determine the bone age for adolescents.[2] Jackson et al.[2] evaluated the hands-on-clavicle vs. hands resting on a support with their arms at 30° and 45°, and found little difference between these positions. Ideally, to allow for comparison between images taken at different times, there should be some standardization in the position and the acquisition method. The images should span the whole spine from the base of the skull to the pelvis and include both femoral heads. This allows for specific spinal alignment parameters to be determined without repeat imaging.

Atlas of Spinal Imaging. https://doi.org/10.1016/B978-0-323-76111-6.00009-2

RADIOGRAPHIC PARAMETERS

Most parameters are either linear measurements or angular measurements. The remainder will involve ratios between angles or a proportion of deformity by level (deformity angular ratio—DAR). These parameters can be useful in understanding a patient's spinal balance, preoperative assessment of the deformity, and operative planning. Postoperatively, these parameters can also be used to determine sagittal and coronal balance restoration as well as to monitor the long-term adjacent deformity. One should, however, be cautious when using linear measurements as they are highly dependent on calibration. The EOS™ images being acquired in a rigid calibrated environment are more precise and less subject to linear measurement errors.

Coronal Parameters

Normal spinal alignment usually refers to a thoracic and lumbar curve devoid of any significant curvature. A deformity is considered significant only when a Cobb angle of more than 10° can be measured on the PA or AP standing radiograph. The Cobb angle[3] measures the maximal curve of a particular region of the spine formed by the most angled superior vertebra and the most angled lower vertebra. Parallel lines to the superior and inferior endplates are used to measure the Cobb angle. Although not always present, a proximal thoracic (PT), main thoracic (MT), and a thoraco-lumbar/lumbar (TL/L) curve can be measured (Fig. 1). The upper-end

vertebra (UEV) and the lower-end vertebra (LEV) are the proximal and distal vertebra composing a structural curve. The center sacral vertical line (CSVL) is a vertical line drawn from the center of S1. It helps in determining the position of the different components of the curve relative to the coronal mid-axis. The neutral vertebra is usually the vertebra that appears to have the least rotation on a coronal radiograph distal to the main structural curve. The stable vertebra (SV) is usually the most cephalad vertebra directly distal to the major curve that is most closely bisected by the CSVL (Fig. 2).

The sagittal balance (C7-plumbline) can be drawn in the both PA and lateral radiographs. In the coronal and the sagittal plane, it is a vertical line drawn from the center of the C7 vertebral body.

The deformity angular ratio (DAR)[4] is an indirect measure of the severity of a curve as it represents a ratio between the total deformity (maximal Cobb angle) divided by the number of levels comprised in a curve. The DAR can be measured globally, in the coronal plane (C-DAR) or in the sagittal plane (S-DAR). It gives a better perspective of the severity of a specific curve with higher DAR being more angular. The DAR may affect the surgical plan (Fig. 3).

Barycenter (centroids) of a vertebra: The centroid of a vertebral body can be identified on a coronal or a sagittal radiograph by determining the barycenter of the vertebra. This can be accomplished by identifying the four corners (2 upper and 2 lower) of a vertebral body

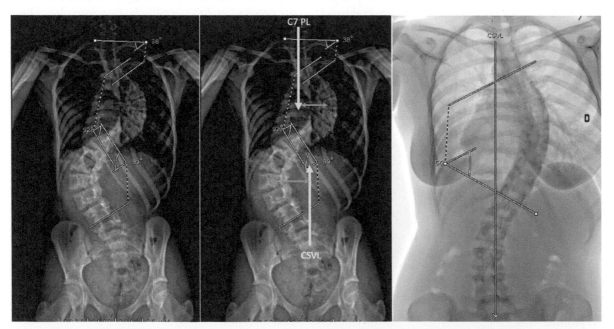

FIG. 1 Radiographs showing an example of the measurements of the Proximal Thoracic (PT), Main Thoracic (MT), and a Thoraco-Lumbar/Lumbar (TL/L) curve in idiopathic scoliosis.

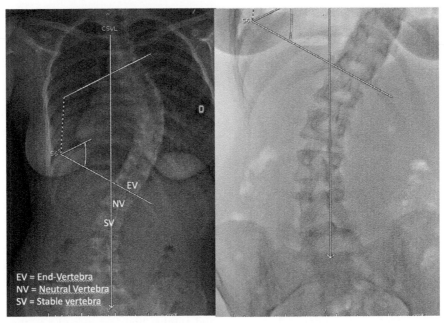

FIG. 2 Radiographs showing an example of end, neutral, and stable vertebrae (EV, NV, SV) in idiopathic scoliosis.

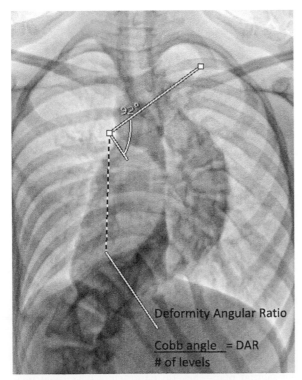

FIG. 3 Radiographs showing an example of the measurement of the Deformity Angular Ratio (DAR), which represents a ratio between the total deformity (maximal Cobb angle) divided by the number of levels comprised in a curve.

and drawing an "X" joining opposite corners. Although this technique is relatively accurate for a rectangular structure, it is not as accurate for a trapezoidal structure. An alternate method of finding the centroid is by using the midpoint of each endplate and each side of the vertebral body and drawing a cross to identify the centroid. These centroids will be commonly used to measure different distances such as trunk shift, apical vertebral translation, retrolisthesis, spondylolisthesis, and rotatory subluxation.

In the coronal plane, the apical vertebral translation (AVT) is determined by identifying the apical vertebra of a curve and measuring the distance from the centroid to the CSVL or C7 plumbline. In the case where the C7 plumbline and CSVL are superimposed, the AVT is the distance from this line for thoracic and lumbar curves. If the two lines do not superimpose, the thoracic AVT will be measured from the centroid of the apical vertebra to the C7 plumbline, while AVT for thoraco-lumbar/lumbar curves will be measured from the CSVL. A right thoracic curve apex is usually to the right of the CSVL and the measurement is by convention positive.

Rotatory subluxation and lateral olisthesis are a hallmark of degenerative scoliosis. They can be measured on coronal plain radiographs. Lateral olisthesis is a lateral translation of a vertebra compared with another (similar to spondylolisthesis in the sagittal plane) with minimal rotation. Rotatory subluxation is translation of the cephalad vertebra accompanied by vertebral rotation. The degree of subluxation is measured in millimeters. To measure, a vertical line will be erected from the superior corner of the caudal vertebra and the inferior corner of the cephalad vertebra. The horizontal distance between these two vertical lines will define the degree of subluxation in millimeters.[5]

Pelvic obliquity can be measured on the full-length spine radiographs. As the identification of specific landmarks on the pelvis can be difficult, several options are available to determine pelvic obliquity. By identifying two corresponding structures on both sides of the pelvis, one can draw a line joining the structures and measuring the angle it forms with the horizontal. The femoral heads, the tips of the sacral ala, the iliac wings, and the acetabula are all structures that can be used to measure pelvic obliquity. Pelvic obliquity can be secondary to leg length discrepancy but can also be secondary to pelvic malformation or spinal deformity.

Nash and Moe[6] proposed a method to measure vertebral rotation on plain radiographs. They divided the vertebral body into 6 equivalent sections with 3 sections on each side of the spinous process in a nonrotated vertebra (neutral). With increasing rotation, the pedicle on the concave side moves toward the edge of the vertebral body, while the convex pedicle moves toward the midline (grade I). In grade II, the concave pedicle is disappearing, while the convex pedicle is now 2/3 toward midline. In grade III, the concave pedicle has disappeared and the convex pedicle is in midline. In grade IV, rotation is so severe that the convex pedicle is located beyond the midline of the vertebral body.

Sagittal Parameters

Thoracic kyphosis and lumbar lordosis are measured in the sagittal plane, and although several measurements have been proposed, it remains challenging to restrict lumbar lordosis and thoracic kyphosis to specific segments of the spine. The challenge with the sagittal profile is that normal individuals present a wide variety of possible sagittal profiles that cannot be reduced to a predefined set of variables. For example, lumbar lordosis is often referred as the angle formed by the upper endplate of T12 to the upper endplate of S1, whereas other authors have defined lumbar lordosis as the angle formed by the upper endplate of L1 to the upper endplate of S1. Similarly, thoracic kyphosis has been reported as the angle formed between T5 and T12 (or T4 to T12) or from T2 to T12. Although many individuals would probably have their kyphosis and lordosis adequately measured according to these arbitrary levels, others may have perfectly normal balanced

spines that do not respect these levels. Berthonnaud et al.[7] have proposed to use arc of circles to represent lordosis and kyphosis and to use the Cobb method between the sacral endplate and the inflection point between the lordosis and kyphosis without relation to the anatomical landmarks. Although this method is attractive, it is not really practical for everyday use. Therefore, the best method is probably to identify the lordotic portion of the spine and measure the lordosis based on the most angled vertebra as identified on the lateral radiograph.

Pelvic parameters are important as they are important determinants of the sagittal profile. Pelvic incidence (PI) is a stable morphological angle present at maturity. It has been shown to evolve during childhood but remains relatively unchanged after maturity. It represents the relationship between the acetabulum and the upper endplate of S1. This relationship can be measured on a lateral view of the spine and pelvis by measuring the angle formed by a line from the center of the bifemoral axis to the center of the upper endplate of S1 and another line perpendicular to the endplate of S1 (Fig. 4). Pelvic tilt (PT) is an angle formed by a line from the center of the upper endplate of S1 to the bifemoral axis and a vertical line drawn from the center of the bifemoral axis (Fig. 4). Finally, sacral slope (SS) is an angle formed by a line drawn parallel to the upper endplate of S1 and a horizontal line. As described by Duval-Beaupère,[8] PI is constant and represents the sum of SS and PT (PI = SS + PT). SS and PT can vary depending on the position of the pelvis in space or with compensatory mechanisms such as pelvic retroversion to compensate for loss of lumbar lordosis, but the PI is not affected by the spatial orientation of the pelvis, which is specific to every individual.

Although the topic of spondylolisthesis will be discussed more in depth in a subsequent chapter, retrolisthesis and degenerative spondylolisthesis can be present on the full-length spine radiographs. They are usually associated with the loss of disc height and adult scoliosis. Degenerative spondylolisthesis is usually not associated with spondylolysis. The anterolisthesis is reported by measuring the distance from the posteroinferior cephalad vertebra to the postero-superior corner of the caudal vertebra.

Global Sagittal Parameters

Considerable work has been done in recent years to better characterize global spinal balance especially in the sagittal plane. Several parameters have been proposed to better correlate sagittal balance and quality of life with the notion that poor sagittal balance correlates

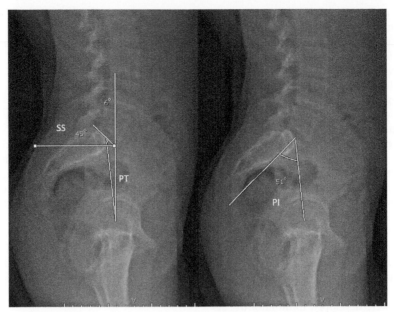

FIG. 4 Lateral view of the spine and pelvis showing an example of Pelvic Parameters. Pelvic Incidence (PI) is the sum of Sacral Slope (SS) and Pelvic Tilt (PT).

with poor quality of life.[9,10] The first global parameter to consider is the C7-plumbline. By convention, when the C7-plumbline lies in front of the hip axis, it is considered positive, and when it lies behind the hip axis, it is considered negative. The sagittal vertical axis (SVA) was defined by Schwab et al. and is the linear measurement between the posterior-superior corner of S1 and the C7-plumbline.[11] They defined 5 cm as an indicator of sagittal imbalance.[12] (Fig. 5). C7 tilt is the angle between a line joining the center of S1 to the center of C7 and the C7 plumbline (Fig. 5). The normal is usually 3° to 5° backward.

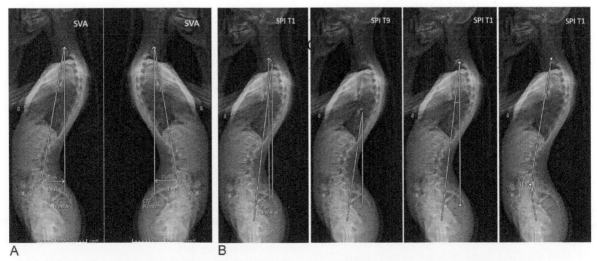

FIG. 5 The C7-plumbline lies in front of the hip axis, it is considered positive and when it lies behind the hip axis, it is considered negative. The Sagittal Vertical Axis (SVA) is the linear measurement between the posterior-superior corner of S1 and the C7-plumbline. C7 tilt is the angle between a line joining the center of S1 to the center of C7 and the C7 plumbline.

The spinopelvic inclination (SPI) is a measure of global sagittal alignment that was initially described by Duval-Beaupère.[13] The T9 SPI is an angle formed by a line between the bifemoral axis and the center (barycenter) of T9 and a vertical line going through the center of T9. The T1 SPI is similarly drawn by using the barycenter of T1 (Fig. 5). The spinopelvis angle (SPA) described by Roussouly et al.[14] is an angle formed by a line joining the center of S1 to the center of C7 and another line joining the bifemoral axis to the center of S1.

Postoperative Radiographic Measurements

The upper instrumented vertebra (UIV) and lower instrumented vertebra (LIV) represent, respectively, the upper and lower extent of the instrumentation. This can change with additional procedures (longer extent of fusion). Most parameters measured preoperatively on the full-length radiographs can usually be measured on postoperative radiographs notwithstanding structures that cannot be identified due to instrumentation.

Some parameters were developed to monitor the behavior of the unfused spine proximally and distally to the fusion. Proximal junctional kyphosis (PJK) is generally defined as an angle between the inferior endplate of the UIV and the upper endplate of the second supra-adjacent vertebra that is greater than 10°-20°. The exact amount of deformity is still debated and varies greatly in the literature. Distal junctional kyphosis (DJK) is similarly measured between the upper endplate of the LIV and the lower endplate of the second distally adjacent vertebra. A value greater than 10-20° is used as a criterion to define DJK.

Distal adding-on usually occurs following surgery for scoliosis and is defined as a progressive increase in the number of vertebrae included distally within the primary curve combined with either an increase of more than 5 mm in deviation of the first vertebra below instrumentation from the CSVL, or an increase of more than 5° in the angulation of the first disc below the instrumentation at the minimum one-year follow-up.[15]

Adding-on is a phenomenon whereby there is distal progression of a spinal deformity following instrumentation and fusion of a spinal deformity. The definition of distal adding-on as proposed by Wang et al.[15] refers to progressive deformity under the LIV with progressive increase in the number of vertebrae included within the primary curve distally to the instrumentation combined with either an increase of more than 5 mm in the deviation of the first vertebra below the instrumentation from the CSVL or an increase of more than 5° in angulation of the first disc below the instrumentation.

Although adjacent segment disease is a clinical entity resulting from the pathologic process associated with disc degeneration resulting in back pain, radiculopathy, and spinal stenosis, disc height can be found to be decreased following instrumentation and fusion.

CONCLUSION

A good understanding of normal spinal anatomy is essential to identify pathologic conditions. Spinal deformities, including scoliosis, kyphosis, and spondylolisthesis, may affect the position and shape of vertebral structures. Although significant work has been done to understand the coronal aspects of the deformity, the focus has shifted in recent years to better understand the sagittal balance both in adolescents and in adults. There is also significant work being done to understand the 3D aspects of spinal deformities, and as 3D reconstructions become more readily available, new knowledge should emerge in the coming years.

REFERENCES

1. Deschênes S, Charron G, Beaudoin G, et al. Diagnostic imaging of spinal deformities: reducing patients radiation dose with a new slot-scanning X-ray imager. *Spine.* 2010;35(9):989–994.
2. Jackson TJ, Miller D, Nelson S, Cahill PJ, Flynn JM. Two for one: a change in hand positioning during low-dose spinal stereoradiography allows for concurrent, reliable sanders skeletal maturity staging. *Spine Deform.* 2018;6(4):391–396.
3. Cobb J. Technique for study of scoliosis. *AAOS Instr Course Lect.* 1948;261–275.
4. Lewis NDH, Keshen SGN, Lenke LG, et al. The deformity angular ratio: does it correlate with high-risk cases for potential spinal cord monitoring alerts in pediatric 3-column thoracic spinal deformity corrective surgery? *Spine.* 2015;40(15):E879–E885.
5. *Radiographic Measurement Manual.* Medtronic Sofamor Danek USA; 2008:91.
6. Nash CL, Moe JH. A study of vertebral rotation. *J Bone Joint Surg Am.* 1969;51(2):223–229.
7. Berthonnaud E, Dimnet J, Roussouly P, Labelle H. Analysis of the sagittal balance of the spine and pelvis using shape and orientation parameters. *J Spinal Disord Tech.* 2005;18(1):40–47.
8. Legaye J, Duval-Beaupère G, Hecquet J, Marty C. Pelvic incidence: a fundamental pelvic parameter for three-dimensional regulation of spinal sagittal curves. *Eur Spine J.* 1998;7(2):99–103.
9. Harroud A, Labelle H, Joncas J, Mac-Thiong J-M. Global sagittal alignment and health-related quality of life in lumbosacral spondylolisthesis. *Eur Spine J.* 2013;22(4):849–856. Springer-Verlag.

10. Glassman SD, Bridwell K, Dimar JR, Horton W, Berven S, Schwab F. The impact of positive sagittal balance in adult spinal deformity. *Spine*. 2005;30(18):2024–2029.

11. Schwab F, Lafage V, Patel A, Farcy J-P. Sagittal plane considerations and the pelvis in the adult patient. *Spine*. 2009;34(17):1828–1833.

12. Schwab FJ, Hawkinson N, Lafage V, et al. Risk factors for major peri-operative complications in adult spinal deformity surgery: a multi-center review of 953 consecutive patients. *Eur Spine J*. 2012;21(12):2603–2610. Springer-Verlag.

13. Duval-Beaupère G, Schmidt C, Cosson P. A Barycentremetric study of the sagittal shape of spine and pelvis: the conditions required for an economic standing position. *Ann Biomed Eng*. 1992;20(4):451–462. Kluwer Academic Publishers.

14. Roussouly P, Pinheiro-Franco JL, Labelle H. *Sagittal Balance of the Spine*. Thieme; 2019 [1 p].

15. Wang Y, Hansen ES, Høy K, Wu C, Bünger CE. Distal adding-on phenomenon in Lenke 1A scoliosis: risk factor identification and treatment strategy comparison. *Spine*. 2011;36(14):1113–1122.

CHAPTER 11

Full-Length Spine CT and MRI in Daily Practice

STEPHANE BOURRET[a] • TAE-KEUN AHN[b] • WENDY THOMPSON[a] •
CECILE ROSCOP[a] • THIBAULT CLOCHÉ[a] • JEAN-CHARLES LE HUEC[a]
[a]Polyclinique Bordeaux Nord Aquitaine, Vertebra Spine Unit, Bordeaux, France, [b]Department of
Orthopedic Surgery, CHA Bundang Medical Center, CHA University, Pocheon-si, South Korea

INTRODUCTION

There are multiple imaging modalities to evaluate the spine. The type of imaging tool for the spine depends on the type of disease, the amount of radiation hazard, as well as contraindications and any allergy to contrast.

Among the multiple imaging strategies, computed tomography (CT) is a reliable method to evaluate the spine and has better sensitivity for bony abnormality than radiography or magnetic resonance imaging (MRI).[1] In the past, the time factor limited the use of CT. However, owing to the development of fast spiral CT and multidirectional CT (MDCT), the whole spine can be examined in a very short time.[2] However, CT is less sensitive to a patient's movement than MRI.[3] Now, it is widely applied to assess trauma, deformity, metastasis, and pre- and postoperative analyses.

MRI is one of the most sensitive and specific modalities to visualize the spine. Furthermore, there are no risks of radiation hazard. It provides information about the spinal neural structures including cord, cauda equina and roots, the vertebral bodies, and intervertebral disc. Multiple sequences can be obtained in different planes and each sequence helps in evaluating various changes of the spine. The most commonly using sequences include sagittal and axial T1 and T2, and a sagittal STIR (short tau inversion recovery). Postcontrast T1-weighted images are useful for evaluating spinal infections, postoperative complications, vascular malformation, primary spinal tumors, and metastases. STIR sequences are beneficial in assessing marrow edema, which demonstrates an increased signal on these sequences.[4]

In most cases, spine CT and MR images are obtained to focus on the region of interest where the pathology exists. However, full-length spine examination can be helpful for a more comprehensive evaluation and early detection of disease and trauma (Fig. 1). Therefore, the aim of this chapter was to describe when and how full-length spine evaluation through CT and MRI is applied.

METHODOLOGY

A literature review using PubMed and Google Scholar was performed. To identify relevant studies, search was conducted on studies in English published between 2000 and February 2020 using various combinations of the following key words: "full-length spine," "entire spine," "whole spine," "imaging," "computed tomography," and "magnetic resonance imaging." Based on this search, 127 studies were initially detected. After excluding articles about rare disease, technical aspects of CT and MRI, measurement, and imaging protocol, 56 articles were selected. After an internal peer review with all the authors of this article and a supplementary search that involved bibliographic screening and citation tracking associated with individual spine pathology, 24 articles of interest were finally selected (Fig. 2). Those articles are categorized as "trauma," "deformity," "infection," "axial spondyloarthropathy," and "spinal metastasis" described in the following sections.

CONTRIBUTIONS OF FULL-LENGTH SPINE CT AND MRI

Trauma

When trauma to the spine occurs, based on physical examination and simple radiography findings, targeted CT and/or MRI is performed specifically at the region of the affected spine for further imaging workup. However, if the patient sustains high-energy trauma or multiple trauma, that regional imaging can be insufficient. In high-energy or polytrauma patients, once the patient's condition is deemed stable, unforeseen injuries to the spine should be delineated accurately as symptoms of

Atlas of Spinal Imaging. https://doi.org/10.1016/B978-0-323-76111-6.00016-X

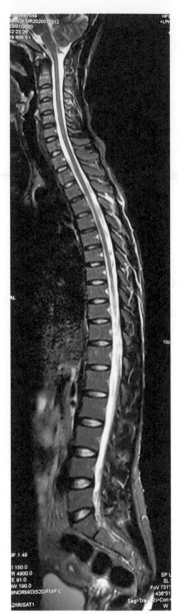

FIG. 1 Normal sagittal T2-weighted magnetic resonance image of full-length spine.

fractures were prevalent in 30.2% of the cases of high-energy trauma. Among patients with a cervical fracture, 37.5% had a fracture that unrevealed on radiographs of the cervical spine but were first diagnosed by a CT scan. Patients with a thoracolumbar fracture did not have clinical symptoms of a fracture in 14% of cases but had a fracture revealed by CT in those 14%. Therefore, Takami et al. postulated that the full-length spine CT should be taken to evaluate all high-energy trauma patients.[6]

The application of full-length MRI in spine trauma patients remains controversial. Atsina et al. described that full-length MRI is not usually recommended in patients with spine trauma. When the full-length MRI is performed in patients with blunt trauma after full-length spinal CT, most additional spinal injuries detected on MRI were bone contusions and mild compression fractures. These additional spinal diagnoses are unlikely to change the management or treatment.[8] Therefore, the targeted MRI is more useful in patients with high-energy blunt trauma. However, Kanna et al. reported that full-length sagittal T2-weighted images help diagnose multilevel noncontiguous spinal injuries in spinal trauma patients and can be performed in approximately 4 min without radiation hazard.[9]

Deformity

Spinal deformity is a complex disease with different three-dimensional abnormalities that often involve the entire spine.[10] In cases with a complex or severe spinal deformity, full-length spine CT should be taken of the entire spine as plain radiography alone is insufficient to visualize complicated abnormalities of the deformity.[11] Furthermore, in comparison with radiography, full-length spine CT scanning provides additional information about extent of rotation of the spine; segmentation defects; three-dimensional reconstruction and detection of bony spurs in diastematomyelia; and associated congenital anomalies of ribs, scapula, and pelvis.[12]

Full-length spine CT is also useful for surgical planning. Current surgical techniques for deformity correction allow surgeons to effectively correct coronal, sagittal, and rotational aspects of spinal deformity.[13] Multiplanar reconstruction of the axial CT images is important, especially when trying to understand the anatomy of deformity, and allows visualizing levels where osteotomies or resections are planned. The CT scan allows surgeons to understand the pedicle anatomy including the width, depth, and trajectory of the pedicles. During a deformity surgery, caution must be placed when placing screws in the pedicles, especially on the concave side of curvature where pedicles are

a spine injury may be masked by concomitant injuries, patient's state of consciousness (Fig. 3), spinal cord injury or shock.[5,6] In these situations, full-length spine evaluations with CT and/or MRI are essential.

In patients with high-energy blunt trauma, Deunk et al. reported that the nontargeted CT detected 8.2% more spine injuries unrevealed by simple radiographs than the targeted CT.[7] In a prospective study, spinal

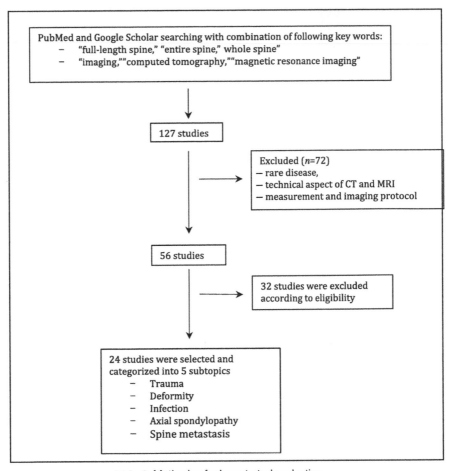

FIG. 2 Methods of relevant study selection.

extremely narrow and the spinal cord is vulnerable to iatrogenic injuries due to restricted epidural space.[14] Preoperative full-length spine CT in this context has been recommended because of the high probability of the presence of narrow pedicles. It also allows surgeons to identify pseudarthroses if the patients underwent previous fusion surgery. Postoperative full-length spine CT is considered for patients with a new neurologic deficit after surgery. Specifically, a postoperative CT can identify potential pedicle screw malposition that may be causing postoperative neurological symptoms.[15]

Full-length spine MRI can be obtained for deformity patients who develop neurologic symptoms or for preoperative planning. The MRI provides visualization of neurological structures, helps determine appropriate levels of surgery, and can assist in the evaluation for adjacent-level pathology when fusion extension is considered.[16] MRI is also essential for the patients with an unusual curve pattern and for those patients who should be assessed on the neural axis. It is important to identify whether syrinx, tethering of the spinal cord, intramedullary tumors, or Chiari malformations are present. The presence of those intraspinal anomalies without neurological findings in idiopathic scoliosis has been estimated between 4 and 26% and associated with neurological complications resulted from correction surgery.[17] Stenosis or cord impingement secondary to severe deformity can be visualized by full-length MRI. In kyphoscoliosis, the level of cord compression should be identified preoperatively and always on the concave pedicle. These regions of compression may require a resection of that pedicle with the remaining body during deformity surgery.[11,15]

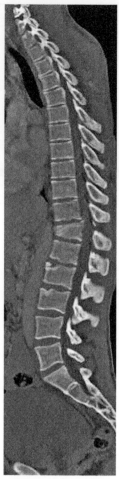

FIG. 3 Sagittal full-length spine computed tomography image showing Denis B-type T12 fracture with widened interspinous space. A 29-year-old man sustained an injury from vehicle-pedestrian accident. The patient was unconscious in the emergency room.

Infection

The diagnosis of spinal infection can be difficult and even delayed because clinical manifestations widely vary and, at times, may be equivocal. Physicians have relied heavily on imaging modalities due to difficulty in detecting spinal infection. Among imaging modalities, MRI plays a pivotal role in the diagnosis and management of spinal infection with a sensitivity, specificity, and accuracy above 90%.[18]

If the spinal infection is likely localized, it may not be necessary to obtain imaging along the full length of the spine. However, identification of one infected site in the spine cannot rule out the infection in multiple regions of the spine. The areas adjacent to anterolateral vertebral endplates have abundant vascular supply and are the most common regions where pyogenic, tuberculous, and other spinal infections can present. Associated edema is commonly pronounced and affects the entire vertebral body and intervertebral disc.[19] If there is epidural involvement associated with neurologic symptoms, it is recommended to obtain full-length spine MRI to assess for epidural abscess spread.[20] Among spinal infections caused by various organisms, *mycobacterium tuberculosis* is notorious for multifocality, and the subligamentous spread of infection to multiple levels is an imaging hallmark of the disease. The infection typically starts in the anterior aspects of the vertebral body adjacent to the intervertebral disc and then spreads to the vertebral bodies under the anterior longitudinal ligaments involving multiple adjacent vertebrae. Through valveless vein system, noncontiguous lesions at additional levels may be impacted.[21]

The incidence of multifocal spinal infection has varied from around 4% to 23%. Mann et al. evaluated 24 patients with spondylitis and found 21 patients had single-level infections, while 1 (4%) had multisegmental infection.[22] Ledermann et al. found 7 (16%) out of 44 patients with disc infection had involvement at several spinal levels.[23] Cox et al. reported that 82 patients with single-level infection performed full-length MRI examination and 19 (23%) patients had additional noncontiguous sites of infection. Remote levels of spondylodiscitis were also present in 11 patients (13%).[20] In cases of multifocal spinal tuberculosis, the reported incidence varies, ranging from 1.1% to 71.4%. Kaila et al. reported a very high incidence of 71.4%,[24] but their data are likely overestimated due to the small number of cases presented. According to a retrospective study, 47 (25.1%) out of 187 patients with spinal tuberculosis had multifocal spinal tuberculosis.[25]

In the setting of spinal infection, full-length spine MRI can be used as a diagnostic screening test to detect multifocal lesions, even if the patients do not have clinical symptoms, and provides early detection of spinal infection, thus preventing progression of osteomyelitis.

In regard to the management and treatment of spinal infection, the detection of an epidural abscess or other infective lesions remote from the site of a known uncomplicated spinal infection may result in a change of management.[26]

Axial Spondyloarthropathy

In the management and treatment of axial spondyloarthropathy(SpA), of great importance is the benefit of early detection before the structural damage begins. However, clinical findings of early axial SpA are not specific and assessment can be challenging. Furthermore, current imaging modalities such as radiographs, CT, and bone scintigraphy have shown limitations for use in early detection of axial SpA. Both CT and bone scintigraphy expose the patients to high levels of ionizing radiation; bone scintigraphy showed low specificity and CT cannot detect until structural bone changes have progressed.[27] On the contrary, MRI has shown high sensitivity and specificity to evaluate prestructural early inflammatory changes, specifically in observation of bone marrow edema adjacent to joints and discs, entheses, and ligaments.[28]

Although MRI of the sacroiliac (SI) joints has traditionally been used in suspected axial SpA, this localized technique may be inadequate. Inflammatory lesions in the spine have been found most commonly in the thoracic spine in addition to the SI joints. Full-length spine MRI can reveal the involvement of the thoracic spine, with emphasis on the most lateral sagittal aspects of vertebral endplates and costovertebral junctions. About 23% of the ankylosing spondylitis patients with the clinically active disease only have inflammatory spinal lesions and no evidence of active inflammatory sacroiliitis, even in very early disease. Cervical spine involvement is also common in ankylosing spondylitis. For these reasons, full-length spine MRI of the whole spine including SI joints is an essential tool in the diagnosis, management, and prognosis of axial SpA.[29]

Full-length spine MRI has been integrated into recommendations for the staging and therapeutic response evaluation in ankylosing spondylitis. It has been used to evaluate the therapeutic response showing the transition from active enthesitis with bone marrow edema to quiescent fatty infiltration of the bone marrow.[30]

Spinal Metastasis

Plain radiography, CT, and MRI comprise the core imaging modalities for patients with vertebral metastases. The CT provides cross-sectional images, allows for entire spine imaging, visualization of cortical and trabecular bone, and is more sensitive than conventional radiography. CT scans can detect a bony metastatic lesion up to 6 months earlier than a plain radiograph. However, when compared to MRI, Buhmann et al. found the diagnostic accuracy of MRI (98.7%) to be significantly superior to MDCT (88.8%) for the detection of osseous metastases. Sensitivity was significantly lower for MDCT (66.2%) than for MRI (98.5%).[31] Moreover, cortical destruction may be difficult to assess on CT when osteoporosis or degenerative changes are present. There is also an inherent associated risk of radiation exposure. Changes in the bone marrow are fundamental to the sensitivity of MRI in the detection of skeletal metastases to the spine. The combination of unenhanced T1-weighted spin echo and STIR sequences has shown to be the most useful for the detection of bone marrow abnormalities and is able to discriminate benign from malignant bone marrow changes.[32]

Therefore, contrast-enhanced MRI of the entire spinal axis is the current standard for the diagnosis and evaluation of spinal column metastases. If the MRI examination is limited to the spine region of interest, and bone marrow metastases outside the image, other areas of spinal disease can be missed. Full-length spine MRI is often imperative to visualize multiple levels of spinal involvement with asymptomatic disease or the large amount of bone destruction on plain radiography. Full-length spine MRI including pelvis has been used to detect bone metastases and hematologic malignancies. In prostate cancer, full-length spine MRI including the pelvis is highly sensitive for the detection of metastases in the axial skeleton (Fig. 4). In multiple myeloma, the axial skeleton approach with entire spine and pelvis is recommended in the staging system.[33]

After radiation therapy, MRI appears to be a powerful tool for differentiating post-therapeutic changes from tumor recurrence. CT is not used routinely during the follow-up but may be necessary for surveying osteoblastic, osteolytic, or mixed lesions. MRI is also useful for the evaluation of paravertebral masses and epidural extension.[34]

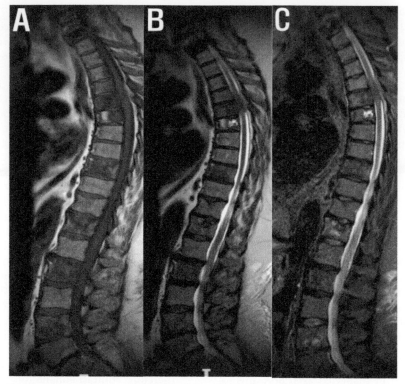

FIG. 4 Sagittal full-length spine T1-weighted (A), T2-weighted (B), and STIR (C) MR images shows multiple spinal metastasis originating from a prostate cancer.

CONCLUSION

In summary, full-length spine examination with CT and/or MRI can be helpful for a more comprehensive evaluation and early detection of disease and trauma. Specifically, CT and MR imaging of the full-length spine are critical in the evaluation and treatment of patients presenting with spine trauma, deformity, infection, spondyloarthropathy, and tumor.

CONFLICTS OF INTEREST

The authors declare no conflicts of interest regarding the publication of this paper.

REFERENCES

1. Døhn UM, Ejbjerg BJ, Hasselquist M, et al. Detection of bone erosions in rheumatoid arthritis wrist joints with magnetic resonance imaging, computed tomography and radiography. *Arthritis Res Ther.* 2008;10:R25.
2. Imhof H, Fuchsjäger M. Traumatic injuries: imaging of spinal injuries. *Eur Radiol.* 2002;12:1262–1272.
3. Linsenmaier U, Krötz M, Häuser H, et al. Whole-body computed tomography in polytrauma: techniques and management. *Eur Radiol.* 2002;12:1728–1740.
4. Balasubramanya R, Selvarajan SK. *Lumbar Spine Imaging.* StatPearls Publishing; 2020.
5. Anderson S, Biros MH, Reardon RF. Delayed diagnosis of thoracolumbar fractures in multiple-trauma patients. *Acad Emerg Med.* 1996;3:832–839.
6. Takami M, Nohda K, Sakanaka J, Nakamura M, Yoshida M. Usefulness of full spine computed tomography in cases of high-energy trauma: a prospective study. *Eur J Orthop Surg Traumatol.* 2014;24:167–171.
7. Deunk J, Brink M, Dekker HM, et al. Routine versus selective computed tomography of the abdomen, pelvis, and lumbar spine in blunt trauma: a prospective evaluation. *J Trauma Acute Care Surg.* 2009;66:1108–1117.
8. Atsina K-B, Rozenberg A, Selvarajan SK. The utility of whole spine survey MRI in blunt trauma patients sustaining single level or contiguous spinal fractures. *Emerg Radiol.* 2019;26:493–500.
9. Kanna RM, Gaike CV, Mahesh A, Shetty AP, Rajasekaran S. Multilevel non-contiguous spinal injuries: incidence and patterns based on whole spine MRI. *Eur Spine J.* 2016;25:1163–1169.

10. Youssef JA, Orndorff DO, Patty CA, et al. Current status of adult spinal deformity. *Global Spine J.* 2013;3:51–62.

11. Sucato DJ. Management of severe spinal deformity: scoliosis and kyphosis. *Spine.* 2010;35:2186–2192.

12. Kalra MK, Quick P, Singh S, Sandborg M, Persson A. Whole spine CT for evaluation of scoliosis in children: feasibility of sub-milliSievert scanning protocol. *Acta Radiol.* 2013;54:226–230.

13. Lafon Y, Lafage V, Dubousset J, Skalli W. Intraoperative three-dimensional correction during rod rotation technique. *Spine.* 2009;34:512–519.

14. Liau KM, Yusof MI, Abdullah MS, Abdullah S, Yusof AH. Computed tomographic morphometry of thoracic pedicles: safety margin of transpedicular screw fixation in Malaysian Malay population. *Spine.* 2006;31:E545–E550.

15. Kim H, Kim HS, Moon ES, et al. Scoliosis imaging: what radiologists should know. *RadioGraphics.* 2010;30:1823–1842.

16. Smith JA. Adult deformity: management of sagittal plane deformity in revision adult spine surgery. *Contemp Spine Surg.* 2002;3:10–16.

17. Ozturk C, Karadereler S, Ornek I, Enercan M, Ganiyusufoglu K, Hamzaoglu A. The role of routine magnetic resonance imaging in the preoperative evaluation of adolescent idiopathic scoliosis. *Int Orthop.* 2010;34:543–546.

18. Kouijzer IJE, Scheper H, de Rooy JWJ, et al. The diagnostic value of 18F–FDG-PET/CT and MRI in suspected vertebral osteomyelitis—a prospective study. *Eur J Nucl Med Mol Imaging.* 2018;45:798–805.

19. Tins BJ, Cassar-Pullicino VN. *MR Imaging of Spinal Infection Seminars in Musculoskeletal Radiology.* Vol 8; 2004:215–229. Copyright\copyright 2004 by Thieme Medical Publishers, Inc., 333 Seventh Avenue.

20. Cox M, Curtis B, Patel M, Babatunde V, Flanders AE. Utility of sagittal MR imaging of the whole spine in cases of known or suspected single-level spinal infection: overkill or good clinical practice? *Clin Imaging.* 2018;51:98–103.

21. Moorthy S, Prabhu NK. Spectrum of MR imaging findings in spinal tuberculosis. *Am J Roentgenol.* 2002;179:979–983.

22. Mann S, Schütze M, Sola S, Piek J. Nonspecific pyogenic spondylodiscitis: clinical manifestations, surgical treatment, and outcome in 24 patients. *Neurosurg Focus.* 2004;17:1–7.

23. Ledermann HP, Schweitzer ME, Morrison WB, Carrino JA. MR imaging findings in spinal infections: rules or myths? *Radiology.* 2003;228:506–514.

24. Kaila R, Malhi AM, Mahmood B, Saifuddin A. The incidence of multiple level noncontiguous vertebral tuberculosis detected using whole spine MRI. *J Spinal Disord Tech.* 2007;20:78–81.

25. Siddiqui MA, Sartaj S, Rizvi SWA, Khan MJ, Khan IA. Role of whole-spine screening magnetic resonance imaging using short tau inversion recovery or fat-suppressed T2 fast spin echo sequences for detecting noncontiguous multiple-level spinal tuberculosis. *Asian Spine J.* 2018;12:686.

26. Spernovasilis N, Demetriou S, Bachlitzanaki M, et al. Characteristics and predictors of outcome of spontaneous spinal epidural abscesses treated conservatively: a retrospective cohort study in a referral center. *Clin Neurol Neurosurg.* 2017;156:11–17.

27. Braun J, Van Der Heijde D. Imaging and scoring in ankylosing spondylitis. *Best Pract Res Clin Rheumatol.* 2002;16:573–604.

28. Barakat E, Kirchgesner T, Triqueneaux P, Galant C, Stoenoiu M, Lecouvet FE. Whole-body magnetic resonance imaging in rheumatic and systemic diseases: from emerging to validated indications. *Magn Reson Imaging Clin N Am.* 2018;26:581–597.

29. Bennett AN, Marzo-Ortega H, Rehman A, Emery P, McGonagle D. The evidence for whole-spine MRI in the assessment of axial spondyloarthropathy. *Rheumatology.* 2010;49:426–432.

30. Song IH, Hermann KG, Haibel H, et al. Effects of etanercept versus sulfasalazine in early axial spondyloarthritis on active inflammatory lesions as detected by whole-body MRI (ESTHER): a 48-week randomised controlled trial. *Ann Rheum Dis.* 2011;70:590–596.

31. Buhmann S, Becker C, Duerr HR, Reiser M, Baur-Melnyk A. Detection of osseous metastases of the spine: comparison of high resolution multi-detector-CT with MRI. *Eur J Radiol.* 2009;69:567–573.

32. Shah LM, Salzman KL. Imaging of spinal metastatic disease. *Int J Surg Oncol.* 2011;2011.

33. Lecouvet FE. Whole-body MR imaging: musculoskeletal applications. *Radiology.* 2016;279:345–365.

34. Guillevin R, Vallee J-N, Lafitte F, Menuel C, Duverneuil N-M, Chiras J. Spine metastasis imaging: review of the literature. *J Neuroradiol.* 2007;34:311–321.

CHAPTER 12

Full-Length Spine—Clinical Correlations With Specific Phenotypes and Measurements With Classification Systems

ANDREW N. SAWIRES[a] • MEGHAN CERPA[b] • LAWRENCE G. LENKE[b]
[a]Department of Orthopaedic Surgery, Lenox Hill Hospital, New York, NY, United States, [b]Department of Orthopaedic Surgery, Columbia University Irving Medical Center, New York, NY, United States

INTRODUCTION

Full-length radiographic spinal imaging is indicated in several clinical scenarios such as screening for congenital abnormalities of the spine, demyelinating processes affecting the spinal cord, scoliosis diagnoses, and trauma as well as many other clinical indications. Abnormalities that arise in early embryologic osseous and neurologic development may foresee the development of spinal deformities. Spinal imaging typically begins with a series of full-length radiographs, including AP, lateral, and supine images. Advanced imaging includes CT scan and MRI imaging, as detailed in earlier sections of this chapter. The purpose of this section is to describe how to accurately perform different radiographic measurements based on plain radiographs, CT imaging, and MRI, and discuss the clinical relevance of these findings.

ANATOMY

A clear and detailed understanding of normal spinal anatomy is important in understanding the possible pathologic entities in spinal deformity. There are four distinct regions of the spine: cervical, thoracic, lumbar, and sacropelvic.[1] In the normal spine, the cervical region consists of seven vertebral segments labeled C1-C7. The thoracic spine has 12 mobile segments: T1-T12. The thoracic ribs from T1 to T10 each have a pair of ribs that are joined anteriorly at the costochondral junction or sternum. T11 and T12 usually have "floating ribs," which are not connected anteriorly to the rib cage. The lumbar spine typically has five mobile segments: L1-L5, except in cases where there is lumbarization or

sacralization of the transitional vertebra.[2] The sacropelvic unit consists of five fused segments of the sacrum that articulate with the ilium through the SI joints bilaterally and the coccyx.

COMMON MEASUREMENTS AND RADIOGRAPHIC PARAMETERS IN FULL-LENGTH SPINE RADIOGRAPHS

Overview of Radiographic and Advanced Spinal Imaging Techniques

Standard full-length spine radiographs for adults are typically taken on 36-in. cassette standing films to assess coronal (AP radiograph) and sagittal plane alignment (lateral radiograph). The patient should be in the standing position with the hips and knees fully extended to limit compensatory realignment from hip and knee flexion.[3] Often, depending on the type of deformity, additional imaging is performed such as supine and/or right and left bending films, which aid in assessing curve flexibility.[4] Assessment of curve flexibility has traditionally been used to select patients who could undergo a selective fusion of only the thoracic component of a double major curve, thus sparing lumbar motion segments.[5] Curve flexibility also allows the surgeon to evaluate structural and nonstructural deformity, and has important implications on deformity classification, which is discussed in more detail later in this chapter. Both supine traction imaging and side bending films are valid methods to assess curve flexibility; side bending films show greater flexibility in the thoracic spine with curves between 50° and 60°, whereas in the lumbar spine both films show equivalent flexibility.[6,7] Additionally, other imaging to assess curve flexibility include push-prone, supine AP, fulcrum-bend (thoracic curve), traction AP, and supine hyperextension crosstable lateral radiographs.[8] Such imaging is important, as patients who had full-length standing spine radiographs preoperatively have been shown to have a significantly lower rate of revision surgery at 5 years postoperatively.[9]

CT scans of the spine provide an excellent visualization of cortical bone and calcifications. Recent techniques to improve the accuracy of screw placement intraoperatively include utilizing low-dose CT scans of the patient's spine to build a virtual model to plan the screw trajectories and a 3D-printed patient-specific guide system to prepare the screw trajectories.[10] Screw misplacement incidence can be as high as 15%–30% in spinal deformity surgery, especially with congenital, revision, or severe deformity cases.[11,12] In patients with severe spinal deformity or multiple prior spinal surgeries, the bony spinal anatomy can be severely altered, which makes freehand pedicle screw placement more challenging. In these cases, 3D-printed spinal models placed in sterile bags and studied intraoperatively have been found to increase the safety of freehand pedicle screw with acceptable accuracy, and no neurological or vascular complications[13]. These patient-specific models can also be used preoperatively to facilitate patient education regarding the specific pathology and planning the surgical procedure.[14,15]

Compared with other modalities, MRI does not use ionizing radiation. MRI also provides better soft tissue contrast and allows direct visualization of the spinal cord, nerve roots, and intervertebral discs. Disorders of the spine that may warrant MRI evaluation include congenital spine and spinal cord malformations, inflammatory disorders, infectious conditions, vascular disorders, degenerative disorders, and neoplastic abnormalities.[16]

Classification Systems
Lenke classification
The spine has a standard characteristic alignment in the coronal and sagittal planes. In the coronal plane, the spine is straight.[17] Scoliosis is defined as the presence of one or more lateral rotatory curves of the spine measured in the coronal and sagittal planes. The most prevalent classification system used for scoliosis is the Lenke classification system. This classification system was developed in 2001 to guide the surgeon in determining appropriate fusion levels by avoiding unnecessary fusion of the nonstructural lumbar or thoracic spine

as well as avoiding undercorrection of the structural secondary curves.[18] This classification scheme improved upon the King classification system by emphasizing the sagittal plane along with the coronal plane while demonstrating good-to-excellent intraobserver and interobserver reliability.[19] The selection of fusion levels is a heavily debated topic in spinal deformity literature. Various measurements taken from the AP radiographs are compared with predetermined numeric values that allow the identification of structural and nonstructural curves. This classification system takes into account the structural, nonstructural curves, shoulder balance, and thoracic kyphosis to determine the upper instrumented and lower instrumented vertebrae. The details of fusion-level selection are beyond the scope of this chapter but can be referred to in the original Lenke et al.'s classification or in subsequent review articles with long-term follow-up discussing the selection of upper and lower instrumented vertebrae for different Lenke curve types.[20-26]

After the Cobb angles (discussed later) are determined for the various curves, the regional curves are then determined, which are defined as the proximal thoracic (PT), main thoracic (MT), and thoracolumbar/lumbar (TL/L) curves. Adult scoliosis in addition to having TL/L curves will often have a fractional lumbosacral (FL) curve below the TL/L curve, defined in the region L4-S1.[27] Identification and treatment of the fractional curve can lead to improved patient outcomes and decreased revision rates in this complicated pathologic process.[27] Each curve is defined by the level of its respective apex. Thoracic curves have the apex located between the T2 and T11-T12 disc, thoracolumbar curves between T12 and L1, and lumbar curves between the L1–2 disc through L4.[28]

To begin classification, the structural or nonstructural quality of each of the three curves must be determined. The major curve will always be the MT or TL/L, whichever is the largest curve. The other two curves in a scoliotic spine are defined as minor curves, which may be defined as structural or nonstructural. Curves are considered structural if they are $\geq 25°$ on the standing AP radiograph and do not bend out to $< 25°$ on the side-bending radiographs.[29,30] Minor curves $< 25°$ on the standing AP radiograph by definition will be nonstructural. However, minor curves may be deemed structural if their regional sagittal profile reveals a kyphosis $\geq +20°$. After determining the structural or nonstructural nature of each regional curve, the Lenke type[1-6] can be assigned according to Fig. 1.

Once the Lenke curve type is assigned, the practitioner can then assign the lumbar modifier (A, B, or C).

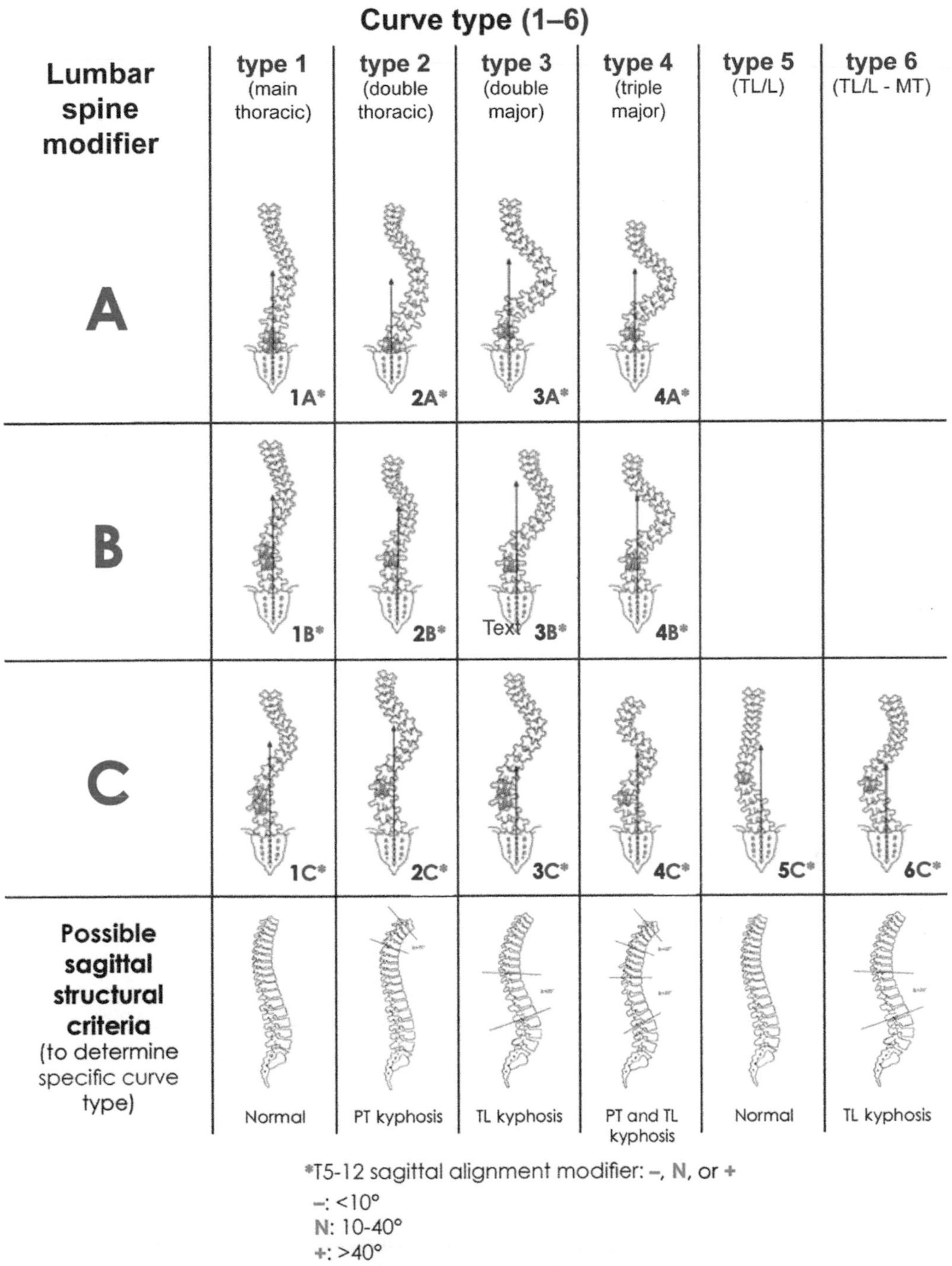

Curve type (1–6)

Lumbar spine modifier	type 1 (main thoracic)	type 2 (double thoracic)	type 3 (double major)	type 4 (triple major)	type 5 (TL/L)	type 6 (TL/L - MT)
A	1A*	2A*	3A*	4A*		
B	1B*	2B*	Text 3B*	4B*		
C	1C*	2C*	3C*	4C*	5C*	6C*
Possible sagittal structural criteria (to determine specific curve type)	Normal	PT kyphosis	TL kyphosis	PT and TL kyphosis	Normal	TL kyphosis

*T5-12 sagittal alignment modifier: –, N, or +

–: <10°
N: 10-40°
+: >40°

FIG. 1 Lenke Curve Classification System.

To perform this assignment, a center sacral vertical line (CSVL) is drawn vertically from the midpoint of S1.[31] If the CSVL passes between the pedicles of the apical lumbar vertebra, the lumbar modifier A is assigned. If the CSVL falls between the medial edge of the pedicle and the lateral edge of the vertebral body, the lumbar modifier B is assigned. If the CSVL does not touch the lateral edge of the apical lumbar vertebra, the lumbar modifier C is assigned.

The thoracic sagittal modifier is added by measuring the sagittal Cobb angle between T5 and T12.[32] If the T5-T12 sagittal Cobb is less than 10 degrees, the sagittal thoracic alignment is considered hypokyphotic and is assigned a minus modifier (−). If the sagittal Cobb is between 10 and 40 degrees, the sagittal alignment is considered normal (N). If the sagittal Cobb measurement between T5 and T12 is greater than 40 degrees, the sagittal alignment is considered hyperkyphotic and is assigned a plus modifier (+).

The Lenke system was developed to guide the practitioner in performing selective fusions, which optimizes mobile segments of the spine in patients with scoliosis. When contemplating fusion levels, radiographic parameters such as curve ratios, Cobb magnitude, apical vertebral translation and rotation, as well as relative flexibility assessments of the two curves, are used.[19,33] In one series looking at selective fusion for Lenke curve types 1–2, minor global imbalance was measured on the long-term follow-up and patients demonstrated good maintenance of curve correction and global balance.[34] However, the benefits of correcting spinal balance must be weighed against the morbidity of performing increasingly extensive surgery. Though thoracolumbar anterior fusions were associated with better radiographic outcomes, SRS-24 Questionnaire data showed no clinical difference between patients fused anteriorly vs. posteriorly.[35]

The Lenke classification system allows for less confusion between surgeons with corresponding surgical fusion guidance and planning. Since the advent of the classification scheme, there has been a significant reduction in the variation of treatment approaches.[36] The reliability of the Lenke curve-type classification is categorized as good-to-excellent by many studies with inter- and intraobserver reliability rates of 86.5% and 87.4%, respectively.[37] Other studies have shown that better radiologic results were achieved through the use of the Lenke classification system for the selection of fusion levels and avoiding undercorrection of the structural secondary curves in Types 2, 3, and 6 Lenke spines.[18]

SRS-Schwab classification

In 2012, Schwab et al. and the SRS published a hybrid classification system which utilized radiographic parameters with patient-reported outcomes to design an adult idiopathic scoliosis classification system[38] (Fig. 2). This hybrid system also includes radiographic pelvic parameters, such as pelvic incidence, lumbar lordosis, pelvic tilt, and sagittal vertical axis, to group the curves into seven curve types and three modifiers accounting for regional sagittal, lumbar degenerative, and global alignment.[38–40] This newer SRS-Schwab classification system improved on the older Schwab classification system by including these spinopelvic parameters linked with pain and disability to establish treatment recommendations.[41] The SRS-Schwab classification system uses frontal and sagittal full-length radiographs to determine coronal curve types and sagittal curve modifiers. This classification scheme is summarized in the table below. The coronal curve types are grouped into one of four types: Type T with a thoracic major curve > 30° and a lumbar curve < 30°, Type L with a lumbar or thoracolumbar major curve > 30°, Type D with a double major curve with each curve > 30°, and Type N (normal) with no coronal curve > 30°.[42]

The first sagittal modifier used in this classification scheme takes into account two radiographic parameters, namely, pelvic incidence and lumbar lordosis, to calculate the difference between the two in order to achieve proper postoperative lumbar alignment.[38] The pelvic incidence minus lumbar lordosis modifier is labeled "0" if the mismatch is < 10°, modifier "+" if it is between 10° and 20°, and modifier "++" if > 20°.

Pelvic tilt is an important sagittal modifier to measure because patients with greater pelvic tilt often need larger corrections to reduce the risk of postoperative failures.[38,41] Patients are classified as pelvic tilt modifier "0" if the measurement is < 20°, modifier "+" if it is between 20° and 30°, and modifier "++" if the pelvic tilt is > 30°.

The last sagittal modifier is the global alignment modifier, which is based off of the sagittal vertical axis (SVA). Patients are classified as having a sagittal vertical axis modifier "0" if the measurement is < 40 mm, modifier "+" if it is 40 to 95 mm, and modifier "++" if > 95 mm.[43]

The SRS-Schwab system focuses on spinopelvic parameters that have been shown to correlate with better health-related quality-of-life (HRQoL) scores after surgery.[41,44] SRS-Schwab classification reflects severity of disease state based on multiple measures of

Coronal curve type	PI mins LL	Global alignment	Pelvic tilt
T: Thoracic only (lumbar curve <30°	0: within 10°	0: SVA <4 cm	0: PT <20°
L: TL/ lumbar only (thoracic curve <30°)	+: moderate 10–20°	+: SVA 4 to 9.5 cm	+: PT 20-30°
D: Double curve (T an TL/L curves >30°)	++ marked >20°	++: SVA >9.5 cm	++: PT>30°
N: No major coronal deformity (all coronal curves <30°)			

FIG. 2 SRS-Schwab Classification System.

(HRQoL); those with worse modifier grades required more extensive surgery to correct the deformity.[45] Recent studies have also shown that the SRS-Schwab classification system can predict patient disability and guide preference for nonoperative versus operative treatment decisions based on the preoperative sagittal spinopelvic alignment.[46,47] Patients with thoracolumbar and primary sagittal deformities had worse outcomes and greater disability than other curve types.[40] These studies also found operative managed patients to have worse spinopelvic modifier grades than nonoperative patients with increasingly worse grades correlating with worsening HRQoL scores. Inter- and intraobserver reliability rates for the SRS-Schwab classification system are high and have been shown to be consistent in predicting prognosis and guiding treatment decisions for surgeons.[44,48] The SRS-Schwab system has great utility in regard to treatment decisions and prognostic information.

Roussouly spinal shape classification
The Roussouly classification developed in 2003 describes four common variants in lumbar lordosis by classifying the sagittal profile and the spinopelvic alignment[49,50] (Fig. 3). Type 1 and 2 spinal shapes have a low sacral slope defined as < 35°. *Type 1* spines are characterized as a nonharmonious back with thoracolumbar kyphosis and short hyperlordosis. *Type 2* is characterized by a longer and flatter distal arch, close to a straight line. It is a harmonious flat back. *Type 3* variants have *a* mean sacral slope between 35° and 45°. It is a harmonious regular back. *Type 4* consists of spines with a high sacral slope > 45°. The distal arch has an increased angle and number of vertebrae; it is a harmonious hypercurved back.

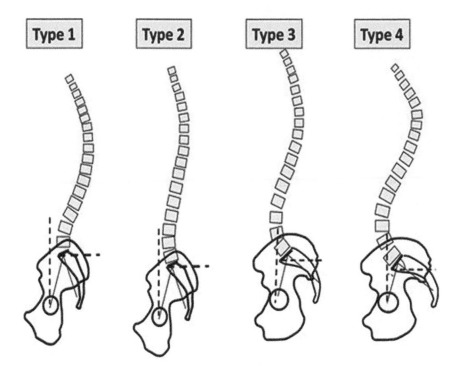

FIG. 3 Subdivision of the sagittal spinal curvatures according to the Roussouly Classification System.

Depending on the type of classification, different degenerative changes of the spine can be predicted based on the mechanical stresses according to the geometry of the lordosis and spine balance. These different stresses include both sliding forces parallel to the endplate and pressure forces perpendicular to the endplate.[49] An understanding of how different types of spinopelvic complexes can lead to different patterns of degenerative spine disease may help the surgeon tailor the treatment strategy for his or her patient.

The Roussouly classification allows the surgeon to form a correlation in shape and positioning, and form and function, between the pelvis and the spine. Patients with a low-grade PI need a restoration of Type 1 or 2 spine type, without increasing the lordosis. With increasing pelvic incidence, additional lumbar lordosis has to be augmented in angle and length, to reduce the posterior tilt of the pelvis.[50] Patients who both matched Roussouly sagittal spinal type and improved in SRS-Schwab modifiers had superior patient-reported outcomes at 1 year. Utilizing both classification systems in surgical decision-making can optimize postop patient outcomes.[51]

Spondylolisthesis classification
Spondylolisthesis is defined as the anterior, posterior, or lateral translation of one vertebral body relative to an adjacent level. When a slipped vertebra is identified, further assessment is warranted to determine the stability between two adjacent levels.[52] To measure the subluxation, the distance technique can be used to measure the degree of subluxation in millimeters. The most prevalent grading system for spondylolisthesis is the Meyerding classification, which divides the superior endplate of the caudal vertebra into four quarters[53] (Fig. 4).

Vertebral rotation classification
Measurement of vertebral rotation is of key significance in the prognosis and treatment of scoliotic curves. This variable has been shown to be related to curve progression, thus being clinically applicable for both preoperative and postoperative assessment.[54,55] Furthermore, knowledge of vertebral rotation can decrease the risk of pedicle screw misplacement, which may lead to spinal cord injury.[56] The different classification methods for vertebral rotation include ones described by Cobb, Nash and Moe, Perdriolle, Stokes, Aaro-Dahlborn, and Ho et al. (Fig. 5). These classification schemes are discussed at length later in this chapter.

In the following sections, various measurements that can be obtained from the full-length spinal radiographs and advanced imaging will be discussed in detail.

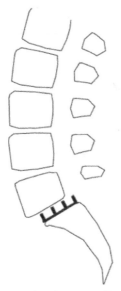

FIG. 4 A depiction of a Meyerding Grade 1 slip of L5 on S1. Note how the sacrum is divided into four quadrants for the five grades of the Meyerding Classification System.

Coronal Alignment and Radiographic Measurements

Cobb angle

The Cobb angle is the most widely used measurement to quantify the magnitude of spinal deformities measured on radiographs.[57] To measure the Cobb angle, the end vertebrae of the curve deformity are chosen for each curve segment that exists. End vertebrae are the most tilted vertebrae at the cephalad and caudal ends of a curve. Lines are then drawn along the endplates, and the angle between the intersection of the two lines is then measured[58] (Fig. 6). In cases where the lines will not intersect on the film or monitor, two lines at right angles to the previous lines can be drawn and the angle between these new lines measured (Fig. 6). Some caution should be used during Cobb angle measurement, which has approximately a 5–10 degree intraobserver and interobserver variation.[59] It is also important to keep rotation in mind, as minor rotation of patients between examinations can significantly change measurements.[60] The severity of thoracic and lumbar Cobb angles is correlated with an increased progression of spinal deformity.[61] Bracing is typically initiated for curves greater than 25 degrees, while surgical intervention is typically pursued for curves measuring more than 45 degrees.[62,63]

Instrumented vertebra tilt angle

The upper instrumented vertebra (UIV) tilt angle is measured by drawing a line along the cephalad endplate of the UIV. A second line is drawn perpendicular to the vertical edge of the radiograph and intersects Line A at the edge of the UIV. When the left edge of the vertebral body is up, the tilt angle is defined as positive.[64] This measurement was found to be an important postoperative radiological parameter that has a significant correlation with postoperative neck and medial shoulder imbalance and measures of T1 tilt and cervical axis measurement.[20] The lower instrumented vertebra (LIV) is measured similarly, using a line drawn along the caudal endplate of the LIV and a line perpendicular to the vertical edge of the radiograph. Smaller UIVDiff (difference between postoperative UIV tilt and preoperative optimal UIV tilt) angles are associated with better lateral shoulder balance.[65]

T1 tilt angle

The T1 tilt angle is an angle formed by a line drawn between a horizontal line and the superior endplate of T1 or along the zenith of both first ribs if the T1 endplate is not well visualized (Fig. 7). This measurement has been found to have a moderate positive correlation with SVA (dens) and can be used as a good predictor of overall sagittal balance.[66] When the T1 tilt was higher than 25°, all patients in the series by Knott et al.[66] had at least 10 cm of positive sagittal imbalance and patients with negative sagittal balance had mostly low T1 tilt values, usually below 13° of angulation.

Clavicle angle

The clavicle angle is an angle drawn between a horizontal reference line and clavicle horizontal reference line (CHRL), which is drawn perpendicular to the lateral edge of the radiograph and touches the most cephalad portion of the elevated clavicle and a line which touches the most cephalad aspect of both the right and left clavicles (clavicle reference line)[67] (Fig. 8). Angles in which the left shoulder up are positive and angles with the right shoulder up are negative. This directionality is consistent with that of the T1 tilt angle described earlier. Clavicle tilt has been shown in some studies to have an association with postoperative shoulder imbalance.[67]

Radiographic shoulder height

Radiographic shoulder height is defined as the distance measured in millimeters between the superior horizontal reference line (SHRL) and the inferior horizontal reference line (IHRL)[68] (Fig. 9). The SHRL passes through

Method	Method description	Diagram
Cobb [24]	The vertebral body is divided into six sections; the region in which the spinous process is sligned determines the grade assigned	Position of spinous process A B C D beyond D Grading 0 1+ 2+ 3+ 4+
Nash-Moe [25]	The percentage displacement of the convex pedicle with respect to the vertebral body width is used to approximate the angle of vertebral rotation	Percentage displacement 0% 50% 100% Approximate rotation angle 0° 50° 100°
Perdriolle [10]	The edges of the nomogram are aligned with innermost points on the vertebral margin (A and B); rotation angle is read from a vertical line drawn through the convex pedicle (C)	
Stokes [27]	The projected distances of both pedicles from the vertebral center (a and b) are measured from the radiographic film; fixed width-to-depth ratios for each vertebral level is applied to Stokes' formula to determine rotation angle	$$\tan \theta = \frac{w}{2d} \times \frac{a-b}{a+b}$$

FIG. 5 A summary of common radiographic methods of vertebral rotation measurement.

Method	Method description	Diagram
Aaro-Dahlborm [38]	Line AB joins the anterior midline of body (A) and dorsal central aspect of vertebral foramen (B); line BC runs through the midline of the vertebral body; rotation angle is the angle between these two lines	
Ho et al. [39]	Inner surface of the junction between the two laminae (C); two points between the pedicle and laminae (B); line AC bisects the angle CBC; rotation angle is that between the biseeting line and the vertical (ACV)	

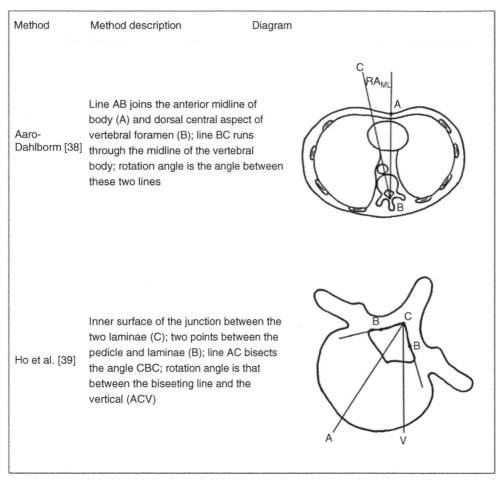

FIG. 5, CONT'D

the intersection of the soft tissue shadow of the shoulder and a line drawn vertically up from the acromial clavicular joint of the cephalad shoulder. The IHRL is a similar line drawn over the caudal acromial clavicular joint. The distance the linear distance between these two reference lines is measured in millimeters and defined as positive if the left shoulder is up and negative if the right shoulder is up. Again, by convention, left up is always positive and right up is always negative.

Thoracic trunk shift
Thoracic trunk shift is measured on standing PA or AP full-length spine films. Once the apical thoracic vertebra is identified, a horizontal reference line is drawn through the center of the vertebra and extending to the right and left rib cages.[69] The midpoint of the reference line is marked and a perpendicular line

is dropped as a vertical trunk reference line (VTRL). Trunk shift is then calculated by measuring the linear distance in millimeters between the VTRL and the CSVL (Fig. 10). A trunk shift to the right of the CSVL is a positive value, and to the left of the CSVL a negative value. Trunk shift is a spinal imbalance in which the thorax is not centered over the pelvis. LIV selection and ratio of MT to TL/L curve are highly correlated with the onset of postoperative trunk shift in Lenke Type 1C curves.[70]

Pelvic obliquity
Pelvic obliquity can be measured using several different reference points and a horizontal reference line. The tips or sulcus of the sacral ala can be used to create the pelvic coronal reference line (PCRL) for the pelvic orientation in the coronal plane. An angle

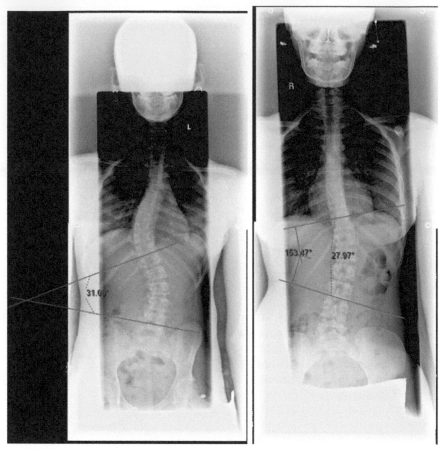

FIG. 6 Cobb angle measurement of a thoracolumbar curve.

between this line and a horizontal reference line is then measured[71,72] (Fig. 11). Alternatively, the top of the ilium may be used to create the PCRL. Leg length discrepancy (LLD) is measured using PA standing radiographs without blocks under the patient's feet and with the knees extended.[73] A femoral horizontal reference line (FHRL) will be created by making a horizontal line that is tangent to the top of the highest femoral head or at the level of the lesser trochanter. The difference between the height of this line and the height of the lower femoral head is then measured as the LLD. If the left hip is up, the value is positive (+). If the right hip is up, then the value will be negative (−). Poorer clinical outcomes have been associated with sagittal (C7-SVA, PT, LL, sagittal LIVDA) and/or coronal imbalance (C7-CSVL, shoulder-tilt, and pelvic obliquity).[74]

Sacral obliquity

Sacral obliquity is defined as a tilt in the sacral endplate secondary to an intrinsic sacral deformity. This deformity, along with pelvic obliquity described earlier and leg length discrepancy, can cause coronal tilting of the sacral endplate and contribute to thoracolumbar/lumbar scoliosis.[72,75] Sacral is measured in relation to the femoral head reference line (FHRL). Once the FHRL is drawn, a line is drawn perpendicular to the FHRL (line 2). Next, a line is drawn along the coronal projection of the S1 endplate on a Ferguson AP of the sacrum. Lastly, a parallel line to the FHRL is drawn at the intersection of the sacral endplate line and its intersection with line 2. The angle subtended between this line and the line drawn along the coronal projection of the S1 endplate is the sacral obliquity angle (a°) (Fig. 12). The angle

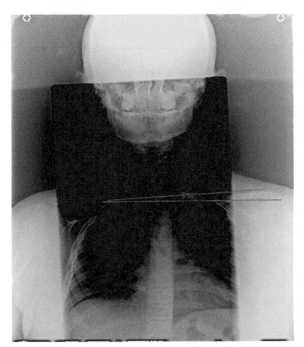

FIG. 7 Alternative Cobb measurement using perpendicular lines.

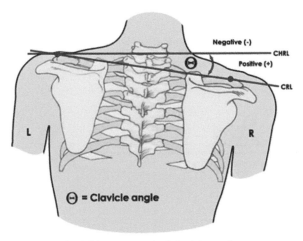

FIG. 8 Measurement of clavicle angle.

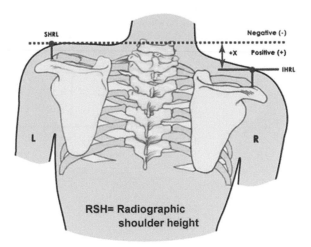

FIG. 9 Measurement of radiographic shoulder height.

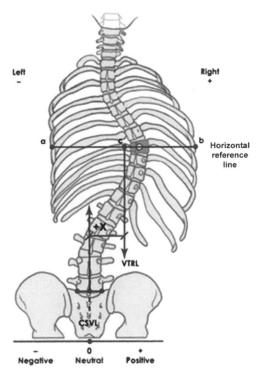

FIG. 10 Measurement of thoracic trunk shift.

Sagittal Alignment and Radiographic Measurements

In the sagittal plane, the spine is lordotic in the cervical and lumbar regions and kyphotic in the thoracic region.[76] Thoracolumbar sagittal alignment is measured from the upper endplate of T10 to the lower endplate of L2. By convention, kyphosis is a positive angle and

is positive if the left side of the sacrum is high and negative if the right side of the sacrum is high. If the FHRL is not horizontal to the floor, the sacral obliquity may be secondary to both leg length discrepancy and intrinsic sacral obliquity.

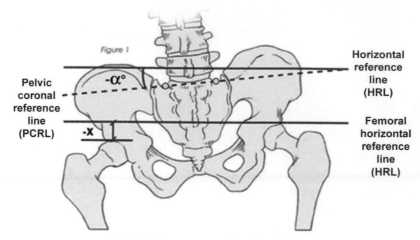

FIG. 11 Measurement of pelvic obliquity.

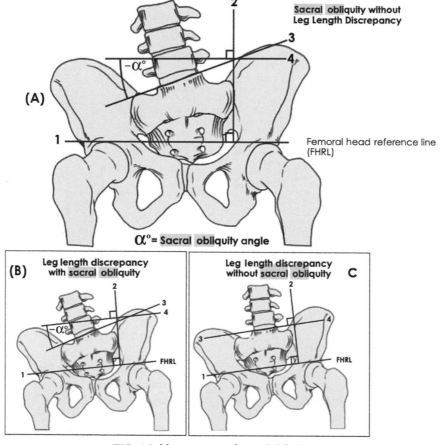

FIG. 12 Measurement of sacral obliquity.

lordosis is a negative angle. Lumbar sagittal alignment is measured from the upper endplate of T12 to the endplate of S1. There is a wide range of normal sagittal profiles for each region. In the cervical spine, acceptable lordosis is 40° ±9.7°.[77] Thoracic kyphosis is approximately between 20° and 50°, and the lumbar spine should have approximately 40 to 60° of lordosis.[78,79] The lumbar spine should have 30° more lordosis than thoracic kyphosis.

Sagittal balance

Imbalance in the sagittal plane is defined as radiographic sagittal imbalance of more than 5 cm.[80] To determine this, a line is drawn from the middle of the body of the C7 vertebra. This line should pass through within 2 cm of the posterosuperior corner of the S1 vertebral body.[81] The position of this line is then termed positive, neutral, or negative. If the plumb line passes more than 2 cm in front of the posterosuperior corner of the S1 vertebral body, the spine has positive (+) sagittal balance, within 2 cm is termed neutral balance, and if plumb line passes more than 2 cm behind the posterosuperior corner of the S1 vertebral body, the spine has a negative sagittal balance (Fig. 13).

Lumbar lordosis

Lumbar lordosis is the measurement of the sagittal Cobb angle between the superior endplate of S1 and the superior endplate of L1. In order to measure this parameter, two parallel lines to these two endplates are drawn and the angle measured between these two lines is calculated (Fig. 14).

Pelvic incidence

Pelvic incidence (PI) is the angle between[1] a line perpendicular to the midpoint of the sacral endplate and[2] the center of the femoral head. In radiographs where the femoral heads are not perfectly superimposed, the center of each femoral head is marked and a line is drawn that connects the centers of the femoral heads. The midpoint of this line is then used instead of the center of the femoral head to determine the pelvic incidence (Fig. 15).

Pelvic tilt

Pelvic tilt is a measure of the degree of pelvic retroversion. To measure this angle, a vertical reference line (VRL) originating from the center of the femoral head is drawn. The angle is defined as the angle between

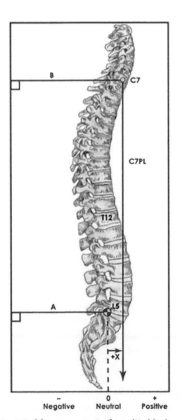

FIG. 13 Measurement of sagittal balance.

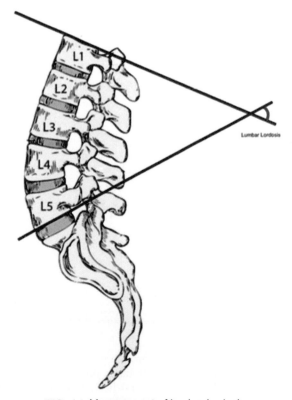

FIG. 14 Measurement of lumbar lordosis.

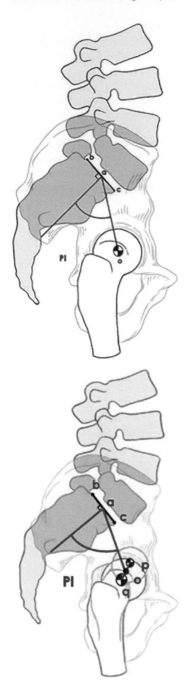

FIG. 15 Measurement of pelvic incidence when femoral heads are not superimposed.

this line and a line drawn through the midpoint of the sacral endplate (Fig. 16). PT has a positive (+) value when line between the femoral head and sacral endplate is posterior to the VRL and a negative (−) value when this line is anterior to the VRL.

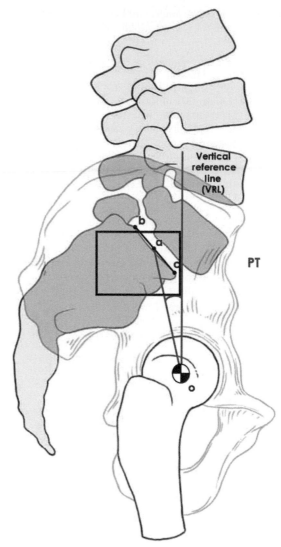

FIG. 16 Measurement of pelvic tilt.

Sacral slope

Sacral slope (SS) is defined as the angle between a horizontal reference line (HRL) and the sacral endplate line. PI is measured from static anatomic structures and does not change with patient position (Fig. 17). PT and SS, on the other hand, vary in relation to patient positions because these measurements are dependent on the angular position of the sacrum/pelvis with the femoral heads.[82,83]

Sagittal vertical axis

The sagittal vertical axis (SVA) is defined as the length of a horizontal line connecting the posterior superior sacral endplate to a vertical plumb line dropped from

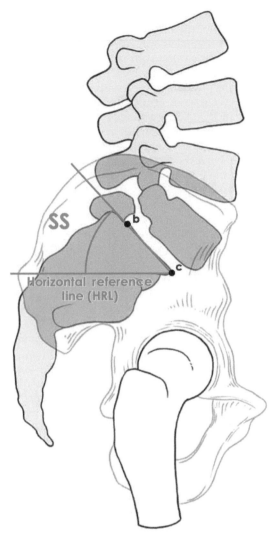

FIG. 17 Measurement of sacral slope.

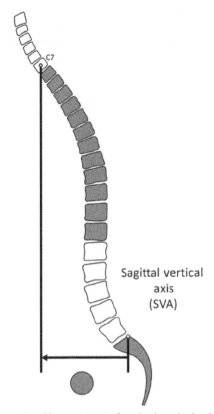

FIG. 18 Measurement of sagittal vertical axis.

the center of the C7 vertebral body[84] (Fig. 18). This measurement is posture dependent.

Spondylolisthesis

Other measurements of vertebral irregularities include subluxations of one vertebra relative to the next. All olistheses (spondylo, retro, rotatory, or lateral) are described relative to the upper vertebra in relation to the lower vertebra.[29,85] In the coronal plane, subluxations are often identified in degenerative scoliosis. Lateral subluxations are measured in millimeters. To measure the subluxation, a vertical line is drawn from the superior corner of the caudal vertebra and the inferior corner of the cephalad vertebra. The horizontal distance between these two vertical lines will define the degree

of subluxation in millimeters. If osteophytes impede this measurement, the waist of the respective vertebrae can be used instead. Sagittal plane subluxations are often identified in degenerative adult scoliosis. These may be spondylolisthesis (anterolisthesis or retrolisthesis). These subluxations are measured in millimeters from the posterior inferior corner of the cephalad vertebra to the posterior superior corner of the caudal vertebra. Anterolisthesis is recorded as a positive number, and retrolisthesis is recorded as a negative number. The most prevalent grading system for anterolisthesis is the Meyerding classification described in 1932.[86] In this grading system, superior endplate of the vertebra below is divided into four quarters. The grade depends on the location of the posteroinferior corner of the vertebra above: grade I: 0%–25%, grade II: 26%–50%, grade III: 51%–75%, grade IV: 76%–100%, and grade V (spondyloptosis): > 100% displacement of the superior vertebra.

Vertebral Rotation

The earliest recorded technique used for measuring vertebral rotation is the Cobb method. Cobb's method is valuable in being simple to use and requiring no additional patient exposure to radiation.[87,88] In this grading scheme, the vertebral body is divided into six sections; the region in which the spinous process is aligned determines the grade assigned.[89] The grading scheme is limited to five grades and does not allow quantification of the angle of axial rotation. Thus, the measurements can be inaccurate for severe scoliotic cases with intravertebral rotation.[55,90] Despite these criticisms, the concept of measuring axial rotation using vertebral landmarks from anteroposterior radiographs was adopted by many newer methods and remains popular in clinical settings.

The most prevalent classification system for pedicle rotation is the Nash and Moe method of determining vertebral rotation clinically.[91] The apical vertebral body is divided into six equal segments longitudinally. When both pedicles are in view, there is no vertebral rotation. It is graded as "0." When the pedicle is at the edge of the vertebral body, it is graded as "1." When the pedicle disappears, it is graded as "2." When the contralateral pedicle is in the midline of the vertebra, it is graded as "3." When it crosses the midline of the vertebra, it is graded as "4." One drawback of this classification technique is that it can only provide a rough approximation of axial rotation. The use of a single anatomical landmark limits accurate measurements to small rotations.[92] This was demonstrated in a study by Ho et al., where Nash and Moe grade 0 vertebra determined by radiograph was measured as a rotation of up to 11° determined by CT scans.[93]

The Perdriolle method for measuring vertebral rotation uses a torsion meter. On an AP radiograph, the edges of a nomogram are directly aligned with the innermost points of the lateral walls of the vertebral body, a vertical line is then drawn through the convex pedicle, and the rotation angle is read from a torsion meter.[89] Advantages of the Perdriolle method using the torsion meter include that it is affordable, noninvasive, and simple to use, making it applicable in clinical settings.[94–96] A single AP radiograph to perform the measurements minimizes patient exposure to harmful radiation. This method has been found to be fairly accurate with an individual observer error of approximately 6° and 98% of intraobserver measurements fell within ± 5°.[97] A 2-mm error in visualizing the pedicles has been found to correlate with 5° of rotation.[94]

The Stokes method involves taking two radiographic images, AP and lateral, to obtain measurement of vertebral dimensions. The distances from both pedicles to the vertebral center are measured from the radiographs, and labeled as width and depth. The fixed width-to-depth ratios for each vertebral level is then applied to Stokes formula shown in the figure to determine the rotation angle. This method allows the interpreter to account for vertebral asymmetry and dimension by determining pedicle offset with respect to a center point rather than the vertebral edges.[98] Stokes method is a well-described technique for measuring vertebral rotation; however, it has a significant deviation for rotation greater than 5°.[99,100] The geometry of scoliotic vertebrae can vary greatly among individuals, and the accuracy of calculations obtained from the Stokes formula can vary significantly in severely distorted vertebrae.

The use of CT technology to grade vertebral rotation began with the Aaro-Dahlborn. In comparison with radiography, CT produces clearer and more detailed images that allow landmarks to be easily identified. To calculate the rotation using this method, a line is drawn along the midline of the body in the sagittal plane. A second line is drawn along the midline of the vertebral body, and the rotation angle is defined as the angle between these two lines.[89] Disadvantages of using CT scan measurements to quantify the degree of rotation include the supine position required for CT scans, which reduces the Cobb angle, rotation angle, and rib hump, which can underrepresent true rotation.[101,102] CT scans also require greater time and involve greater patient exposure to ionizing radiation, particularly in the thoracolumbar region.[103] Among other CT methods discussed later, the Aaro-Dahlborn method reached measurements with greater correlation with the actual rotation value, even with tilt in the sagittal and coronal planes.[102] In separate studies, the Aaro-Dahlborn method was found to be more difficult to use for inexperienced observers with higher intraobserver and interobserver errors when compared with other CT measurement techniques.[101,104]

The method by Ho et al. determines rotation from CT scans using the laminae and laminae junction. To calculate the vertebral rotation using this method, the inner surface of the junction between the two laminae is marked. Two lines are then drawn along the pedicles and laminae to this point. A bisecting line is drawn between these three points. The rotation angle is the angle formed between the bisecting line and the vertical.[105] Ho et al.'s method has showed results reported as high as a 95% clinical success rate and 1.2° error ratio compared with the methods described earlier.[106] While both Aaro-Dahlborn and Ho et al.'s methods proved clinically applicable and accurate, the study also showed that interobserver reliability was significantly better in the latter technique.[104]

Corrections in vertebral rotation have been associated with postoperative coronal balance and improved clinical outcomes.[107] Koller et al. demonstrated that C7-CSVL, shoulder-tilt, pelvic obliquity, and vertebral rotation (measured by the Nash and Moe method) were correlated with clinical outcomes.[74]

CLINICAL CORRELATIONS IN SPINAL PHENOTYPES

Classification systems have many useful clinical benefits, including standardizing diagnoses across practices, guiding surgical management, and also allowing physicians to predict clinical outcomes. The added benefit of many of these classification systems discussed in this chapter is that there is strong data showing that the severity of the deformity measured on diagnostic imaging is associated with adverse clinical outcomes. Many of these clinical correlations have been described in detail in the previous text.

In general, postoperative pain is related to alterations of sagittal balance and spinopelvic angulation.[108] Increasing SVA in standing subjects leads to a posterior pelvic shift in relation to the feet.[109] A SVA greater than 4.7 cm has been found to be associated with significantly increased disability.[110] SRS-24 Questionnaire results showed inferior pain, self-image, and function subset scores for patients with postoperative coronal imbalances, indicating that postoperative balance is important in improving patient outcomes.[35] Other studies have shown global sagittal balance and loss of lumbar lordosis to be independent predictors of disability and pain associated with deformity in adults.[111,112] In addition, a high pelvic incidence has been shown to be a predicting factor of sagittal imbalance after spinal fusion and requires more lumbar correction for sagittal balance.[113,114]

Individual vertebral relationships also have been found to have an impact on clinical outcomes. High-grade spondylolisthesis and the resulting spinopelvic misalignment in the sagittal plane can result in global sagittal imbalance of the whole body in the upright standing position.[115] Vertebral slip results in compensatory chances in pelvic version, contributing to sagittal imbalance.[41] Correction of the vertebral slip and sagittal imbalance results in favorable impacts on patient-reported pain levels.[108,116] Vertebral rotation and lateral spondylolisthesis have been established to be sources of mechanical lower back pain in these patients as well.[117]

One must also keep in mind the impact of age on spinopelvic alignment. In one study looking at age-specific ideal alignment, it was found that older patients had greater compensation, more degenerative loss of lordosis, and were more pitched forward.[118] The authors concluded that younger patients require more

stringent alignment objectives. This is a recent finding, and more research needs to be performed in this domain in order to improve outcomes in postoperative alignment and clinical outcomes.

CONCLUSION

Given the prevalence of spinal deformity in modern spine surgery, an understanding of appropriate imaging techniques and the clinical relevance of classification schemes can assist the surgeon in preoperative surgical planning and postoperative follow-up. The methods outlined in this chapter are useful for routine clinical practice and have applications in research as well. At this present point in time, the sheer volume of imaging techniques highlights the importance of imaging assessments and the amount of information provided through plain radiographs. It is likely that the techniques outlined here will see continued use in deformity spine surgery and that new approaches will continue to emerge in the future.

REFERENCES

1. Thieme E-Books & E-Journals. Accessed January 22, 2020 https://www.thieme-connect.de/products/ebooks/book/10.1055/b-002-44926.
2. Castellvi AE, Goldstein LA, Chan DP. Lumbosacral transitional vertebrae and their relationship with lumbar extradural defects. *Spine (Phila Pa 1976)*. 1984;9:493–495. PubMed - NCBI. Accessed January 22, 2020 https://www.ncbi.nlm.nih.gov/pubmed/6495013.
3. Woodhull AM, Maltrud K, Mello BL. Alignment of the human body in standing. *Eur J Appl Physiol Occup Physiol*. 1985;54(1):109–115. SpringerLink. Accessed April 10, 2020 https://link.springer.com/article/10.1007/BF00426309.
4. Bunch JT, Glassman SD, Underwood HR, et al. Preoperative full-length standing radiographs and revision rates in lumbar degenerative scoliosis. *J Neurosurg Spine*. 2018;28(6):581–585. https://doi.org/10.3171/2017.10.SPINE17638.
5. King HA, Moe JH, Bradford DS, Winter RB. The selection of fusion levels in thoracic idiopathic scoliosis. *J Bone Joint Surg Am*. 1983;65:1302–1313. PubMed - NCBI. Accessed April 3, 2020 https://www.ncbi.nlm.nih.gov/pubmed/6654943.
6. Hirsch C, Ilharreborde B, Mazda K. Flexibility analysis in adolescent idiopathic scoliosis on side-bending images using the EOS imaging system. *Orthop Traumatol Surg Res*. 2016;102(4):495–500. https://doi.org/10.1016/j.otsr.2016.01.021.
7. Polly DWJ, Sturm PF. Traction versus supine side bending: which technique best determines curve flexibility? *Spine*. 1998;23(7):804–808.

8. Chapman MW, James MA. *Chapman's Comprehensive Orthopaedic Surgery: Four Volume Set.* JP Medical Ltd; 2019.

9. Preoperative full-length standing radiographs and revision rates in lumbar degenerative scoliosis. *J Neurosurg Spine.* 2018;28(6). https://thejns.org/spine/view/journals/j-neurosurg-spine/28/6/article-p581.xml. Accessed 4 March 2020.

10. Cecchinato R, Berjano P, Zerbi A, Damilano M, Redaelli A, Lamartina C. Pedicle screw insertion with patient-specific 3D-printed guides based on low-dose CT scan is more accurate than free-hand technique in spine deformity patients: a prospective, randomized clinical trial. *Eur Spine J.* 2019;28(7):1712–1723. https://doi.org/10.1007/s00586-019-05978-3.

11. Bhagat S, Vozar V, Lutchman L, Crawford RJ, Rai AS. Morbidity and mortality in adult spinal deformity surgery: Norwich Spinal Unit experience. *Eur Spine J.* 2013;22:42–46. SpringerLink. Accessed April 3, 2020 https://link.springer.com/article/10.1007/s00586-012-2627-y.

12. Sciubba DM, Yurter A, Smith JS, et al. A comprehensive review of complication rates after surgery for adult deformity: a reference for informed consent. *Spine Deform.* 2015;3(6):575–594. https://doi.org/10.1016/j.jspd.2015.04.005.

13. Tan LA, Yerneni K, Tuchman A, et al. Utilization of the 3D-printed spine model for freehand pedicle screw placement in complex spinal deformity correction. *J Spine Surg.* 2018;4(2):319–327. https://doi.org/10.21037/jss.2018.05.16.

14. Liew Y, Beveridge E, Demetriades AK, Hughes MA. Full article: 3D printing of patient-specific anatomy: a tool to improve patient consent and enhance imaging interpretation by trainees. *Br J Neurosurg.* 2015;29:712–714. Accessed April 3, 2020 https://www.tandfonline.com/doi/full/10.3109/02688697.2015.1026799.

15. Pacione D, Tanweer O, Berman P, Harter DH. The utility of a multimaterial 3D printed model for surgical planning of complex deformity of the skull base and craniovertebral junction. *J Neurosurg.* 2016;125(5):1194–1197. https://doi.org/10.3171/2015.12.JNS151936.

16. American College of Radiology. ACR practice parameter for performing and interpreting magnetic resonance imaging (MRI). 2011. Available at: https://www.acr.org/-/media/ACR/Files/Practice-Parameters/MR-PerfInterpret.pdf.

17. Vrtovec T, Pernuš F, Likar B. A review of methods for quantitative evaluation of spinal curvature. *Eur Spine J.* 2009;18:593–607. SpringerLink. Accessed February 23, 2020 https://link.springer.com/article/10.1007/s00586-009-0913-0.

18. Puno RM, An K-C, Puno RL, Jacob A, Chung S-S. Treatment recommendations for idiopathic scoliosis: an assessment of the Lenke classification. *Spine.* 2003;28(18):2102–2114. discussion 2114-2115 https://doi.org/10.1097/01.BRS.0000088480.08179.35.

19. Lenke LG, Betz RR, Harms J, et al. Adolescent idiopathic scoliosis: a new classification to determine extent of spinal arthrodesis. *J Bone Joint Surg Am.* 2001;83(8):1169–1181.

20. Chan CYW, Chiu CK, Ler XY, et al. Upper instrumented vertebrae (UIV) tilt angle is an important postoperative radiological parameter that correlates with postoperative neck and medial shoulder imbalance. *Spine.* 2018;43(19):E1143–E1151. https://doi.org/10.1097/BRS.0000000000002645.

21. Oba H, Takahashi J, Kobayashi S, et al. Upper instrumented vertebra to the right of the lowest instrumented vertebra as a predictor of an increase in the main thoracic curve after selective posterior fusion for the thoracolumbar/lumbar curve in Lenke type 5C adolescent idiopathic scoliosis: multicenter study on the relationship between fusion area and surgical outcome. *J Neurosurg Spine.* 2019;1–8. https://doi.org/10.3171/2019.5.SPINE181469. Published online August 23.

22. Chan CYW, Chiu CK, Kwan MK. Assessing the flexibility of the proximal thoracic segments above the "potential upper instrumented vertebra" using the cervical supine side bending radiographs in Lenke 1 and 2 curves for adolescent idiopathic scoliosis patients. *Spine.* 2016;41(16):E973–E980. https://doi.org/10.1097/BRS.0000000000001516.

23. Ketenci IE, Yanik HS, Ulusoy A, Demiroz S, Erdem S. Lowest instrumented vertebrae selection for posterior fusion of lenke 5C adolescent idiopathic scoliosis: can we stop the fusion one level proximal to lower-end vertebra? *Indian J Orthop.* 2018;52(6):657–664. https://doi.org/10.4103/ortho.IJOrtho_579_16.

24. Bai J, Chen K, Wei Q, et al. Selecting the LSTV as the lower instrumented vertebra in the treatment of lenke types 1A and 2A adolescent idiopathic scoliosis: a minimal 3-year follow-up. *Spine.* 2018;43(7):E390–E398. https://doi.org/10.1097/BRS.0000000000002375.

25. Cao K, Watanabe K, Kawakami N, et al. Selection of lower instrumented vertebra in treating Lenke type 2A adolescent idiopathic scoliosis. *Spine.* 2014;39(4):E253–E261. https://doi.org/10.1097/BRS.0000000000000126.

26. Ishikawa M, Nishiyama M, Kamata M. Selective thoracic fusion for king-moe type II/lenke 1C curve in adolescent idiopathic scoliosis: a comprehensive review of major concerns. *Spine Surg Relat Res.* 2018. PubMed - NCBI. Accessed April 2, 2020 https://www.ncbi.nlm.nih.gov/pubmed/31435563.

27. Campbell PG, Nunley PD. The challenge of the lumbosacral fractional curve in the setting of adult degenerative scoliosis. *Neurosurg Clin N Am.* 2018;29(3):467–474. https://doi.org/10.1016/j.nec.2018.02.004.

28. Benzel EC. *Spine Surgery 2-Vol Set E-Book: Techniques, Complication Avoidance, and Management (Expert Consult - Online).* Elsevier Health Sciences; 2012.

29. Oref, Sdsg-Radiographic-Measuremnt-Manual.pdf. n.d. Accessed April 10, 2020. https://www.oref.org/docs/default-source/default-document-library/sdsg-radiographic-measuremnt-manual.pdf.

30. Jada A, Mackel CE, Hwang SW, et al. Evaluation and management of adolescent idiopathic scoliosis: a review. *Neurosurg Focus.* 2017;43(4). https://thejns.org/focus/view/journals/neurosurg-focus/43/4/article-pE2.xml. Accessed 10 April 2020.

31. Kubat O, Ovadia D. Frontal and sagittal imbalance in patients with adolescent idiopathic deformity. *Ann Transl Med.* 2020;8. Accessed April 11, 2020 https://www.ncbi.nlm.nih.gov/pmc/articles/PMC6995921/.

32. El-Fiky T, Elsagheer H, Darwish M, et al. The sagittal thoracic modifier component of the lenke classification system in moderate and severe adolescent idiopathic scoliosis. *Clin Spine Surg.* 2019;32:E266–E271. Accessed April 11, 2020 https://journals.lww.com/jspinaldisorders/Citation/2019/07000/The_Sagittal_Thoracic_Modifier_Component_of_the.8.aspx.

33. Sanders AE, Baumann R, Brown H, Johnston CE, Lenke LG, Sink E. Selective anterior fusion of thoracolumbar/lumbar curves in adolescents: when can the associated thoracic curve be left unfused? *Spine.* 2003;28:706–713. Abstract - Europe PMC. Accessed April 8, 2020 https://europepmc.org/article/med/12671359.

34. Lenke LG, Edwards CCI, Bridwell KH. The lenke classification of adolescent idiopathic scoliosis: how it organizes curve patterns as a template to perform selective fusions of the spine. *Spine.* 2003;28(20S):S199. https://doi.org/10.1097/01.BRS.0000092216.16155.33.

35. Haher TR, Gorup JM, Shin TM, et al. Results of the scoliosis research society instrument for evaluation of surgical outcome in adolescent idiopathic scoliosis: a multicenter study of 244 patients. *Spine.* 1999;24(14):1435.

36. Clements DH, Marks M, Newton PO, et al. Did the lenke classification change scoliosis treatment? *Spine.* 2011;36(14):1142–1145. https://doi.org/10.1097/BRS.0b013e318207e9c4.

37. Qiu G, Li Q, Wang Y, et al. Comparison of reliability between the PUMC and lenke classification systems for classifying adolescent idiopathic scoliosis. *Spine.* 2008;33:836–842. Accessed June 21, 2020 https://journals.lww.com/spinejournal/Abstract/2008/10150/Comparison_of_Reliability_Between_the_PUMC_and.27.aspx.

38. Schwab F, Ungar B, Blondel B, et al. Scoliosis Research Society-Schwab adult spinal deformity classification: a validation study. *Spine.* 2012;37(12):1077–1082. PubMed - NCBI. Accessed April 14, 2020 https://www.ncbi.nlm.nih.gov/pubmed/22045006.

39. Lowe T, Berven SH, Schwab FJ, Bridwell KH. The SRS classification for adult spinal deformity: building on the King/Moe and Lenke classification systems. *Spine.* 2006;31(19 Suppl):S119–S125. https://doi.org/10.1097/01.brs.0000232709.48446.be.

40. Mundis GM, Turner JD, Deverin V, et al. A critical analysis of sagittal plane deformity correction with minimally invasive adult spinal deformity surgery: a 2-year follow-up study. *Spine Deform.* 2017;5(4):265–271. https://doi.org/10.1016/j.jspd.2017.01.010.

41. Lafage V, Schwab F, Patel A, Hawkinson N, Farcy JP. Pelvic tilt and truncal inclination: two key radiographic parameters in the setting of adults with spinal deformity. *Spine.* 2009;34:E599–E606. PubMed - NCBI. Accessed April 5, 2020 https://www.ncbi.nlm.nih.gov/pubmed/19644319/.

42. Slattery C, Verma K. Classification in brief: SRS-Schwab classification of adult spinal deformity. *Clin Orthop.* 2018;476(9):1890–1894. https://doi.org/10.1007/s11999.0000000000000264.

43. Makhni MC, Shillingford JN, Laratta JL, Hyun SJ, Kim YJ. Restoration of sagittal balance in spinal deformity surgery. *J Korean Neurosurg Soc.* 2018;61–167. Accessed April 11, 2020 https://www.ncbi.nlm.nih.gov/pmc/articles/PMC5853192/.

44. Ames CP, Smith JS, Scheer JK, et al. Impact of spinopelvic alignment on decision making in deformity surgery in adults: a review. *J Neurosurg Spine.* 2012;16(6):547–564. https://doi.org/10.3171/2012.2.SPINE11320.

45. Terran J, Schwab F, Shaffrey CI, et al. The SRS-Schwab adult spinal deformity classification assessment and clinical correlations based on a prospective operative and nonoperative cohort. *Neurosurgery.* 2013;73(4):559–568. https://doi.org/10.1227/NEU.0000000000000012.

46. Schwab F, Lafage V, Shaffrey CI, et al. 138; The Schwab-SRS adult spinal deformity classification. *Neurosurgery.* 2012;71:E556. ProQuest. Accessed April 8, 2020 https://search.proquest.com/openview/3f5be-3d1ae805127550950eb0f367061/1?pq-origsite=gscholar&cbl=2046368.

47. Smith JS, Shaffrey CI, Berven S, et al. Operative versus nonoperative treatment of leg pain in adults with scoliosis: a retrospective review of a prospective multicenter database with two-year follow-up. *Spine.* 2009;34(16):1693–1698. https://doi.org/10.1097/BRS.0b013e3181ac5fcd.

48. Schwab F, Patel A, Ungar B, Farcy J-P, Lafage V. Adult spinal deformity-postoperative standing imbalance: how much can you tolerate? An overview of key parameters in assessing alignment and planning corrective surgery. *Spine.* 2010;35(25):2224–2231. https://doi.org/10.1097/BRS.0b013e3181ee6bd4.

49. Roussouly P, Berthonnaud E, Dimnet J. Geometrical and mechanical analysis of lumbar lordosis in an asymptomatic population: proposed classification. *Rev Chir Orthop Reparatrice Appar Mot.* 2003;89(7):632–639.

50. Roussouly P, Pinheiro-Franco JL. Biomechanical analysis of the spino-pelvic organization and adaptation in pathology. *Eur Spine J.* 2011;20(Suppl 5):609–618. https://doi.org/10.1007/s00586-011-1928-x.

51. Passias PG, Pierce KE, Bortz C, et al. P102. Does matching Roussouly spinal shape and improvement in SRS-Schwab modifier contribute to improved patient-reported outcomes? *Spine J.* 2019;19(9):S205–S206. https://doi.org/10.1016/j.spinee.2019.05.527.

52. Kwon BK, Albert TJ. Adult low-grade acquired spondylolytic spondylolisthesis: evaluation and management. *Spine.* 2005;30:S35–S41. LWW https://doi.org/10.1097/01.brs.0000155561.70727.20.

53. Niggemann P, Kuchta J, Grosskurth D, Beyer HK, Hoeffer J, Delank KS. Spondylolysis and isthmic spondylolisthesis: impact of vertebral hypoplasia on the use of the Meyerding classification. *Br J Radiol*. 2012;85(1012):358–362. Accessed April 11, 2020 https://www.birpublications.org/doi/full/10.1259/bjr/60355971.

54. Perdriolle R, Vidal J. Thoracic idiopathic scoliosis curve evolution and prognosis. *Spine*. 1985;10(9):785–791. https://doi.org/10.1097/00007632-198511000-00001.

55. Drerup B. Improvements in measuring vertebral rotation from the projections of the pedicles. *J Biomech*. 1985;18(5):369–378. https://doi.org/10.1016/0021-9290(85)90292-1.

56. Sugimoto Y, Tanaka M, Nakanishi K, Misawa H, Takigawa T, Ozaki T. Predicting intraoperative vertebral rotation in patients with scoliosis using posterior elements as anatomical landmarks. *Spine*. 2007;32(25):E761–E763. https://doi.org/10.1097/BRS.0b013e31815b7e87.

57. Srinivasalu S, Modi HN, SMehta S, Suh S-W, Chen T, Murun T. Cobb angle measurement of scoliosis using computer measurement of digitally acquired radiographs-intraobserver and interobserver variability. *Asian Spine J*. 2008;2(2):90–93. https://doi.org/10.4184/asj.2008.2.2.90.

58. Langensiepen S, Semler O, Sobottke R, et al. Measuring procedures to determine the Cobb angle in idiopathic scoliosis: a systematic review. *Eur Spine J*. 2013;22(11):2360–2371. PubMed - NCBI. Accessed March 10, 2020 https://www.ncbi.nlm.nih.gov/pubmed/23443679.

59. Kim H, Kim HS, Moon ES, et al. Scoliosis imaging: what radiologists should know. PubMed - NCBI. Accessed March 10, 2020, *Radiographics*. 2010;30:1823–1842. https://www.ncbi.nlm.nih.gov/pubmed/21057122.

60. Ylikoski M, Tallroth K. Measurement variations in scoliotic angle, vertebral rotation, vertebral body height, and intervertebral disc space height. *J Spinal Disord*. 1990;3(4):387–391.

61. Weinstein SL, Ponseti IV. Curve progression in idiopathic scoliosis. *JBJS*. 1983;65(4):447–455.

62. Maruyama T, Takeshita K. Surgical treatment of scoliosis: a review of techniques currently applied. *Scoliosis*. 2008;3(1):6. https://doi.org/10.1186/1748-7161-3-6.

63. Karavidas N. Bracing in the treatment of adolescent idiopathic scoliosis: evidence to date. *Adolesc Health Med Ther*. 2019;10:153–172. https://doi.org/10.2147/AHMT.S190565.

64. Elfiky TA, Samartzis D, Cheung W-Y, Wong Y-W, Luk KDK, Cheung KMC. The proximal thoracic curve in adolescent idiopathic scoliosis: surgical strategy and management outcomes. *Glob Spine J*. 2011;1(1):27–36. https://doi.org/10.1055/s-0031-1296054.

65. Kwan MK, Chan CYW. Is there an optimal upper instrumented vertebra (UIV) tilt angle to prevent postoperative shoulder imbalance and neck tilt in Lenke 1 and 2 adolescent idiopathic scoliosis (AIS) patients? *Eur Spine J*. 2016;25(10):3065–3074. https://doi.org/10.1007/s00586-016-4529-x.

66. Knott PT, Mardjetko SM, Techy F. The use of the T1 sagittal angle in predicting overall sagittal balance of the spine. *Spine J*. 2010;10(11):994–998. https://doi.org/10.1016/j.spinee.2010.08.031.

67. Ono T, Bastrom TP, Newton PO. Defining 2 components of shoulder imbalance: clavicle tilt and trapezial prominence. *Spine*. 2012;37:E1511–E1516. Accessed April 11, 2020 https://cdn.journals.lww.com/spinejournal/Fulltext/2012/11150/Defining_2_Components_of_Shoulder_Imbalance_.15.aspx?casa_token=aoTxN-2PKkIAAAAA:gjic7MDjE7erTye1R6Dq8QeaUAdZYeIkaS12bMW5RH4dViTfMKeYivz4Jtlw4q5grV2FMlaeEq4AOPRFFlyiU89H.

68. Hong J-Y, Suh S-W, Yang J-H, Park S-Y, Han J-H. Reliability analysis of shoulder balance measures: comparison of the 4 available methods. *Spine*. 2013;38(26). https://doi.org/10.1097/BRS.0b013e3182a18486, E1684.

69. Richards BS, Scaduto A, Vanderhave K, Browne R. Assessment of trunk balance in thoracic scoliosis. *Spine*. 2005;30:1621–1626. https://doi.org/10.1097/01.brs.0000170298.89145.b4. LWW.

70. Wang Y, Bünger CE, Wu C, Zhang Y, Hansen ES. Postoperative trunk shift in lenke 1C scoliosis: what causes it? How can it be prevented? *Spine*. 2012;37:1676–1682. LWW https://doi.org/10.1097/BRS.0b013e318255a053.

71. Fann AV, Lee R, Verbois GM. The reliability of postural x-rays in measuring pelvic obliquity. *Arch Phys Med Rehabil*. 1999;80(4):458–461. https://doi.org/10.1016/S0003-9993(99)90286-1.

72. Fann AV. Validation of postural radiographs as a way to measure change in pelvic obliquity. *Arch Phys Med Rehabil*. 2003;84(1):75–78. https://doi.org/10.1053/apmr.2003.50067.

73. Sabharwal S, Kumar A. Methods for assessing leg length discrepancy. *Clin Orthop Relat Res*. 2008;466:2910–2922. SpringerLink. Accessed April 11, 2020 https://link.springer.com/article/10.1007/s11999-008-0524-9.

74. Koller H, Pfanz C, Meier O, et al. Factors influencing radiographic and clinical outcomes in adult scoliosis surgery: a study of 448 European patients. *Eur Spine J*. 2016;25(2):532–548. https://doi.org/10.1007/s00586-015-3898-x.

75. Dulhunty J. A preliminary study of sacral base obliquity measured on erect radiographs taken in a clinical setting. *Chiropr J Aust*. 2004;34(2):68.

76. Legaye J, Duval-Beaupère G. Sagittal plane alignment of the spine and gravity a radiological and clinical evaluation. *Acta Orthop Belg*. 2005;71:8.

77. Hardacker JW, Shuford RF, Capicotto PN, Pryor PW. Radiographic standing cervical segmental alignment in adult volunteers without neck symptoms. *Spine*. 1997;22:1472–1479. PubMed - NCBI. Accessed April 11, 2020 https://www.ncbi.nlm.nih.gov/pubmed/9231966/.

78. Barrett E, McCreesh K, Lewis J. Reliability and validity of non-radiographic methods of thoracic kyphosis measurement: a systematic review. *Man Ther*. 2014;19(1):10–17. https://doi.org/10.1016/j.math.2013.09.003.

79. Kim D, Menger RP. Spine sagittal balance. In: *StatPearls.* StatPearls Publishing; 2020. http://www.ncbi.nlm.nih.gov/books/NBK534858/. Accessed 11 April 2020.

80. Savage JW, Patel AA. Fixed sagittal plane imbalance. *Glob Spine J.* 2014;4(4):287–296. https://doi.org/10.1055/s-0034-1394126.

81. Roussouly P, Nnadi C. Sagittal plane deformity: an overview of interpretation and management. *Eur Spine J.* 2010;19(11):1824–1836. https://doi.org/10.1007/s00586-010-1476-9.

82. Le Huec JC, Aunoble S, Philippe L, Nicolas P. Pelvic parameters: origin and significance. *Eur Spine J.* 2011;20(5):564. https://doi.org/10.1007/s00586-011-1940-1.

83. Lazennec J-Y, Brusson A, Rousseau M-A. Hip–spine relations and sagittal balance clinical consequences. *Eur Spine J.* 2011;20(5):686. https://doi.org/10.1007/s00586-011-1937-9.

84. Van Royen BJ, Toussaint HM, Kingma I, et al. Accuracy of the sagittal vertical axis in a standing lateral radiograph as a measurement of balance in spinal deformities. *Eur Spine J.* 1998;7:408–412. SpringerLink. Accessed April 11, 2020 https://link.springer.com/article/10.1007/s005860050098.

85. Wiltse LL, Winter RB. Terminology and measurement of spondylolisthesis. *J Bone Joint Surg Am.* 1983;65(6):768–772.

86. Meyerding HW. Spondylolisthesis. *Surg Gynecol Obstet.* 1932;54:371–377.

87. Stokes IA, Wilder DG, Frymoyer JW, Pope MH. 1980 Volvo award in clinical sciences. Assessment of patients with low-back pain by biplanar radiographic measurement of intervertebral motion. *Spine.* 1981;6(3):233–240. https://doi.org/10.1097/00007632-198105000-00005.

88. Brown RH, Burstein AH, Nash CL, Schock CC. Spinal analysis using a three-dimensional radiographic technique. *J Biomech.* 1976;9(6):355–365. https://doi.org/10.1016/0021-9290(76)90113-5.

89. Lam GC, Hill DL, Le LH, Raso JV, Lou EH. Vertebral rotation measurement: a summary and comparison of common radiographic and CT methods. *Scoliosis.* 2008;3:16. Accessed March 29, 2020 https://www.ncbi.nlm.nih.gov/pmc/articles/PMC2587463/.

90. Drerup B. Principles of measurement of vertebral rotation from frontal projections of the pedicles. *J Biomech.* 1984;17:923–935. PubMed - NCBI. Accessed March 29, 2020 https://www.ncbi.nlm.nih.gov/pubmed/6520140.

91. Nash CL, Moe JH. A study of vertebral rotation. *J Bone Joint Surg Am.* 1969;51(2):223–229.

92. Mehta MH. Radiographic estimation of vertebral rotation in scoliosis. *J Bone Joint Surg (Br).* 1973;55(3):513–520.

93. Ho EK, Upadhyay SS, Chan FL, Hsu LC, Leong JC. New methods of measuring vertebral rotation from computed tomographic scans. An intraobserver and interobserver study on girls with scoliosis. *Spine.* 1993;18(9):1173–1177. https://doi.org/10.1097/00007632-199307000-00008.

94. Barsanti CM, deBari A, Covino BM. The torsion meter: a critical review. *J Pediatr Orthop.* 1990;10(4):527–531.

95. Omeroğlu H, Ozekin O, Biçimoğlu A. Measurement of vertebral rotation in idiopathic scoliosis using the Perdriolle torsionmeter: a clinical study on intraobserver and interobserver error. *Eur Spine J.* 1996;5(3):167–171. https://doi.org/10.1007/bf00395508.

96. Yazici M, Acaroglu ER, Alanay A, Deviren V, Cila A, Surat A. Measurement of vertebral rotation in standing versus supine position in adolescent idiopathic scoliosis. *J Pediatr Orthop.* 2001;21(2):252–256.

97. Richards BS. Measurement error in assessment of vertebral rotation using the Perdriolle torsionmeter. *Spine.* 1992;17(5):513–517. https://doi.org/10.1097/00007632-199205000-00008.

98. Stokes IA, Bigalow LC, Moreland MS. Measurement of axial rotation of vertebrae in scoliosis. *Spine.* 1986;11(3):213–218. https://doi.org/10.1097/00007632-198604000-00006.

99. Russell GG, Raso VJ, Hill D, McIvor J. A comparison of four computerized methods for measuring vertebral rotation. *Spine.* 1990;15(1):24–27. https://doi.org/10.1097/00007632-199001000-00007.

100. Weiss H.R. Technical error of vertebral rotation measurements Three-Dimensional Analysis of Spinal Deformities. Studies in Health Technology and Informatics. Google Scholar, n.d. Accessed March 29, 2020. https://scholar.google.com/scholar_lookup?journal=Studies+in+Health+Technology+and+Informatics:+Three-Dimensional+Analysis+of+Spinal+Deformities&title=Technical+error+of+vertebral+rotation+measurements&author=HR+Weiss&volume=15&publication_year=1995&pages=243-249&.

101. Aaro S, Dahlborn M, Svensson L. Estimation of vertebral rotation in structural scoliosis by computer tomography. *Acta Radiol Diagn (Stockh).* 1978;19(6):990–992. https://doi.org/10.1177/028418517801900614.

102. Skalli W, Lavaste F, Descrimes JL. Quantification of three-dimensional vertebral rotations in scoliosis: what are the true values? *Spine.* 1995;20(5):546–553. https://doi.org/10.1097/00007632-199503010-00008.

103. Birchall D, Hughes DG, Robinson L, Williamson JB. Analysis of intravertebral axial rotation in adolescent idiopathic scoliosis using three-dimensional MRI. *Spine (Phila Pa 1976).* 1997;22:2403–2407. Google Scholar. Accessed March 29, 2020 https://scholar.google.com/scholar_lookup?journal=Studies+in+Health+Technology+and+Informatics:+Research+into+Spinal+Deformities+2&title=Analysis+of+intravertebral+axial+rotation+in+adolescent+-idiopathic+scoliosis+using+three-dimensional+MRI&author=D+Birchall&author=DG+Hughes&author=L+Robinson&author=JB+Williamson&volume=59&publication_year=1999&pages=61-64&.

104. Krismer M, Chen AM, Steinlechner M, Haid C, Lener M, Wimmer C. Measurement of vertebral rotation: a comparison of two methods based on CT scans. *J Spinal Disord.* 1999;12(2):126–130.

105. Merolli A, Leali PT, Aulisa L, Guidi PL, Impagnatello M. A new method for clinical measurement of vertebral rotation. In: *Studies in Health Technology and Informatics*; 1997. Google Scholar. Accessed March 29, 2020 https://scholar.google.com/scholar_lookup?journal=Studies+in+Health+Technology+and+Informatics:+Research+into+Spinal+Deformities+1&title=A+new+method+for+clinical+measurement+of+vertebral+rotation&author=A+Merolli&author=PT+Leali&author=L+Aulisa&author=PL+Guidi&author=M+Impagnatello&volume=37&publication_year=1997&pages=147-149&.

106. Göçen S, Aksu MG, Baktiroğlu L, Ozcan O. Evaluation of computed tomographic methods to measure vertebral rotation in adolescent idiopathic scoliosis: an intraobserver and interobserver analysis. *J Spinal Disord.* 1998;11(3):210–214.

107. Hong J-Y, Suh S-W, Easwar TR, Modi HN, Yang J-H, Park J-H. Evaluation of the three-dimensional deformities in scoliosis surgery with computed tomography: efficacy and relationship with clinical outcomes. *Spine.* 2011;36(19). https://doi.org/10.1097/BRS.0b013e318205e413, E1259.

108. Lazennec JY, Ramaré S, Arafati N, et al. Sagittal alignment in lumbosacral fusion: relations between radiological parameters and pain. *Eur Spine J.* 2000;9:47–55. PubMed - NCBI. Accessed April 8, 2020 https://www.ncbi.nlm.nih.gov/pubmed/10766077?dopt=Abstract.

109. Lafage V, Schwab F, Skalli W, et al. Standing balance and sagittal plane spinal deformity: analysis of spinopelvic and gravity line parameters. *Spine.* 2008;33(14):1572–1578. https://doi.org/10.1097/BRS.0b013e31817886a2.

110. ScienceDirect, Sagittal Vertical Axis—An Overview. ScienceDirect Topics | n.d. Accessed April 8, 2020. https://www.sciencedirect.com/topics/nursing-and-health-professions/sagittal-vertical-axis.

111. Glassman SD, Berven S, Bridwell K, Horton W, Dimar JR. Correlation of radiographic parameters and clinical symptoms in adult scoliosis. *Spine.* 2005;30(6):682–688. https://doi.org/10.1097/01.brs.0000155425.04536.f7.

112. Schwab FJ, Smith VA, Biserni M, Gamez L, Farcy J-PC, Pagala M. Adult scoliosis: a quantitative radiographic and clinical analysis. *Spine.* 2002;27(4):387–392. https://doi.org/10.1097/00007632-200202150-00012.

113. Cho KJ, Suk SI, Park SR, et al. Risk factors of sagittal decompensation after long posterior instrumentation and fusion for degenerative lumbar scoliosis. *Spine.* 2010;35:1595–1601. PubMed - NCBI. Accessed April 8, 2020 https://www.ncbi.nlm.nih.gov/pubmed/20386505.

114. Gottfried ON, Daubs MD, Patel AA, Dailey AT, Brodke DS. Spinopelvic parameters in postfusion flatback deformity patients. *Spine J.* 2009;9(8):639–647. https://doi.org/10.1016/j.spinee.2009.04.008.

115. Roussouly P, Gollogly S, Berthonnaud E, Dimnet J. Classification of the normal variation in the sagittal alignment of the human lumbar spine and pelvis in the standing position. *Spine.* 2005;30:346–353. PubMed - NCBI. Accessed April 8, 2020 https://www.ncbi.nlm.nih.gov/pubmed/15682018.

116. Chaléat-Valayer E, Mac-Thiong J-M, Paquet J, Berthonnaud E, Siani F, Roussouly P. Sagittal spino-pelvic alignment in chronic low back pain. *Eur Spine J.* 2011;20(Suppl 5):634–640. https://doi.org/10.1007/s00586-011-1931-2.

117. Tsutsui S, Kagotani R, Yamada H, et al. Can decompression surgery relieve low back pain in patients with lumbar spinal stenosis combined with degenerative lumbar scoliosis? *Eur Spine J.* 2013;22(9):2010–2014. https://doi.org/10.1007/s00586-013-2786-5.

118. Lafage R, Schwab F, Challier V, et al. Defining spino-pelvic alignment thresholds: should operative goals in adult spinal deformity surgery account for age? *Spine.* 2016;41(1):62–68. https://doi.org/10.1097/BRS.0000000000001171.

CHAPTER 13

Lumbosacral Spine Plain Radiographs

DOMINGO MOLINA, IV[a] • SCOTT BLUMENTHAL[b]
[a]Texas Back Institute, Plano, TX, United States
[b]Center for Disc Replacement at Texas Back Institute, Plano, TX, United States

INTRODUCTION

The lumbosacral spine consists of five large vertebrae that make up the lumbar spine and five fused vertebrae that make up one single bone which articulate on each side of pelvis called the sacrum.[1] Overall, spinal balance is determined by a mixture of kyphosis and lordosis throughout the spine. Lumbar lordosis is an important factor in overall sagittal balance, which contributes to bipedalism posture and upright gait.[2,3] Approximately 40–60 degrees of lordosis is present in the lumbar spine.[4] Although there is inherent variability between patients, there is an increase in lumbar lordosis from the upper to lower segments with approximately two-thirds of lumbar lordosis occurring at the L4-S1 levels.[5] The balance, alignment, and motion of the spine are determined by lumbopelvic alignment and pelvic compensation for sagittal alignment in the thoracic and lumbar spine.[3,6]

Ultimately lumbopelvic parameters have an important impact on the pathogenesis of lumbar degenerative conditions and spinal deformity. The relationship between the lumbosacral spine and the pelvic morphology stresses the importance of plain radiographs in overall spinal alignment. The present chapter discusses the importance of plain radiographs in determining the relationship between the lumbosacral spine and the pelvis with an emphasis on clinical relevance and techniques when performing these measurements.

SPECIFIC RADIOGRAPHIC PARAMETERS

During examination of the lumbosacral spine, indications for full-length or isolated posteroanterior and lateral radiographs may differ upon the presenting complaints. Standing full-length 36-inch posteroanterior and lateral radiographs are the baseline imaging studies to evaluate sagittal balance, which has been described in depth in a previous chapter. The hips and knees should be extended

during standing radiographs to negate any compensatory mechanisms. The use of posteroanterior projection decreases patient radiation exposure by 41% in comparison with the use of anteroposterior projection.[7] If a practitioner chooses to obtain isolated standing lumbosacral radiographs, the femoral heads should be included to adequately assess the relationship between lumbosacral and pelvic parameters. All measurements are made using lateral radiographs unless otherwise specified.

General Lumbar Spine
Coronal balance
When evaluating overall spinal balance, coronal alignment should be assessed with full-length 36-inch standing posteroanterior radiographs with the hips and knees extended. The presence of deformity, pelvic obliquity, and leg length discrepancy can be noted on posteroanterior radiographs. If a leg length discrepancy greater than 2 cm is already known, then a leg lift can be placed under the shorter leg during radiographic evaluation.

Coronal regional alignment
Coronal lumbar and lumbosacral curves are defined as having an apex from L1 to L5 and L5 to S1, respectively, as measured by the Cobb method from the end vertebrae.[2] The cephalad end vertebra is the first vertebra in the cephalad direction whose superior endplate is tilted maximally toward the concavity of the curve. The caudad end vertebra is the first vertebra in the caudad direction whose inferior endplate is tilted maximally toward the concavity of the curve. Apical vertebral translation (AVT) is defined as the horizontal distance measured from the C7 plumb line to the center of the central sacral vertical line (CSVL) for lumbar and lumbosacral curves.[2] The central sacral vertical line is defined as a vertical line drawn through the center of the S1 endplate.[2] Coronal spinal balance is defined

Atlas of Spinal Imaging. https://doi.org/10.1016/B978-0-323-76111-6.00009-2

from the center of C7 and the midpoint of the thoracic trunk to the sacrum. Coronal imbalance of greater than 4 cm has been correlated with deterioration in pain and function scores in unoperated patients but not in patients with surgery.[8] This suggests that sagittal correction may be more important than coronal correction and will be discussed later in this chapter.

Coronal pelvic alignment

Coronal pelvic alignment can be defined by leg length discrepancy and pelvic obliquity. Pelvic obliquity is measured by the angle created by a horizontal line and a line tangential to the top of the sacral ala. Pelvic obliquity can be seen as a compensatory mechanism from lumbar or lumbosacral deformity, leg length deformity, or both. Leg length discrepancy is defined as the vertical distance measured between horizontal lines drawn tangential to the top of each femoral head. It is important to note the etiology of the pelvic obliquity as compensatory lumbar or lumbosacral curves can be mistaken for true deformity in the setting of an undiagnosed leg length discrepancy greater than 2 cm.

Spinopelvic Parameters

Overall sagittal balance and the relationship between the lumbosacral spine and the pelvis are evaluated from the lateral radiograph. Key components of spinopelvic parameters include lumbar lordosis (LL), pelvic incidence (PI), pelvic tilt (PT), and sacral slope (SS). The influence of the cervical spine on the overall sagittal balance is worth mentioning here and is measured by the C7–S1 sagittal vertical axis (SVA) (Fig. 1).

- C7–S1 sagittal vertical axis
  - Draw a vertical plumb line centered at the midline of the C7 vertebral body to the posterior-superior corner of the S1 endplate
  - Measure the horizontal distance from the vertical plumb line
  - SVA has a (+) value when anterior to the sacral reference point and a (−) value when posterior to the sacral reference point.

There is an association between the loss of lordosis and an anterior shift of the SVA.[4] Spinopelvic harmony exists when the SVA < 50 mm. Restoration of the SVA achieves level gaze and has been found to lead to better Health Related Quality of Life (HRQoL) scores.[9]

Lumbar lordosis

There is a relationship between thoracic kyphosis and lumbar lordosis as well as a relationship between lumbar lordosis and pelvic incidence.[10,11] Different patterns of lordosis have been reported, each defined by the

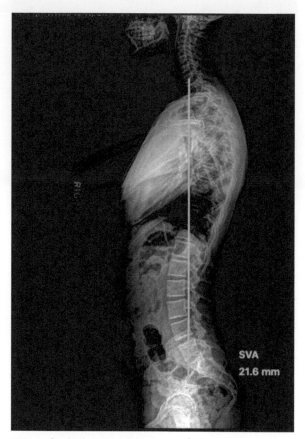

FIG. 1 Sagittal vertical axis.

patient's pelvic incidence.[10] Defining lumbar lordosis is important when evaluating sagittal balance (Fig. 2).

- Cobb angle
  - Draw a line along the superior endplate of L1
  - Draw a perpendicular line intersecting the first line
  - Draw a line along the superior endplate of S1
  - Draw a perpendicular line intersecting the second line
  - The angle formed by the intersection of the two perpendicular lines is the Cobb angle measurement for lumbar lordosis.

In spinopelvic harmony, the LL will match PI within 11 degrees.[9,11] Normal values of lumbar lordosis can be seen within 60 degrees ± 12 degrees.[10,12] The majority of lumbar lordosis resides within L4-S1. Degenerative changes within the spine such as loss of disc height can lead to a decrease in lordosis as patients age. Trauma such as compression fractures can also lead to a loss of lumbar lordosis. Iatrogenic flatback deformity from spinal fusions can create a hypolordotic spine and lead

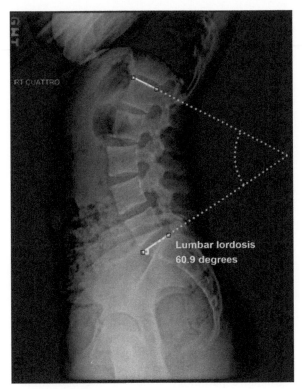

FIG. 2 Lumbar lordosis.

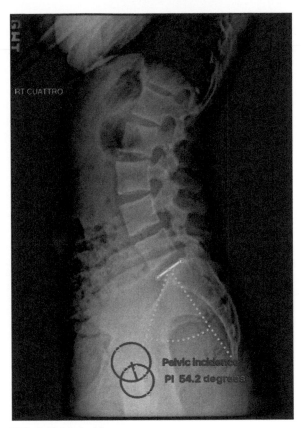

FIG. 3 Pelvic incidence.

to the overall sagittal imbalance. Understanding the etiology of a patient's lordosis in the lumbar spine is important as lumbar lordosis is the most readily changed spinopelvic parameter with surgery.

Pelvic incidence

Pelvic incidence is an anatomic value that is constant and unique to each patient, and does not change with spatial orientation of the pelvis (Fig. 3). As stated previously, PI can influence LL as well as thoracic and cervical sagittal contours.[11]

- Pelvic incidence
  - Draw a line from the center of the femoral head to the midpoint of the sacral endplate
    - If the femoral heads are not overlapping, then choose a point equidistant between the femoral heads.
  - Draw a line orthogonal to the sacral endplate
  - The angle formed between the two lines is defined as pelvic incidence and is also the sum of the sacral slope and pelvic tilt. (PI = SS + PT) (Fig. 4).

Pelvic incidence is a fixed value for patients; therefore, we must evaluate its relationship with lumbar

lordosis. The impact of the relationship between PI and LL has been studied extensively, and a value of greater than 11° (PI-LL) was associated with disability in terms of the Oswestry Disability Index (ODI) scores.[9,11,12] Pelvic incidence can be increased in patients with high-grade spondylolisthesis. While the value itself cannot be changed, it is important to note PI when evaluating the amount of correction needed in the lumbar spine during sagittal correction.

Pelvic tilt

Now that we have assessed the relationship between lumbar lordosis and pelvic incidence, we can evaluate the patient's compensatory mechanism for PI-LL mismatch and positive SVA by the use of pelvic tilt. Pelvic tilt is a variable spinopelvic parameter and is used to compensate for the loss of lumbar lordosis by extending through the pelvis to maintain a normal sagittal balance (Fig. 4).

- Pelvic tilt
  - Draw a vertical line through the center of the femoral heads

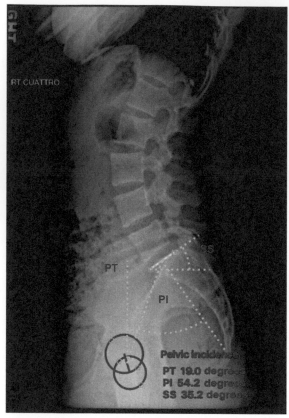

FIG. 4 Sagittal pelvic parameters.

- Draw a line from the center of the femoral heads to the midpoint of the sacral endplate
- The angle between the two lines is defined as pelvic tilt
- Normal value < 25 degrees.

Increasing PT or pelvic retroversion reflects the patient's need to compensate for sagittal imbalance. Significant correlation has been noted between SVA and PT. In addition, pain and disability scores are increased in patients that are found to have PT > 25 degrees and a high SVA > 50 mm.[13] The ability of a patient to compensate for sagittal imbalance via PT can vary and can be limited in patients with joint stiffness and muscle tightness. As a patient exhibits positive SVA, he or she will compensate by retroverting the pelvis and flexing the knees to maintain horizontal gaze and center the head over the pelvis. This method of compensation requires increased energy expenditure and has been noted with decreased HRQoL scores.[9]

Pelvic tilt is not changed by surgical intervention but should be assessed during the evaluation of the lumbosacral spine in order to identify a patient that is compensating for sagittal imbalance. Patients with flatback deformity who have increased posterior pelvic tilt have been found to have little change in posterior pelvic tilt from a standing to sitting position.[14] This lack of change in posterior tilt can lead to femoroacetabular impingement in patients undergoing total hip arthroplasty.

Sacral slope

While PI, PT, and LL receive much attention in regard to spinopelvic parameters, there is a high correlation between lumbar lordosis and sacral slope. Sacral slope is not a fixed angle and depends on the position of the pelvis relative to the hip axis. Pelvic incidence is the sum of sacral slope and pelvic tilt creating an inverse relationship between PT and SS (Fig. 4).

- Sacral slope
  - Draw a line along the sacral endplate
  - Draw a line from the posterosuperior endplate to the horizontal
  - The angle formed between the two lines is defined as sacral slope.

Patients with a lower lumbar lordosis and a more horizontal sacrum are more likely to develop lumbar degenerative pathology, including disc herniation.[10] Patients with a higher SS and correlating PI and a lumbar lordosis apex of L3 or above are more likely to develop spinal stenosis.[3] Patients with a high pelvic incidence and sacral slope shift their center of axis anteriorly creating higher shear forces in the lumbosacral spine. This can lead to pathologies such as developmental spondylolisthesis. While there is no normal value for sacral slope, it is important to take into account its value in the overall sagittal balance. Patients who are fused in a positive sagittal balance with a high sacral slope are more likely to develop adjacent segment degeneration. Correcting a PI-LL mismatch will establish a normal pelvic tilt and normalization of the SS.

Degenerative Lumbar Spine

When evaluating the degenerative lumbosacral spine, it is important to obtain standing posteroanterior and lateral radiographs. If there is concern for spondylolisthesis, standing flexion and extension lumbar radiographs should be obtained as well. The femoral heads should always be included in case a provider wishes to evaluate spinopelvic parameters in the degenerative lumbar patient. All radiographs should be evaluated for signs of osteophytes, foraminal narrowing, endplate sclerosis, disc space narrowing, and vacuum phenomenon within the disc.

Spondylosis

Lumbar spondylosis is broadly defined as the degenerative destruction or remodeling of the spine, intervertebral discs, and facet joints. Facet arthrosis, decreased disc height, foraminal narrowing, and subchondral sclerosis are radiographic signs of degeneration. As the intervertebral disc degenerates, decreased disc height occurs. Decreased disc height alters the biomechanics of the facet joints which can lead to arthrosis, which is often a cause of radiculopathy. Facet arthrosis is best seen on MRI or CT but can also be visualized on standard oblique radiographs. Foraminal stenosis can also be caused by facet hypertrophy, which is indicative of facet arthrosis.

Contour lines

There is no literature regarding the use of contour lines in the lumbar spine radiography, but it is important to note the alignment of the anterior and posterior bodies in the lumbosacral spine. It is also important to note the spinolaminar line as well as the spinous process line. We will discuss pathologies related to contour lines later in this chapter.

Disc height/foraminal height

Disc height (DH) is an important parameter to evaluate the degenerative lumbar spine for both diagnostic purposes and surgical planning. Restoration of DH is a mainstay in lumbosacral spine surgery. Disc height and foraminal height are directly related to each other. The use of interbody cages allows for a change in disc height, which in turn affects foraminal height. Chapter 6 outlines a detailed explanation of DH measurement in the cervical spine that can be applicable to the lumbar spine. For our purposes in the lumbar spine, we will discuss a general measurement of DH and foraminal height used in diagnostic evaluations and surgical planning (Fig. 5).

- Disc height
  - Measure the distance from the superior endplate of the caudal vertebra to the interior endplate of the rostral vertebra at the most anterior aspect of the disc space
  - Measure the distance as stated earlier at the midline of the disc space
  - Measure the distance as stated earlier at the most posterior aspect of the disc space
  - The average of these three measurements is defined as the disc height.
- Foraminal height
  - Measure the distance between the inferior pedicle wall and the superior pedicle wall of the inferior level.

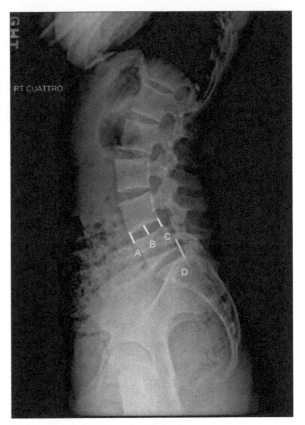

FIG. 5 Disc height/foraminal height.

Restoration of DH and segmental LL are important factors in preventing adjacent segment disease (ASD). Restoration of DH is also known to increase foraminal height after interbody placement, as well as providing indirect decompression of neuroforamina.[15] As artificial disc replacements become more widely used, it will be important to understand and evaluate the relationship between DH and facet joint biomechanics. Each 1-mm increase in DH above its normal position can lead to a decrease in the facet joint articulation overlap by 6% at the L4-L5 level.[16] Appropriate DH is important as over distraction of the disc height can lead to facet joint subluxation.

While we have discussed DH in relation to the facet joints, it is important that we also understand the relationship between DH and ASD. During restoration of DH, the overall spinal column is not increased in height. Kaito et al. have found that an over distraction of DH has led to symptomatic ASD.[17]

Spondylolisthesis

Wiltse classified spondylolisthesis into five categories: dysplastic, isthmic, degenerative, traumatic, and pathologic. Spondylolisthesis is the anterior or posterior displacement of one vertebral body over another. While many etiologies for spondylolisthesis exist, this chapter will focus on radiographic parameters and grading of slippage present. The provider should also note any dysplastic features such as a trapezoidal L5 vertebra, deficient inferior articular process, spondylolysis, and sacral doming that can lead to the pathogenesis of spondylolisthesis.

Spondylolysis refers to a defect in the pars interarticularis. These defects in the pars interarticularis can either be dysplastic in origin or be acquired. If a pars defect is suspected and not elucidated via lateral radiographs, 30-degree oblique lumbar views should be obtained.[18,19] A Ferguson view, X-ray beam angled 30 degrees to 35 degrees cephalad parallel to the L5-S1 disc space can also be used to evaluate L5 transverse process pathology such as fusion to the sacrum as well as the posterior elements of L5 and S1.[19] Flexion and extension views can be used to evaluate instability and grade spondylolisthesis (Fig. 6).

- Instability
  - Obtain flexion/extension views of the lumbar spine
  - Evaluate any disruption of the anterior and posterior contour lines during flexion/extension
  - Instability is defined as listhesis > 2 mm.[20]
- Meyerding classification technique
  - As mentioned earlier, identify a potentially spondylolisthetic level through the initial radiographic examination
  - Measure the entire width of the caudal "normally aligned" vertebral endplate

- As with the distance technique, measure the magnitude of spondylolisthesis between the two adjacent vertebrae
- Divide this distance by the total distance of the "normal" endplate
- This value defines the percentage of translation relative to an adjacent normal level to generate Meyerding grades:
  - Grade I: ≤ 25%
  - Grade II: 25%–50%
  - Grade III: 50%–75%
  - Grade IV: 75%–100%
  - Grade V: > 100%

As we have seen before, pathology within the lumbar spine has a close relationship with spinopelvic parameters. Patients with high-grade spondylolisthesis are found to have an increased pelvic incidence.[19] Low-grade slips that have a low PI (e.g., < 45 degrees) or normal PI (e.g., 45 degrees to 60 degrees) are at low risk for progression and those that have a PI > 60 degrees have a high risk of progression and should be followed closely.[19]

Traumatic Lumbar Spine

Evaluation of the traumatic lumbar spine is most often performed by CT or MRI in the trauma setting but the parameters of measurement via these modalities were first established in plain radiographs. It is important to review these parameters in order to have a thorough understanding of management of thoracolumbar fractures. We will focus on the methods that have been shown to be reliable and reproducible. The radiographic measurement parameters that will be discussed

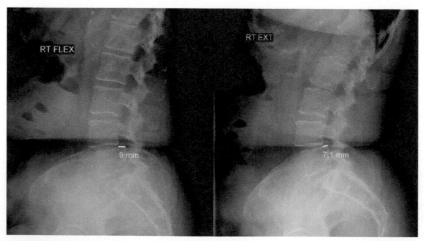

FIG. 6 Spondylolisthesis—flexion/extension.

in evaluating thoracolumbar trauma include sagittal alignment and vertebral body compression.

In contrast to literature in the cervical spine, the amount of vertebral body translation in the thoracolumbar spine is often due to degenerative conditions and inherently applies instability. If a provider suspects translation in the thoracolumbar spine to be from an acute injury, then further evaluation via CT and/or MRI should be performed.

Sagittal alignment

Sagittal alignment in thoracolumbar fractures encompasses evaluating segmental kyphosis at the injured level. There have been a variety of methods of measurement proposed to guide treatment when evaluating sagittal alignment.[21,22]

- The Cobb angle
  - Draw a line parallel to the superior endplate of one vertebra above the fracture
  - Draw a line parallel to the inferior endplate of one vertebra below the fracture
  - The angle formed between these two lines is the Cobb angle.

The Cobb angle has been shown to be most reproducible and reliable along other methods of measurement for sagittal alignment.[22] Sagittal alignment or more specifically segmental kyphosis is important when evaluating for thoracolumbar burst fractures. Segmental kyphosis > 25 degrees is a strong indicator of disruption of posterior osteoligamentous structures that implies instability.[23] Further imaging via CT and MRI should be performed to fully elucidate the integrity of all columns and to evaluate the spinal canal for stenosis caused by retropulsion of fragments.

Vertebral body compression

In addition to segmental kyphosis in a thoracolumbar fracture, the provider must also assess anterior vertebral body compression percentage. The amount of anterior vertebral body compression is another indicator used in determining the need for operative management of thoracolumbar fractures. The fractured thoracolumbar anterior vertebral body is compared with the cranial and caudal intact anterior vertebral body (Fig. 7).

- Anterior vertebral body compression percentage
  - Measure the anterior vertebral body height of the cranial and caudal intact vertebra to a fractured vertebra
  - Apply the formula [(V1 + V3/2 − V2]/(V1 + V3)/2.

The index calculated from the formula for the anterior vertebral body compression gives an indication of the relative compression of the fractured vertebra

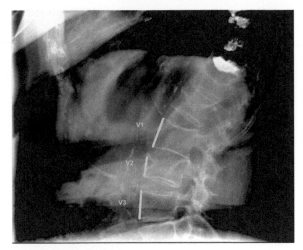

FIG. 7 Anterior vertebral body compression percentage.

compared with that of an intact vertebra. When this index exceeds 50%, operative treatment should be considered when also taking into account the amount of segmental kyphosis as discussed earlier.[21–23]

Postoperative Lumbar Spine

Postoperative radiographic assessment of the lumbar spine is necessary to evaluate the integrity of hardware and status of attempted fusion, and monitor adverse postoperative outcomes. Plain radiography is also used to evaluate adjacent segment disease that can occur around fusion levels. It is important to understand the following pathologies as they present on plain radiographs in order to know when to order further imaging to better elucidate potential pathology.

Fusion/pseudoarthrosis

There is much debate on the most adequate method of imaging to employ when evaluating for pseudoarthrosis. Plain radiography, dynamic radiography, and helical CT scan are the most common methods of imaging used to evaluate pseudoarthrosis. The popularity of using a variety of materials for interbody fusion, bone graft substitutes, and biologic agents has complicated the assessment of fusion in spine surgery. Despite the various methods of imaging, plain radiography continues to be used as the first line of postoperative evaluation of fusion (Fig. 8).

- Classification of Interbody Fusion Success: Brantigan, Steffee, Fraser (BSF)[24,25]
  - BSF-1: *Radiographical pseudarthrosis* is indicated by collapse of the construct, loss of the disc height, vertebral slip, broken screws, displacement of the

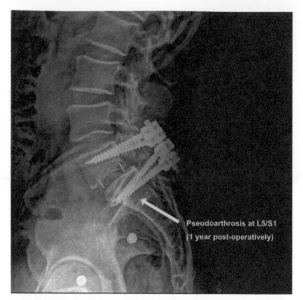

FIG. 8 Radiographic evidence of nonunion/
pseudoarthrosis.

carbon cage, or significant resorption of the bone graft, or lucency visible around the periphery of the graft or cage.

- BSF-2: *Radiographical locked pseudarthrosis* is indicated by lucency visible in the middle of the cages with solid bone growing into the cage from each vertebral endplate.
- BSF-3: *Radiographical fusion:* Bone bridges at least half of the fusion area with at least the density originally achieved at surgery. Radiographical fusion through one cage (half of the fusion area) is considered to be mechanically solid fusion even if there is lucency on the opposite side.

Plain radiography and dynamic radiography are two methods that are routinely used in the postoperative phase to assess thoracolumbar fusion. Dynamic radiography is used to detect motion within a grafted segment. On lateral flexion-extension radiographs, movement > 1–2 mm between spinous processes across the fused segment is indicative of a pseudoarthrosis.[24] A change in the Cobb angle of > 2 degrees between flexion and extension radiographs is another parameter that is used in dynamic radiography.[24,26]

Fogel et al. found no difference in plain radiographs and helical computed tomography when accurately assessing fusion in the thoracolumbar spine.[27] Their studies used the classification system created by Brantigan, described earlier, which is useful with widespread use of interbody cages.[25] Plain radiography and dynamic

radiography are useful and practical in assessing thoracolumbar fusion; however, a provider may choose to order CT or MRI for further evaluation if pseudoarthrosis is suspected after initial imaging.

Adjacent segment degeneration

For the purpose of this chapter, we will distinguish adjacent segment degeneration (ASDeg) from adjacent segment disease (ASD) as the radiographic deterioration of adjacent segments near a thoracolumbar fusion. Identifying the following features on plain radiographs during routine follow-up can assist the provider in evaluating symptomatic patients or those at risk for future degeneration after a thoracolumbar fusion (Fig. 9).

- Assessment of Adjacent Segment Degeneration
  - Identify the levels proximal and distal to a previously operated segment
  - Examine these levels for any of the following by making comparisons to previous radiographs:
    - New or enlarged adjacent level vertebral body osteophytes
    - Anterior longitudinal ligament calcification
    - Spondylolisthesis with displacement ≥ 2 mm
    - Disc space narrowing greater than 30% of the preoperative height
    - New or worsening endplate sclerosis.

The rate of ASDeg after thoracolumbar fusion has been found to be between 2% and 30% at 5 years.[28] In addition to the degeneration of adjacent segments around a thoracolumbar fusion, sagittal balance can

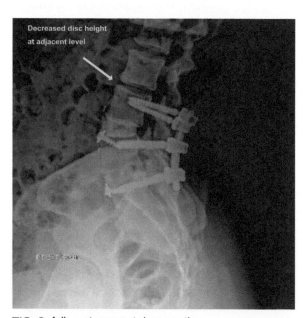

FIG. 9 Adjacent segment degeneration.

be affected as well. Hypolordosis can occur in patients with adjacent segment degeneration and on average has been found to be approximately 8 degrees less than in control patients.[29]

Conclusion

As spine surgery continues to evolve, an understanding of plain radiography is important to adequately evaluate the thoracolumbar spine. The methods outlined here have important clinical applications as our understanding of sagittal balance continues to evolve. As a variety of interbody cages are now being used, we can apply the methods discussed here to adequately assess fusion and the risk of adjacent segment degeneration. It is important to understand the importance of plain radiography and the information it can provide as new and innovate techniques continue to emerge in spine surgery.

REFERENCES

1. Drake LR, Vogl AW, Mitchell A. *Gray's Basic Anatomy.* 2nd ed. Philadelphia, PA: Elsevier; 2018.
2. Steinmetz MP, Benzel EC. *Benzel's Spine Surgery.* 4th ed. Philadelphia, PA: Elsevier; 2017.
3. Berven S, Wadhwa R. Sagittal alignment of the lumbar spine. *Neurosurg Clin N Am.* 2018;29:331–339.
4. Joseph Jr SA, Moreno AP, Brandoff J, Casden AC, Kuflik P, Neuwirth MG. Sagittal plane deformity in the adult patient. *J Am Acad Orthop Surg.* 2009;17(6):378–388.
5. Bernhardt M, Bridwell KH. Segmental analysis of the sagittal plane alignment of the normal thoracic and lumbar spines and thoracolumbar junction. *Spine.* 1989;14(7):717–721.
6. Dubousset J. *The Pediatric Spine.* New York: Raven Press; 1994.
7. Green C, Karneti G, Thomson K, Subramanian A. Lumbar spine radiographs—is it time for widespread adoption of posteroanterior projection? *Br J Radiol.* 2019;92(1103), 20190386.
8. Glassman SD, Sigurd B, Bridwell KH, Horton W, Dimar JR. Correlation of radiographic parameters and clinical symptoms in adult scoliosis. *Spine.* 2005;30:682–688.
9. Schwab F, Patel A, Ungar B, Farcy J, Lafage V. Adult spinal deformity-post operative standing imbalance. *Spine.* 2010;35:2224–2231.
10. Roussouly P, Nnadi C. Sagittal plane deformity: an overview of interpretation and management. *Eur Spine J.* 2010;19:1824–1836.
11. Celestre PC, Dimar JR, Glassman SD. Spinopelvic parameters: lumbar lordosis, pelvic incidence, pelvic tilt, and sacral slope. *Neurosurg Clin N Am.* 2018;29:323–329.
12. Schwab F, Lafage V, Boyce R, Skalli W, Farcy J. Gravity line analysis in adult volunteers: age related correlation with spinal parameters, pelvic parameters, and foot position. *Spine.* 2006;31:E959–E967.
13. Lafage V, Schwab F, Patel A, Hawkinson NP, Farcy J. Pelvic tilt and truncal inclination. *Spine.* 2009;34(17):E599–E606.
14. Buckland AJ, Abotsi EJ, Vasquez-Montes D, Ayres EW, Varlotta CG, Vigdorchik JM. Lumbar spine degeneration and flatback deformity alter sitting standing spinopelvic mechanics-Implications for total hip arthroplasty. *J Arthroplasty.* 2019;19.
15. Kukkar N, Gupta A, Banerjee D, Bedi N, Main BJ, Freitag P. Alterations in disc height, foraminal height and foraminal width following one and two level AxiaLIF-a radiological analysis. *J Spine.* 2013;S5:008.
16. Liu J, Nabil AE, Haman SP, et al. Effect of the increase in the height of lumbar disc space on facet joint articulation area in sagittal plane. *Spine.* 2006;31(7):E198–E202.
17. Kaito T, Hosono N, Mukai Y, Makino T, Fuji T, Yonenobu K. Induction of early degeneration of the adjacent segment after posterior lumbar interbody fusion by excessive distraction of lumbar disc space. *J Neurosurg Spine.* 2010;12(6):671–679.
18. Jones TR, Rao RD. Adult isthmic spondylolisthesis. *J Am Acad Orthop Surg.* 2009;17:609–617.
19. Li Y, Hresko MT. Radiographic analysis of spondylolisthesis and sagittal spinopelvic deformity. *J Am Acad Orthop Surg.* 2012;20(4):194–205.
20. Majid K, Fischgrund JS. Degenerative lumbar spondylolisthesis: trends in management. *J Am Acad Orthop Surg.* 2008;16:208–215.
21. Dai LY, Jiang SD, Wang XY, Jiang LS. A review of the management of thoracolumbar burst fractures. *Spine.* 2007;67:221–231.
22. Keynan O, Fisher CG, Vaccaro AR, et al. Radiographic measurement parameters in thoracolumbar fractures: a systematic review and consensus statement of the spine trauma study group. *Spine.* 2006;31(5):E156–E165.
23. Wood KB, Weishi L, Lebl DS, Ploumis A. Management of thoracolumbar spine fractures. *Spine.* 2014;14:145–164.
24. Selby MD, Clark SR, Hall DJ, Freeman BJ. Radiologic assessment of spinal fusion. *J Am Acad Orthop Surg.* 2012;20(11):694–703.
25. Brantigan JW, Steffee AD. A carbon fiber implant to aid interbody lumbar fusion. *Spine.* 1993;18(14):2106–2117.
26. Raizman NM, O'Brien JR, Kl P-M, Warren D. Pseudoarthrosis of the spine. *J Am Acad Orthop Surg.* 2009;17:494–503.
27. Fogel GR, Toohey JS, Neidre A, Brantigan JW. Fusion assessment of posterior lumbar interbody fusion using radiolucent cages: X-ray films and helical computed tomography scans compared with surgical exploration of fusion. *Spine.* 2008;8:570–577.
28. Radcliff KE, Kepler CK, Jakoi A, et al. Adjacent segment disease in the lumbar spine following different treatment interventions. *Spine.* 2013;13(10):1339–1349.
29. Djurasovic M, Carreon L, Glassman SD, Dimar JR, Puno RM. Sagittal alignment as a risk factor for adjacent level degeneration: a case-control study. *Orthopedics.* 2008;31(6):546.

CHAPTER 14

Lumbosacral Spine MRI

MARTINE VAN BILSEN • RONALD BARTELS
Department of Neurosurgery, Radboud University Medical Center, Nijmegen, The Netherlands

INTRODUCTION

The lumbosacral spine consists on average of 5 lumbar vertebrae, the sacrum, and coccyx. An MRI scan of this area is used to accurately depict soft tissue in and around the lumbosacral spine. Measurements mainly focus on a change in signal intensities and less on absolute distances or angles. Various pathologies affect the configuration of the soft tissue, which can lead to clinical symptoms such as neural compression syndromes, most commonly due to degeneration, congenital disorders, and benign or malignant neoplasms. Structures visible on MRI include neural structures, meninges, cerebrospinal fluid, blood vessels, fat, ligaments, bone and joints, discs, muscles, and organs. Knowledge of normal anatomy and the systematic assessment of these structures will help to generate the most accurate and clinically relevant scan interpretation. In addition, it is important to have a clinical question in mind before requesting and assessing a lumbosacral MRI, since, for example, degenerative abnormalities are common and asymptomatic in the majority of people.[1] More importantly, among patients without clinical signs pointing toward a specific condition, imaging does not improve patient outcomes and may lead to worse outcomes, unnecessary harm, and increased costs.[2, 3]

The focus of this chapter will be on normal anatomical configuration and signal intensities on MRI, but will also expand on the disruption of normal anatomy with various pathologies and their clinical correlations.

GENERAL ANATOMICAL STRUCTURES OF THE LUMBAR SPINE ON MRI

Various lumbar spine MRI scanning protocols exist, each with its own advantages and disadvantages. In this chapter, the main focus will be on sagittal and axial T2-weighted images and T1-weighted images with and without gadolinium and fat-suppressed T1- and T2-weighted images. Axial images should be scanned parallel to the endplates, while keeping in mind that the scanning direction must change as little as possible in order to facilitate the assessment of the course of the nerve roots.

The choice for specific sequences depends on the structures and pathology that need to be assessed. Table 1 shows normal T1, T2, and T1 with gadolinium enhancement (T1-G) intensities on MRI. On T1-weighted images, tissues with short T1 times like fat and bone marrow appear bright, while tissues with long T1 times, such as fluid and cortical bone appear dark. On T2-weighted images, tissues with short T2 times appear dark, as, for example, tendons, ligaments, nerves, and bone. Tissues with long T2 times are bright, as, for example, fluid in the thecal sac and joint effusions. Fat appears bright on both T1- and T2-weighted images and, therefore, fat suppression techniques are often utilized to improve visualization of structures otherwise masked by fat.[4] Furthermore, areas with hyperpermeable blood vessels as tumors, areas of inflammation and infection can show enhancement after gadolinium administration. As it has the highest number of unpaired electrons of all elements, gadolinium can be given as a contrast fluid to evaluate the accumulation of contrast. Often, these postcontrast T1 sequences are fat-suppressed to make this enhancement more distinguishable.

MR images provide a wealth of visible structures. To be complete without losing oneself in a lengthy and unnecessary maze of findings, a structured way of assessing an MRI study is useful. For this purpose, we use a modification of the ABCDE-method (Table 1).[5]

Later, the normal anatomy of these structures will be discussed first, according to the ABCDE-structure. Following the normal anatomy, various pathologies and their appearances on MRI will be explained.

Alignment

Assessment of alignment should include the presence of normal lumbar lordosis and proper positioning of each vertebra on top of the other. MRI of the lumbar spine is normally obtained with the patient in supine position. Previous studies have shown that MR images taken with the patient in supine position and legs straight out were comparable with standing MRI; however, a supine position with bent hips was found to significantly reduce lumbar lordosis by approximately

Atlas of Spinal Imaging. https://doi.org/10.1016/B978-0-323-76111-6.00006-7

TABLE 1		
ABCDE-Method for Structured Assessment of the Lumbar Spine on MRI.		
A	Alignment	Lumbar lordosis, number of lumbar vertebrae, listhesis
B	Bone	Vertebral body, arch, spinous processes, endplates, fractures, lesions, and ligaments (including ligamentum flavum)
C	Canal	Cord, conus, cauda equina, cerebrospinal fluid, epidural fat
D	Discs	Discs, neuroforamina, facet joints
E	Enhancement and extraspinal structures	Organs, muscles, fat, skin, contrast enhancement

TABLE 2
Castellvi Classification[11].
Type I: Enlarged and dysplastic transverse process in coronal view (at least 19 mm)
• **Ia:** Unilateral • **Ib:** Bilateral
Type II: Pseudoarticulation of the transverse process and sacrum with incomplete lumbarization/sacralization; enlargement of the transverse process with pseudoarthrosis
• **IIa:** Unilateral • **IIb:** Bilateral
Type III: Transverse process fuses with the sacrum and there is complete lumbarization or sacralization, enlarged transverse process with complete fusion
• **IIIa:** Unilateral • **IIIb:** Bilateral
Type IV: Type IIa on the one side and Type IIIa on the contralateral side

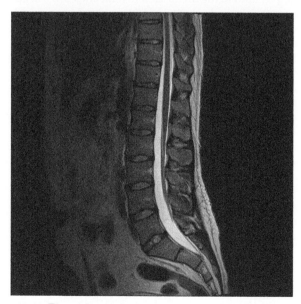

FIG. 1 T2-weighted images of a normal lumbosacral spine.

6.3° (14%).[6, 7] Spinal alignment should be judged on sagittal T1- or T2-weighted images (Fig. 1). It should be emphasized that instability cannot be assessed on a supine MRI. Deviation of vertebrae from the midsagittal plane may indicate scoliosis; however, as previously stated, MRI is not the imaging modality of choice to categorize the scoliosis, to measure angles and to make a treatment plan.

The most common number of lumbar vertebrae is five. In up to 20% of the general population lumbosacral transitional vertebrae (LSTV) are seen, of which the sacralization of L5 is the most common (~ 17%) and the lumbarization of S1 is rarer (~ 2%).[6, 8, 9] Recognition of these anomalies is important as it can influence clinical decision making and help to avoid wrong-level surgery.[10] The Castellvi classification[11] (Table 2) can be used to classify LSTV, but does not replace an accurate description of the anomaly. LSTV may be best visualized in a coronal view, because of the depiction of possible enlarged transverse processes of the lowest lumbar vertebra and the connection with the superior sacrum.[8] However, coronal images are not routinely included in a standard lumbosacral MRI protocol. Ways to recognize LSTV on sagittal images are the recognition of the iliolumbar ligament as this is found to arise from L5 in more than 95% of people[8] (Fig. 2) and a complete S1–2 intervertebral disc. If a LSTV is seen or suspected, aforementioned characteristics should be noted, including where the lowest well-formed intervertebral disc can be found, as this can be recognized at fluoroscopy during invasive treatments.

Bone

Bony and bone-related structures that need to be assessed are vertebral body, arch, spinous processes, endplates, fractures, lesions, and ligaments. The

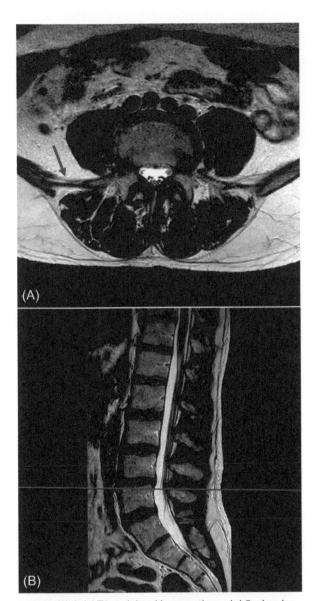

FIG. 2 (A) Axial T2-weighted images through L5, showing the iliolumbar ligament (arrow); (B) sagittal T2-weighted images of the same patient with the blue line indicating the level of the axial image (A) at the level of the L5 vertebra.

the lower boundary is formed by the lower endplate, which are normally symmetrically concave-shaped and without disruptions in young people. With age and degenerative processes, endplates can become thinner and even completely absent.[12] Whether the endplate belongs to the disc or the vertebral body is still debated, since it encompasses both an osseous component as well as a hyaline cartilage component.[13] In young patients, mainly under the age of 25, areas of focal fat deposition are common in the posterior elements of the vertebral body, as well as areas of high vascularity, due to conversion and reconversion processes. These areas include the subendplates and subcortical zones and also the area surrounding the basivertebral vein in the middle of the vertebral body[14, 15] (Fig. 1). This is a normal aging process of conversion and reconversion, expressed by the replacement of red marrow by yellow marrow, and should not raise suspicions when encountered. Other frequent and usually not pathological lesions in vertebral bodies are hemangiomas and vertebral enostosis.

The most important ligaments of the lumbar spine are the anterior longitudinal ligament (ALL) running in front of the vertebral bodies and intervertebral discs from the pelvic surface of the sacrum inferiorly to the anterior tubercle of C1 and basilar portion of the occipital bone superiorly,[16] the posterior longitudinal ligament (PLL) running posteriorly over the vertebral bodies and discs from the sacrum to C2. It then extends as the tectorial membrane at the level of the odontoid.[16] The ligamentum flavum connects the inner lamina, interspinous ligaments, and supraspinous ligaments. Ligaments and also cortical bone appear hypointense on both T1 and T2 and exhibit a slim and regular appearance.

Spinal Canal

The vertebral arches surround the spinal canal. This canal contains the thecal sac with the spinal cord above the L1-L2 level, cauda equina below this level and the conus at the interface of spinal cord and cauda equina floating in cerebrospinal fluid. Cerebrospinal fluid is hyperintense on T2 and hypointense on T1. However, flow voids can mimic a hypointense signal on T2. The neural structures are normally iso- to hypointense on T1- and T2-weighted images. Nerves of the cauda equina can be followed along their course running from the thecal sac through the lateral recess and foramen intervertebralis to the neural plexus. The nerve is normally running just below the pedicle. This is above

vertebral body is the largest part of the vertebral column and in its upper part arise two pedicles, which are connected to two laminae. These, together, form the vertebral arch, connected to a spinous process in a normal situation. The vertebral body is oval-shaped in the axial plain and square in the sagittal plane. Its upper boundary is formed by the upper endplate and

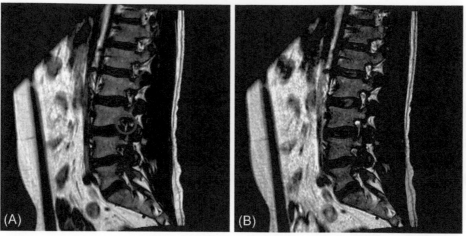

FIG. 3 (A) T1-weighted image through lumbar foramina (circle); (B) T2-weighted image through same lumbar foramina.

the level of the discus in the foramen intervertebralis. The nerve is surrounded by fat, which makes it assume the shape of an oval fried egg on sagittal images. This is best visible on a T1-weighted sequence (Fig. 3), when no compression is present. Normal presence of epidural fat is also seen on the dorsal side of the thecal sac anterior to the ligamentum flavum. Furthermore, a venous plexus is present in the canal and normally shows enhancement on a T1 with gadolinium.

There are various ways to measure spinal canal diameter, without consensus in literature nor uniform appliance in practice. As a result, various quantitative and qualitative measurements exist for the measurement of spinal canal diameter. In an international consensus meeting[17] between radiologists, consensus was reached about the use of five radiological criteria for lumbar spinal stenosis (LSS), which are all qualitative measurements related to LSS and therefore further described later in this chapter. Canal diameter can be quantitatively measured on axial T2, sagittal T1, and sagittal T2 images, as the mid-diameter of the thecal sac at the level of the intervertebral disc and midvertebral level (Fig. 3).

Intervertebral Discs

Intervertebral discs connect the vertebral bodies and together with ligaments buffer and support the spine from the distribution of forces that arise from axial compression and movement. The discs consist of a soft gelatinous core, which is named nucleus pulposus and firm rim, composed of concentric lamellae of fibrocartilage named annulus fibrosus.[16, 18] These

can be seen on an MRI T2 as a relatively hyperintense nucleus pulposus and hypointense annulus fibrosus. Degeneration of discs is a common finding in symptomatic and asymptomatic subjects,[2] which leads to dehydration of discs, visible as lower intensities on T2-weighted images. Herniated discs will be discussed further on in this chapter. When looking at discs, one should also judge the ligamentum flavum, neuroforamina, lateral recesses, and facet joints with their synovium. Figs. 1 and 2 show the normal anatomy of these structures, in relation to adjacent nerve roots. Knowledge of this anatomy is compulsory, as it determines the different levels of neural compression and related clinical symptoms. For example, the L4 root exits just below the pedicle of L4 and therefore will be only compressed by a far lateral disc herniation of the L4-L5 disc.

Enhancement and Extraspinal Structures

As a lumbar spine MRI also shows the abdominal area, visible extraspinal structures should also be assessed. These include organs as bladder, kidneys, uterus, bowel, aorta, muscles, subcutaneous tissue, and skin. Furthermore, enhancement after gadolinium administration should be assessed. Normal areas of contrast enhancement are epidural venous plexus, basivertebral veins, dorsal nerve root ganglion, and veins over the surface of the conus and cord. This enhancement can be differentiated from pathological enhancement by its expected anatomical location and flat and regular appearance in contrast to, for example, leptomeningeal metastasis, which are more nodular (Fig. 4).[19-21]

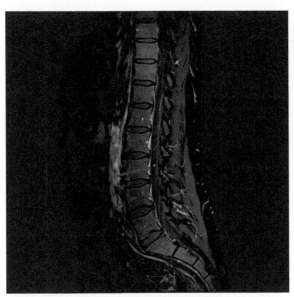

FIG. 4 T1-weighted image after administration of gadolinium. Nodular enhancement at the L3 level (arrow) in a patient with anaplastic ependymoma, suspect of leptomeningeal metastases.

ABNORMAL FINDINGS OF THE LUMBAR SPINE ON MRI

Trauma

MRI is not the imaging modality of choice for lumbosacral spinal trauma, as it does not show bone and vertebral fractures as well as CT imaging or plain radiographs.[22, 23]

However, its role is reserved for cases with neurological deficits. The differential diagnosis would be, for example, intervertebral traumatic disc rupture into the spinal canal, traumatic hematomas compressing the thecal sac or disco-ligamentous injury.[23, 24] This is different in occipitocervical, cervical, and thoracic trauma. However, these are not the subject of this chapter.

In the evaluation of a posttrauma, lumbosacral MRI scan attention must be paid to T2 signal hyperintensities due to edema or extravasation of blood, while ligaments are usually hypointense on all MRI sequences on T2-weighted images. Furthermore, bone marrow edema caused by a fracture or trabecular contusion and soft tissue edema or ligaments or disc disruption can be visualized on MRI (Fig. 5).

The differentiation between benign and malignant compression fractures can sometimes be difficult, especially in the case of osteoporotic fractures, because acute or subacute benign vertebral compression fractures can also show enhancement, large areas of low signal intensity on T1- and high signal intensity on T2-weighted images and even increased metabolism on nuclear imaging modalities, due to intertrabecular hemorrhage, edema, and healing processes.[25] Differentiating signs are a normal posterior element signal intensity and dislodged bony fragments in benign vertebral column fractures, with no epidural or paravertebral soft tissue mass and no expansion of the posterior vertebral contours. Furthermore, in benign vertebral column fractures, margins are more regular, and no diffusion restriction is visible[25, 26] (Fig. 6).

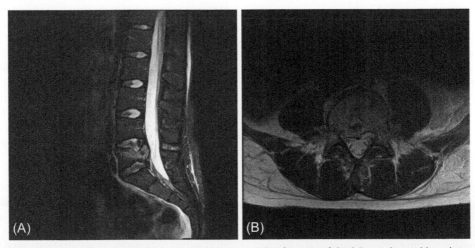

FIG. 5 T2-weighted sagittal (A) and axial (B) images of a compression fracture of the L5 vertebra, with an intraspinal osseous fragment compromising the right L5 rootlet, visible on the axial image (B). There is a discontinuation of the L4–5 intervertebral disc and endplate and a hyperintense signal in the interspinous ligaments between L4 and L5, suspect for discoligamentous injury.

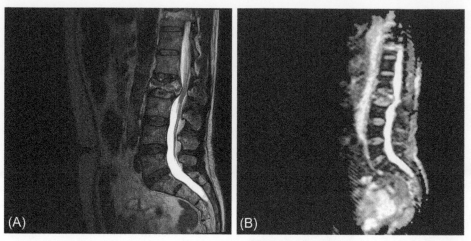

FIG. 6 (A) T2-weighted sagittal image of a fracture of the vertebral body of L2 suspect of a traumatic burst fracture; (B) normal ADC values support the finding of a nonmalignant traumatic fracture.

Degenerative Changes on Lumbosacral MRI

As previously stated, the presence of degeneration in a lumbar spine is a common finding and by no means an indicator of symptoms.[1-3] The etiology of these common degenerative changes is multifactorial: mechanical, traumatic, nutritional, inflammatory, and genetic factors are involved.[3, 27] In asymptomatic individuals, the prevalence of disc degeneration ranges from 37% at the age of 20 years to 96% at the age of 80 years. Facet degeneration has a prevalence of 4%–9% in asymptomatic individuals between 20 and 30 years of age, but its prevalence rises to 83% at the age of 80. Even spondylolisthesis is present in 50% of asymptomatic individuals of 80 years old, Table 3.[1]

Symptomatology can result from degenerative changes leading to the compression of neural structures and inflammatory changes.[3, 28] However, it is understandable that the findings of MRI should be interpreted based on the clinical presentation of the patient and not vice versa. It is of paramount importance that the clinical reason leading to the request of the MRI is stated on the application form in order to ensure proper judgment of a lumbar spinal MRI.

Radicular syndromes, neurogenic claudication, and lateral recess syndrome are frequently encountered. The compression of a nerve root by a herniated intervertebral disc is the most common cause of a radicular syndrome. Other possibilities are a tumor or inflammation causing compression. Neurogenic claudication or Verbiest's syndrome is due to narrowing of the lumbosacral spinal canal by an absolute stenosis and/or a listhesis, which may be due to degeneration of the spine, or more seldom a space-occupying mass, for example, a tumor or epidural lipomatosis. A neurogenic claudication occurring in just one leg, called lateral recess syndrome, can be caused by lateral recess stenosis or a foraminal stenosis.[29]

Intervertebral disc degeneration

Degenerative discs can be described according to the Pfirrmann classification[30] and the accompanying endplate changes according to the Modic classifications.[31] However, a study by Zehra et al.[32] showed great variation exists when it comes to endplate nomenclature and etiology when assessed on MRI and another study conducted by this group showed that a more multidimensional perspective in the assessment of endplate changes is needed in the assessment of endplate changes in MRI, this includes the measurement of depth and width of each endplate defect on MRI. The added values of these endplate defects in a cumulative endplate defect score are correlated with Oswestry Disability Index scores in literature.[33] However, correlation of clinical symptoms with these findings is difficult, even with hopeful research efforts, and controversies remain in literature and clinical practice about the role of endplate changes and disc degeneration when it comes to back pain.[33-35]

The posterior herniation of intervertebral discs must be described by location: central/median, paramedian, foraminal, or extraforaminal (Fig. 7), and kind of herniation can be described by the terms protrusion; extrusion; sequestration, migration, and bulging (Fig. 8). The size of the herniated disc can be mentioned, but most importantly, compression of nerves by the herniated disc must be explicitly named.

TABLE 3
Prevalence of Degenerative Findings on MRI in Asymptomatic Individuals.

	20 Years	30 Years	40 Years	50 Years	60 Years	70 Years	80 Years
Disc height loss	24%	34%	45%	45%	67%	76%	84%
Disc protrusion	29%	31%	33%	36%	38%	40%	43%
Facet degeneration	3%	9%	18%	32%	50%	69%	83%
Spondylolisthesis	3%	5%	8%	14%	23%	35%	50%

Modified and adapted from Brinjikji et al. Used with permission from AJNR.

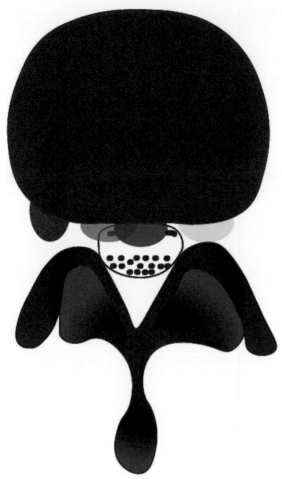

FIG. 7 Location of posterior intervertebral disc herniation. Purple is central/median; orange is paramedian; yellow is foraminal, and blue is extraforaminal.

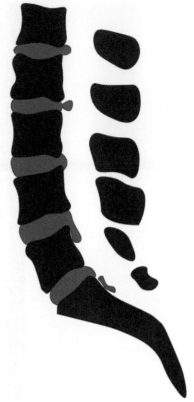

FIG. 8 Terminology of intervertebral disc herniation. L1–2 protrusion; L2–3 extrusion; L3–4 bulging; L4–5 sequestration; L5-S1 migration.

Signal intensity of the herniated disc must be noted. Herniated discs with high signal intensity and free fragmentated disc material have a high change of resolution with conservative therapy.[36] Obviously, conservative management is contraindicated in the case of a cauda equina syndrome.

Degenerative spinal stenosis

Degenerative spinal stenosis includes the narrowing of the central spinal canal, lateral spinal canal, or neuroforamina due to degenerative changes of the vertebral body, facet joints, intervertebral discs, and/or ligaments. Furthermore, epidural lipomatosis can be a contributing factor or an isolated cause in degenerative spinal stenosis. When performing measurements of the spinal canal diameters, one should realize that spinal canal diameter will vary between individuals[17, 37] and quantitative measurements are not sufficient and can even be mystifying when describing the amount of stenosis. As a substitute, qualitative measures should be used to indicate the severity of the stenosis, in other words: the radiographic consequences of the stenosis.[3, 17, 37] Furthermore, we recommend describing the cause of the stenosis, as this influences and supports surgical strategy.[38] Moreover, a variation in normal spinal canal diameter exists in the general population. As described by Singh et al.,[39] congenital stenotic patients are the patients with a shorter pedicular length and with that a smaller cross-sectional spinal canal area with mean critical values of 6.5 mm and 213 mm, respectively. This predisposes these patients to symptomatic neurogenic claudication and potential need for multilevel treatment.

Qualitative measures at the level of the stenosis include compromise of the central zone, visibility of cerebrospinal fluid, possibility to distinguish rootlets, amount of epidural fat, broadening of the ligamentum flavum, hypertrophy of facet joints, presence of synovial cysts, presence of disc pathology, and above the level of the stenosis the presence of redundant roots. The lateral canal and neuroforamina also need to be assessed for nerve root compression in the lateral recess, size, and shape of the foramen. This should include nerve root compression in the neuroforamen and the presence of intraforaminal perineural fat.

Fig. 9 shows a degenerative spinal stenosis. Note the enlargements of both facet joints in the axial plane, as well as the broadening of the ligamentum flavum and the bulging of the intervertebral disc. On the sagittal plane, the impingement of the central canal is clearly visible, the hyperintense signal of the cerebrospinal fluid is diminished, and redundant roots are visible above the level of stenosis. Furthermore, a decreased height of the intervertebral disc space is visible, which leads to infolding of the flaval ligament, sometimes incorrectly called hypertrophy. Furthermore, a noninvasive MR myelography can be helpful to assess the spinal stenosis (Fig. 9c).[40–42] This is done by making a heavy T2-weighted image and using a fast spine echo long-TR/long-TE sequence. With this sequence, CSF signal will be very bright and bone and ligaments are no longer visible.

As stated earlier, epidural lipomatosis can be a contributing factor of spinal stenosis or the solitary cause of the stenosis. It can be due to metabolic diseases as obesity, diabetes mellitus, or alcohol abuse. It can best be visualized on T1-weighted images in both sagittal and axial planes, as it can be hard to distinguish from cerebrospinal fluid and compression of the canal can be missed. The thecal sac will form a typical Y-sign[43] (Fig. 10).

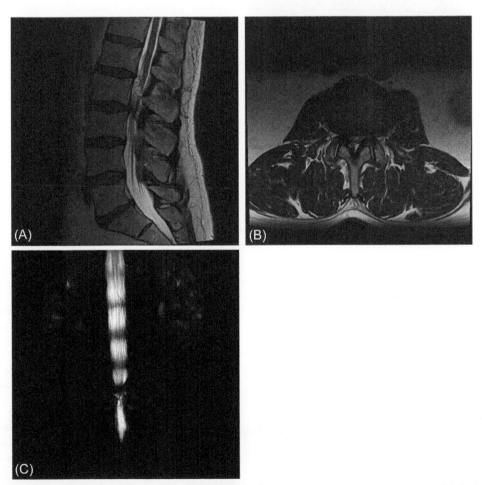

FIG. 9 (A) T2-weighted sagittal image and (B) T2-weighted axial image of a degenerative lumbar spinal stenosis. Redundant roots proximal to stenosis are seen. (C) MR myelography of a different patient shows a stenosis of the L4–5 level.

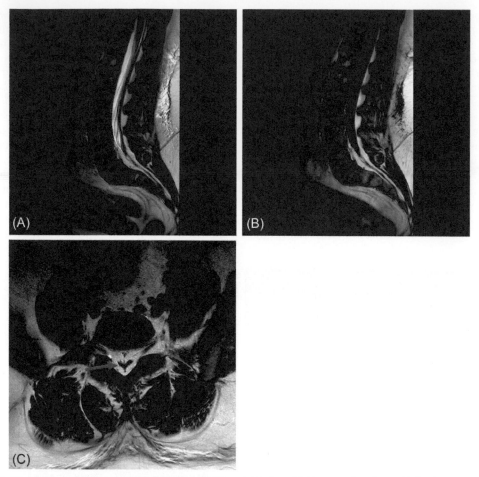

FIG. 10 (A) T2-weighted sagittal image and (B) T1-weighted sagittal image of patient with lumbar lipomatosis of the L5-S1 level, as well as (C) T2-weighted axial image with Y-sign in the same patient (arrow).

In up to 40% of the patients suffering from lumbar spinal stenosis, a phenomenon called "redundant roots" is visible on MRI (Fig. 9).[44] It includes a winding course of nerve rootlets above the level of the stenosis, which was, together with the clinical symptomatology of spinal stenosis, first described by Verbiest in 1954.[29] Its etiology remains still unclear; however, patients who show redundant roots on MRI have poorer clinical outcome than their counterparts without redundant roots on MRI.[44–47] Some findings suggest that a shortening of the lumbar spine due to degeneration is an etiological factor.[44] In addition, a shift of the nerve roots of the cauda equina from the posterior half of the dural sac to either side on T2-weighted images is called "sedimentation sign," which is an indicator of spinal stenosis .[48, 49]

Low back pain and lumbosacral MRI findings

Low back pain is an unspecific finding, and in about 95% of people with low back pain, no physical cause will be demonstrable.[50] When indicating a patient for lumbar MRI scanning, clinical assessment is of the upmost importance to look for concordance on MRI, for example, one should distinguish inflammatory back pain, myofascial pain, and chronic back pain syndrome, each with a different presentation.[51]

Furthermore, MRI scanning is indicated to rule out malignant causes of low back pain in patients with alarm symptoms as nocturnal back pain, progressive back pain, history of cancer, pain after pressure or percussion at the level of the spine, moderate patient condition or cachexia, severe pain in every position, pain between the shoulder blades or concomitant fever.

Inflammatory and Infectious Diseases of the Lumbar Spine on MRI

Infections of the lumbar spine may affect various different anatomical structures, including intervertebral discs, vertebral body, paraspinal tissues, epidural spaces, meninges, and intradural structures as nerve roots and the spinal cord itself. Spinal infections involving intervertebral discs and vertebral bone are most common and are therefore named spondylodiscitis.[52-54] However, this term is used more widely, since, as the infection spreads into the surrounding structures, it will still be referred to as spondylodiscitis. Moreover, the invasion of soft tissue helps in the differentiation from other entities as Modic type I changes of the endplates. Risk factors for spondylodiscitis include a remote infection, prior spinal instrumentation or spinal trauma, intravenous drug use, immunosuppression, steroid use, diabetes mellitus, malnutrition, or cancer. Patients typically present with back pain together with, less frequently, associated fever. Causative bacteria usually originate from hematologic spread and come from sources such as endocarditis or IV drug use. The causative agent is mostly *Staphylococcus aureus* (60%), but *Streptococcus viridans* and gram-negative organisms, such as Enterobacter species and *E. Coli*, are also commonly encountered. The spinal infection with *Mycobacterium tuberculosis* is called Pott's disease (Fig. 11). After blood cultures and biochemical markers are obtained, MRI is the imaging modality of choice, because of its high sensitivity and specificity. Furthermore, it is more cost-effective and faster compared to alternatives such as positron emission tomography.

Typical findings of spondylodiscitis on MRI are destructive lesions in usually two adjacent vertebrae with the involvement of the intermediate intervertebral disc (Fig. 12). Involvement of an intervertebral disc is frequently not seen in malignant disease. On T1-weighted images, changes in bone and disc are hypointense, whereas on T2-weighted images, they are hyperintense. After intravenous gadolinium administration enhancement of these changes will be seen. Additionally, invasion of paravertebral soft tissue and sometimes epidural empyema or abscess formation will be visible.

Sparing of disc spaces is suggestive of Pott's disease, as is subligamentous spread of abscess, vertebral body collapse, and a large abscess with thin abscess wall. A combination of these is highly suggestive.[55] Because these findings can also occur in metastatic disease of the spine, differentiation can be made with certainty by the finding of abscesses, which unfortunately does not occur in all cases of Pott's disease. Other differentiating but not pathognomonic findings are more concentric collapses, skip lesions, and solitary lesions in metastatic cases.[56]

Lumbosacral Neoplasms on MRI

Spinal tumors can be divided into intradural and extradural tumors. Intradural tumors are further divided into intra- or extramedullary tumors. Since the spinal cord normally ends above L1-L2, most of the tumors in the lumbosacral area will be extramedullary. Occasionally,

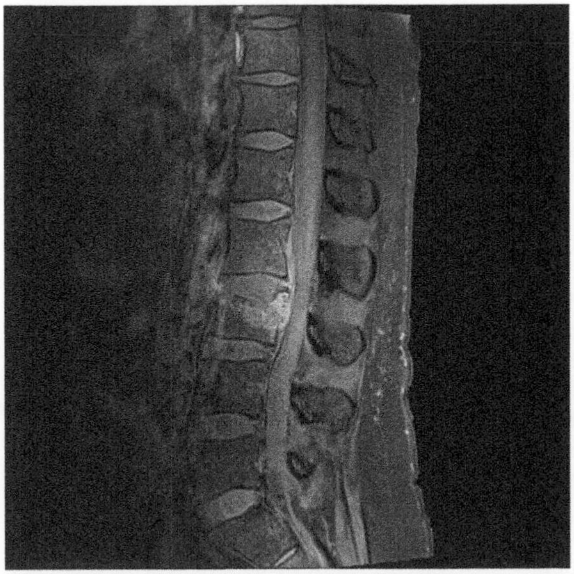

FIG. 11 T1-weighted sagittal image after the administration of gadolinium in a patient with Pott's disease.

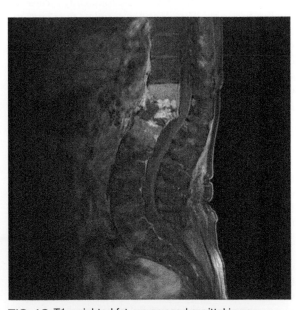

FIG. 12 T1-weighted fat-suppressed sagittal image after the administration of gadolinium in a patient with *Staphylococcus aureus* spondylodiscitis Th12-L2.

they originate from the terminal ligament. Extradural tumors are either primary or secondary. Primary tumors are tumors originating from any of the tissues contributing to the spine (i.e., bones and bone marrow, cartilage that protects the joints in the vertebrae, blood vessels, nerves, meninges, fat, and spinal cord). Secondary spinal tumors are metastatic tumors, these are more common, and their incidence is expected to further increase with improving cancer survival rates. Primary tumors of the spine are far less common than metastatic spinal disease and include a heterogeneous group of tumors with different behavioral patterns. Chordomas, chondrosarcomas, osteosarcomas, and Ewing's sarcomas are the most common malignant types of primary vertebral tumors. As their treatment is highly specialized and challenging and outcomes, such as survival and local recurrence, are dependent on proper and timely treatment, proper recognition and referral is of utmost importance.

Metastatic spinal disease

Up to 70% of the patients with metastatic disease will get spinal metastases.[57] Mostly, these arise from hematogenous spread[58] and their location in the spine is therefore correlated with the relative bone mass and blood flow to the different spinal regions. Location can vary between osseous components of the vertebral column (85%) to paravertebral regions (10%–15%) or epidural or intradural spaces (< 5%).[59] Tumor emboli initially tend to seed to the posterior half of the vertebral body and metastases are therefore most frequently located in the lumbar spine. This does not correlate to symptomatic cord compression, as this most often occurs in the thoracic spine due to the relatively small thoracic spinal canal.[57] Intervertebral discs are mostly spared. MRI is a good imaging modality to diagnose spinal metastatic disease, specify levels of involvement, and assess compression of neural structures and spinal stability.[60]

The signal characteristics of the metastatic lesion vary with the imaging sequences used and need to be differentiated from normal bone marrow and from the conversion and reconversion processes and benign compression fractures, as explained previously. Furthermore, signal intensity varies with the mineralization of the bone and lesion and therefore osteoblastic and osteolytic lesions have different signal intensities. Normal bone marrow is hypointense on T1 imaging and normally becomes more intense with age. Metastatic lesions are hypointense as well and sclerotic lesions are even more hypointense. Hemorrhagic metastasis, however, can appear hyperintense on T1. T1 sequences after administration of gadolinium can improve the visibility of spinal metastasis. However, metastatic lesions, especially sclerotic ones, do

not necessarily show enhancement and, thus, T1 without gadolinium remains necessary for comparison. In the case of a great amount of fatty bone marrow, a fat suppression technique or short tau inversion recovery (STIR) can improve the distinguishability of lesions[61] (Fig. 13).

On T2-weighted images, intensity in metastatic lesions is more variable.[60, 61] Osteoblastic malignant lesions are usually hypointense on T2 compared to normal bone marrow, but can become iso- to hyperintense if the lesion is more osteolytic in nature. Metastatic lesions often show a hyperintense rim surrounding the lesion on T2-weighted images. This is called a halo sign, which is, with a sensitivity of 75% and specificity of 99.5% an indicator of metastatic disease. A hyperintensity visible in the middle of the lesion on T2, on the contrary, is an indicator of normal hematopoietic marrow and has a sensitivity of 75% and specificity of 99.6%.[60, 62] As described earlier in the differentiation between osteoporotic fractures and malignant fractures, ADC can be used, diffusion restriction can occur in malignant lesions as a result of a large amount of intra- and intercellular membranes.[25, 26, 60] Furthermore, the precise location of the pathological signal intensity must be described, as well as any paraspinal extension, collapse, and compression of neural structures.

Vertebral sarcomas of the lumbosacral spine on MRI

Sarcomas of the spine are malignant primary bone tumors and relatively rare entities. They include, among others, osteosarcomas, chondrosarcomas, Ewing's sarcomas, undifferentiated/undefined soft tissue sarcomas, and fibrosarcomas.[63, 64] MRI signal changes are not always specific in differentiating sarcomas. However, MRI is a very good imaging modality for defining the extent of the lesion, relationship with surrounding structures, and evaluating a postoperative status.

Spinal *osteosarcomas* are rare, derive from the vertebral bone, and are divided into primary and secondary osteosarcomas, with different histologic forms.[65] Primary osteosarcomas typically occur in the patients of a young age (10–20 years), whereas secondary osteosarcomas occur in older patients, following, for example, bony infarction, Paget's disease, or radiotherapy. They account for < 5% of primary spinal tumors. Also < 5% of osteosarcomas arise in the spine.[66-68] They can be found in all spinal regions, but are most common in the lumbosacral spine. They can occur in the vertebral body as well as in the posterior elements of the spine, and literature is contradictory about its preferred localization.[66, 67] Occurrence in the posterior elements can make them hard to distinguish from benign osteoblastomas.

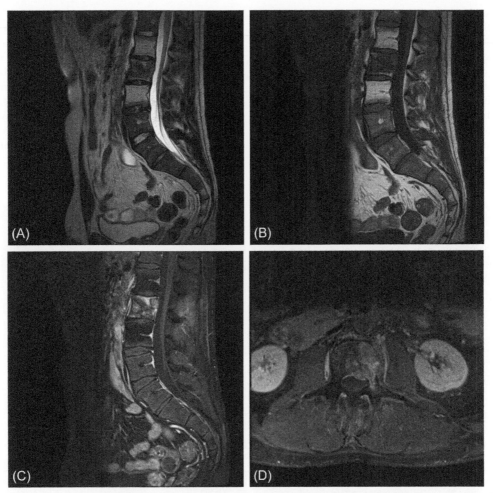

FIG. 13 MR images of a patient with metastatic lesion of melanoma, with prior radiotherapy on metastatic lesions in the L1 and L3 vertebra. (A) Sagittal T2-weighted image with a hyperintense signal change in the L1 and L3 vertebrae as a result of postradiation therapy fatty changes, inhomogeneous signal in the L2 corpus, suggestive of a metastatic lesion. (B) The sagittal T1-weighted image supports the finding of fatty changes in the vertebral body of L1 and L3. (C) Sagittal T1-weighted image after gadolinium administration and fat suppression technique shows enhancement of the L2 vertebral body that supports the suspicion of a metastatic lesion in L2 and fatty conversion after radiotherapy of L1 and L3. (D) Axial T1-weighted image at the level of the L2 vertebra after gadolinium administration shows a lesion suspect for metastasis in the vertebral body expanding in the left pedicle and cortical bone and slightly in the spinal canal.

Osteosarcomas are often highly mineralized, bulky, expansive, and inhomogeneous tumors, which results in a hypointense lesion on both T1- and T2-weighted images, with the areas of more hyperintensity and enhancement of the more solid tumor parts. There can be some hemosiderin deposits and surrounding edema. The disc space is usually, but not always preserved.[64, 67, 68]

Chondrosarcomas arise in about 10% of the cases in the spine[64, 67] and may form cartilage. The mean age of presentation is 45 years, and there is a male predominance.[64]

Most chondrosarcomas are primary lesions, but they can be secondary to an osteochondroma. On MRI, the tumor is often bulky, hypointense on T1 and heterogeneous with both hyperintensities and hypointensities on T2. Ring-and-arc calcifications can best be seen on CT, but are also visible on T2-weighted MRI as hypointense rims, with also on T1 with gadolinium ring-and-arc enhancement (Fig. 14). These ring-and-arc patterns correspond with fibrovascular bundles surrounding hyaline cartilage lobules.[69]

Ewing's sarcomas are, like PNET tumors, considered as a round cell sarcoma and part of Ewing's sarcoma family of tumors.[65, 70] Three to ten percentage of Ewing's sarcomas are located in the spine,[66, 71] but Ewing's sarcoma metastasis of a different primary location can metastasize to the spine, and are more common than primary spinal Ewing's sarcomas. Ewing's sarcoma is a high grade, undifferentiated tumor, consisting of uniform small blue round cells and necrosis is often present.[71] The sacrum is the most common spinal localization, in which the ala is the most frequently involved sacral

site.[67] By far the most lesions are lytic (93%), but they may also be sclerotic or mixed. They exhibit a soft tissue mass that is larger than the intraosseous lesion, and in 91% of the cases, there is an invasion of the spinal canal. They appear iso- to hypointense on T1-weighted images and have a clear contrast enhancement after administration of gadolinium. On T2-weighted images, they appear somewhat heterogeneous, but overall more hyperintense[64, 66] (Fig. 15). Classification from osteosarcomas can be difficult. The appearance of mineralization is the hallmark of osteosarcomas.

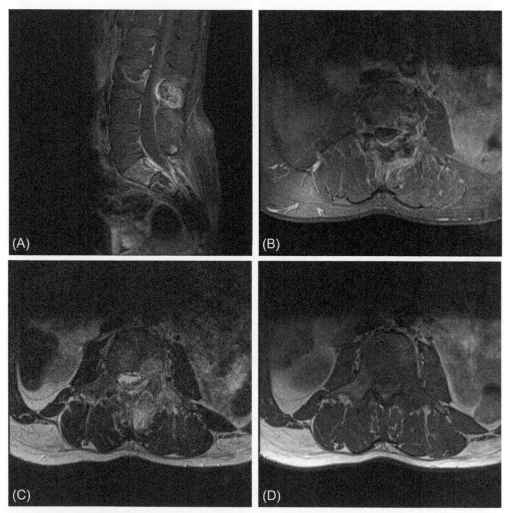

FIG. 14 MRI scan of a patient with metastasis of chondrosarcoma originating from the femur head. (A) Sagittal fat-suppressed T1-weighted image after the administration of gadolinium shows lesions in the L3 vertebral body and spinous process, as well as in the sacrum. Typical ring-and-arc enhancement can best be seen in the L3 spinous process. (B) Axial fat-suppressed T1-weighted image after the administration of gadolinium shows the L3 lesion. (C) Axial T2-weighted image of the L3 lesion shows a heterogeneous signal intensity of the lesion. (D) Axial T1-weighted image of the L3 lesion shows a hypointense signal of the lesion.

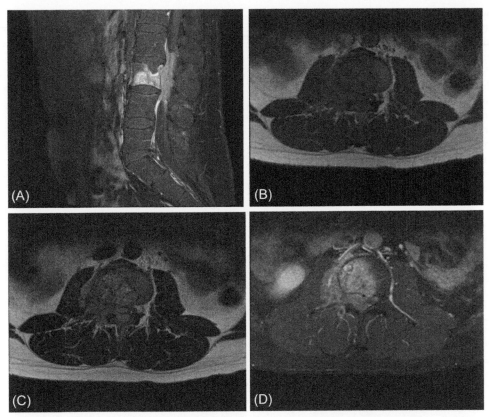

FIG. 15 MRI scan of a patient with Ewing's sarcoma of the L3 vertebra. (A) Fat-suppressed sagittal T1-weighted image after the administration of gadolinium shows a clear contrast enhancement of the lesion as well as intraspinal expansion. (B) Axial T1-weighted image shows an iso- to hypointense lesion. (C) Axial T2-weighted image shows a somewhat heterogeneous lesion. (D) Axial T1-weighted fat-suppressed image after the administration of gadolinium shows also clear contrast enhancement.

Undifferentiated/undefined soft tissue sarcomas previously included a wide spectrum of soft tissue sarcomas called *malignant fibrous histiocytomas* and, before that, fibrosarcomas. The tumors classified in these former categories are nowadays often reclassified in different subcategories of soft tissue sarcomas and the term undifferentiated soft tissue sarcoma is now reserved for a remaining group of tumors that do not have further differentiating characteristics and remain undefined.[72] Soft tissue sarcomas can occur in the entire body, but are most commonly in soft tissues of the extremities. However, 1%–5% do arise in or around bone and can appear as destructive lesions that have a signal intensity similar to muscle. They are iso- to hypointense on T1-weighted images and iso- to hyperintense on T2-weighted images. They often exhibit signs of bleeding, calcification, or necrosis, which will make them more heterogeneous in appearance. After the administration of gadolinium, the T1-weighted images will show, mostly peripheral, enhancement of these lesions.[73]

Other malignant bone tumors

Multiple myeloma is the most common form of primary bone cancer. It is the malignant monoclonal proliferation of plasma cells from red marrow. It can affect any bone in the body and spinal involvement is seen in 65% of the cases.[64] It leads to osteolytic changes in bone induced via a cytokine reaction and results in increased blood calcium, anemia, and decreased kidney function. Plasmacytoma is a precursor of multiple myeloma, as it presents as a solitary bone lesion but without the systemic effects. It has better prognosis but may evolve into multiple myeloma as well. Multiple myeloma typically appears as a hypointense lesion on T1-weighted images and an isointense to hyperintense lesion on T2-weighted images. Fat suppression can help in detecting these lesions, to depress normal bone marrow. After contrast administration multiple myeloma lesions show enhancement in more than 40% of the cases.[74] Furthermore, five appearances of infiltrated vertebral bone marrow on MRI are commonly seen and described by Stäbler et al.,[75] namely normal appearance, diffuse infiltration, and focal lesion(s), combined focal and diffuse infiltration and a salt-and-pepper appearance.

Primary *spinal lymphomas* are relatively rare as spinal lymphoma metastases from other sites of the body are much more common. Most lymphomas involve the anterior part of the spine. However, no specific hallmark of lymphoma exists on MRI. Lesions can be either lytic or mixed and are seldom sclerotic. Intensities are highly heterogeneous, and enhancement is variable. Pathological fractures can be seen.[64]

Chordomas are malignant neoplasms arising from the remnants of the notochord, and therefore, their consistency mimics the annulus of the intervertebral disc. They arise predominantly in the clivus and sacral spine, but can also be seen in the cervical, thoracic, and lumbar spine as well. Their appearance on MRI is also similar to nucleus pulposus of the intervertebral disc, but this is not specific. It is hypo- to isointense on T1-weighted images and hyperintense on T2-weighted images. It has a mushroom-like appearance on coronal images, mostly expands across several segments, and spares intervertebral discs. It enhances heterogeneously after gadolinium administration to the patient, and the enhancement pattern can be septal[76] (Fig. 16).

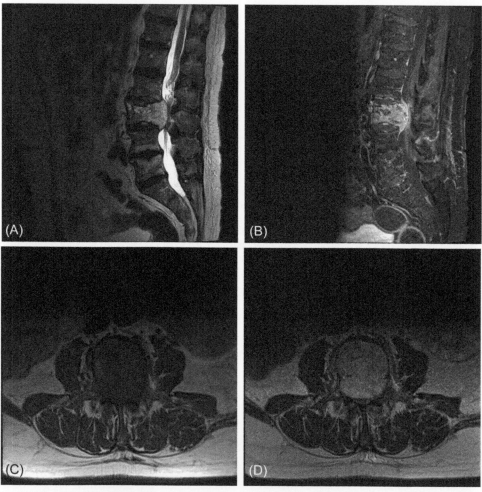

FIG. 16 MRI scan of a patient with a chordoma of the L3 vertebra. (A) Sagittal T2-weighted image shows a hyperintense lesion, which is protruding into and partially obliterating the spinal canal, note the "mushroom" shaped appearance. (B) Sagittal fat-suppressed T1-weighted image after the administration of gadolinium shows an irregular, almost septal enhancement pattern. (C) Axial T1-weighted image shows a hypointense lesion. (D) Axial T2-weighted image shows a hyperintense lesion.

Benign vertebral bone tumors

Vertebral hemangiomas are the most common benign vertebral bone tumors with an estimated incidence of 10%–12%. They appear as high-intensity lesions on T2-weighted images and STIR, due to low blood flow. On T1-weighted images, they also appear as high-intensity lesions, due to a high-fat content. Hemangiomas can show varying patterns of enhancement. When in doubt, correlation with X-ray and CT can help to identify these lesions. They are asymptomatic, save for about 1% of the cases they cause symptoms. Then, they will be called aggressive spinal hemangioma, defined as spinal hemangioma with significant expansion causing neurological damage or spinal instability[77] (Fig. 17).

Eosinophilic granuloma is an idiopathic lytic lesion of the bone that occurs most often in flat bones and long bones, but can occur in the spine as well. It is considered a benign form of Langerhans cell histiocytosis. In children, it presents as a complete flattening of a vertebra, with the preservation of disc spaces, called vertebra plana, and typically involves the thoracic and lumbar spine. In adults, this rare disease is even more uncommon and smaller portions of the vertebral body are involved, preventing the vertebral body from collapsing, cervical involvement is more common. No pathognomonic findings on MRI can be described and most often histopathology identifies these lesions. On MRI, T2-weighted images show a hyperintense lesion with a hypointense rim. This dense rim is also enhancing

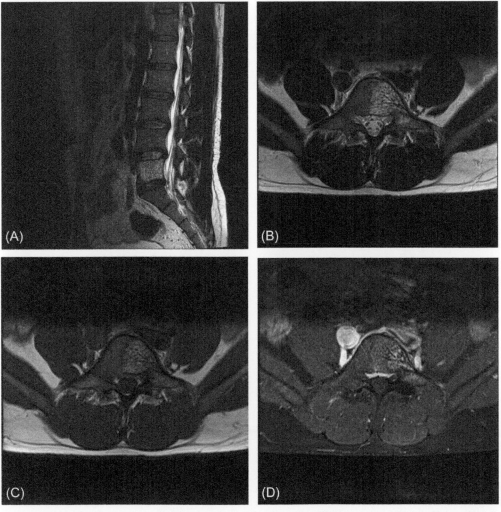

FIG. 17 Vertebral hemangioma of L5.

on T1-weighted images with gadolinium with a central hypointensity.[78, 79]

Osteoid osteoma usually presents with back pain that occurs at night and is accompanied by a painful scoliosis. The osteoid osteoma is then located at the apex of the concavity of the curve. It consists of a 1–2-mm big vascular fibrous nidus with mineralization, enclosed by a variable amount of reactive sclerotic bone and surrounded by edema. CT is the imaging modality of choice, as it is more specific in detecting the nidus. MRI appearance varies with the amount of calcification in the lesion and lesion can enhance after gadolinium administration. As they mostly occur in the posterior elements, a hyperin-

tense signal within these elements is a possible indicator of an underlying osteoid osteoma.[80–82]

Osteoblastomas are histologically similar to osteoid osteomas, except for the fact that they are larger than 1.5-2 cm, do not have a large surrounding sclerotic area, and are more vascular. Furthermore, they do not improve clinically after nonsteroidal anti-inflammatory drugs and do not present with pain that is worse at night. Their aspect on MRI is thus quite similar to osteoblastomas; they can expand into larger areas of bone and even soft tissue and have a more diffuse mineralization pattern (Fig. 18). In 10%–15% of the cases, they are more aggressive and show features of osteosarcoma,

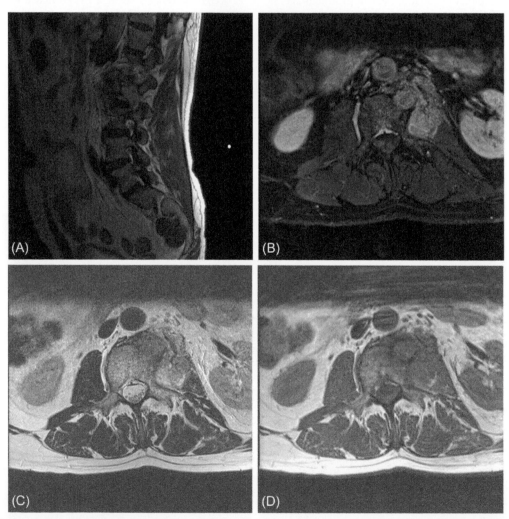

FIG. 18 Osteoblastoma. (A) Sagittal T1-weighted image after gadolinium administration showing a lesion at the left vertebral body and pedicle of L2, expanding into soft tissue. (B) Axial T1-weighted image with fat suppression after gadolinium administration showing the lesion at the L2 level. (C) Axial T2-weighted image showing the lesion at the L2 level. (D) Axial T1-weighted image without fat suppression showing the lesion at the L2 level.

and these lesions are consequently called aggressive osteoblastomas.[81, 82] Transformation into osteosarcoma is very rare and perhaps a misdiagnosis, but has been described in literature.

Osteochondromas, also known as exostosis, are commonly benign bone tumors that are rare in the spinal area. They originate in the periosteal layer and grow because of endochondral bone formation starting from a cartilage cap at the periphery of the lesion. They are often asymptomatic, but if they do occur in the spine, they can cause compression of neural structures.[83] Pathognomonic for these lesions on imaging is their continuity with bony cortex and medullary cavity.[84] These lesions can deteriorate into malignancies, generally osteosarcomas. MRI risk factors for malignant transformation are a cartilage cap thicker than 2 cm in adults and thicker than 3 cm in children.[83, 84] Signal intensities on MRI can vary and mimic normal bone intensities, the cortical areas are of low intensities on both T1- and T2-weighted images, and marrow demonstrates higher T1 signal intensities and is isointense on T2-weighted images. Enhancement pattern can vary, but normally, enhancement is seen in peripheral and septal areas.[84]

Giant cell tumors mostly occur in the sacrum. They consist of osteoclastic giant cells in a spindle cell stroma. They have cystic areas and can have areas that had previously bled and hemosiderin depositions, which makes them heterogeneous on MRI. They are often large and lytic, and grow more aggressive, which makes them less benign. On MRI, they appear hypointense on T2-weighted images, which is in contrast to other bone tumors and is isointense on T1-weighted images. They can enhance and the pattern of enhancement is inhomogeneous.[85, 86]

Aneurysmal bone cysts are most common in the thoracic spine. They consist of multiple bone-filled cavities that are not delineated with endothelium. They probably originate from local disturbances in blood flow due to trauma or other lesions like giant cell tumors, osteoblastomas, or chondrosarcomas and therefore often occur simultaneously. On MRI, fluid levels can be seen. Aneurysmal bone cysts are hypointense on T1-weighted images; on T2-weighted images, they are hyperintense. Moreover, a hypointense rim, coming from periosteum, is also visible sometimes. After administration of gadolinium, T1-weighted images show characteristic thin septal enhancement[87, 88] (Fig. 19).

Intradural lesions

Meningiomas and *schwannomas* are both intradural lesion that can mimic each other on MRI. Meningiomas originate from arachnoid cells and schwannomas orig-

inate from Schwann cells. They are both round- and oval-shaped lesions that are sharply delineated. MRI confers precise measurement, configuration, and anatomical relationships. Furthermore, it can help in differentiating these two lesions, which helps in preoperative planning. Schwannomas can, given their origin, grow into and enlarge the neuroforamen and have a dumbbell-like shape (Fig. 20). The origin of meningiomas makes that they can show a so-called dural tail sign, showing their meningeal adherence. The intensity of the lesions on MRI can differ from hypointense to hyperintense or heterogeneous for both lesions. Meningiomas, however, more often show a hyperintense signal on T2-weighted images and isointense signal on T1-weighted images, whereas schwannomas often show a hypo- to isointense signal on T1-weighted images and an isointense signal on T2-weighted images.[89, 90] Both lesions enhance after the administration of gadolinium. The most common pattern of enhancement is diffuse, but is at times rim-like, indicating a relatively hypovascular lesion core, which is more common in schwannomas. Both schwannomas and meningiomas are benign lesions and a wait and scan policy can be followed safely, as primary malignant peripheral nerve sheath tumors in the intradural lumbosacral region are very rare. However, in the case of a patient with neurofibromatosis type 1, or a fast-growing tumor, this differential diagnosis should be kept in mind.[91]

Spinal neurofibromas are generally located cervically, where they arise along the dorsal sensory rootlets. They are associated with neurofibromatosis type 1 and can have a malignant deterioration into a malignant peripheral nerve sheath tumor. They may also occur in the lumbar region and are on MRI undistinguishable from foraminal schwannomas, as their signal intensity is similar. The intradural location of neurofibroma is a rare entity.[92, 93] As stated before, *malignant peripheral nerve sheath tumor (MPNST)* has to be considered in the case of a fast-growing tumor. Additionally, a large lesion or a lesion with irregular borders should raise the suspicion of a malignant lesion. MPNST shows usually an isointense signal on T1 that is often heterogeneous. On T2, they can appear hypointense and normally show contrast enhancement.[94]

Myxopapillary ependymoma accounts for more than 80% of primary tumors of the conus medullaris region. These tumors are mucoid tumors and arise from glial cells of the filum terminale and in 43% of the cases, multiple lesions are present. On MRI, they regularly appear well delineated as they are usually

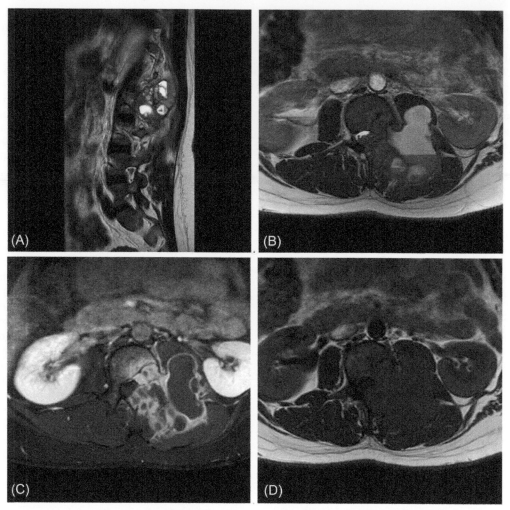

FIG. 19 Aneurysmal bone cyst. (A) Sagittal T2-weighted image at the L2 level, showing typical cysts and fluid levels. (B) Axial T2-weighted image at the L2 level, showing typical cysts and fluid levels. (C) Fat-suppressed T1-weighted image at the L2 level, showing septal enhancement after gadolinium administration. (D) Axial T1-weighted image at the L2 level.

encapsulated (Fig. 21). They appear sausage-shaped and are somewhat heterogeneous and hypointense on T1-weighted images and hyperintense on T2-weighted images. They show diffuse, intense enhancement.[95] Their differential diagnosis includes paragangliomas, which are uncommon, but not rare, in this region. Myxopapillary ependymomas are neuroendocrine tumors that are vascular and often encapsulated. Often, a feeding vessel can be differentiated. They are isointense on T1-weighted images and heterogeneous and of varying intensity on T2-weighted images. There can be intralesional hemorrhage and the lesion shows strong enhancement after gadolinium administration.[96]

Hemangioblastomas are highly vascularized tumors most commonly found in the central nervous system. Lumbosacral spinal hemangioblastomas are generally found in the conus medullaris or spinal cord, but they are described in the cauda equina as well.[97] Hemangioblastomas originate in vascular stromal cells and are associated with von Hippel–Lindau disease. They are composed of a highly vascular nodule and often surrounded by a cyst. This nodule is hypointense on T1-weighted images and hyperintense on T2-weighted images and brightly enhancing after gadolinium. The wall of the cyst may enhance as well.[98]

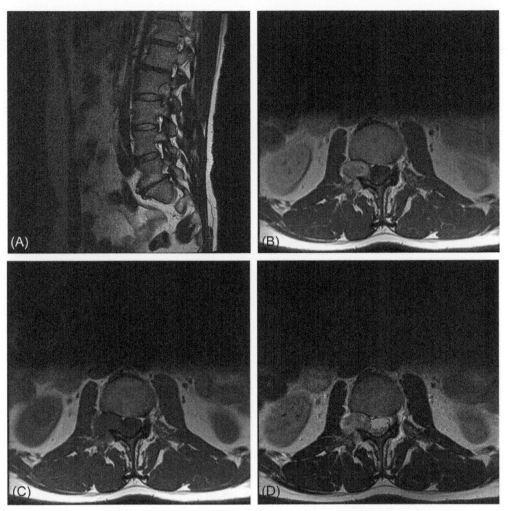

FIG. 20 MRI of an intraforaminal schwannoma of the right L2 nerve root. (A) Sagittal T2-weighted image. Note the enlargement and filling of the neuroforamen of the L2 root. (B) Axial T1-weighted image after the administration of gadolinium; the tumor is dumbbell-shaped, and a diffuse intense enhancement pattern is seen. (C) Axial T1-weighted image. (D) Axial T2-weighted image.

Inclusion cysts are mostly congenital aberrations and include d*ermoid and epidermoid cysts.* They are associated with anomalies such as dermal sinus track, (occult) spinal dysraphism, and Currarino syndrome. Dermoid and epidermoid cysts result from an embryogenic inclusion of ectodermal cells within the neural groove and can thus be located intradurally, intramedullary, extramedullary, or even extradurally in the midline. They grow from the desquamation of keratin from cystic wall cells into the cystic cavity and are therefore not true neoplasms. Both dermoid and epidermoid cysts are delineated by stratified squamous epithelial cells, but epidermoid cysts also contain skin appendages as

sebaceous glands, sweat glands, and sometimes even hair follicles. This results in a more fatty hyperintense signal on T1- and T2-weighted images, although MRI cannot reliably distinguish these two entities. Inclusion cysts are hyperintense on T2-weighted images and hypo- or hyperintense on T1-weighted images. Their FLAIR signal is hyperintense compared to cerebrospinal fluid. Diffusion restriction is common, but not a rule, and mild rim enhancement can be visible[99] (Fig. 22). Differential diagnosis also includes a spinal *teratoma* and *arachnoid cysts.* A spinal teratoma can include hair, teeth, or even bone and is therefore often more heterogeneous on MRI. It has the same signal intensities as dermoid

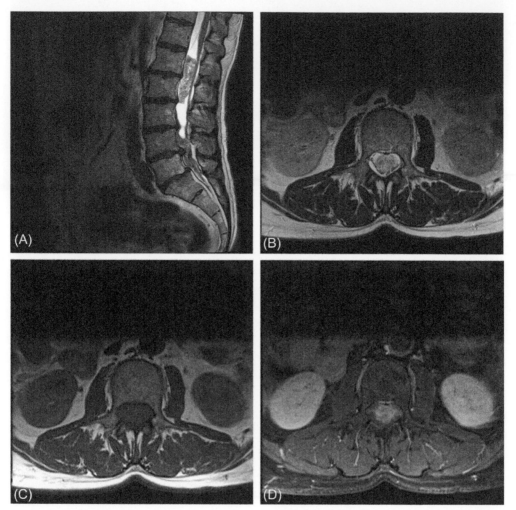

FIG. 21 Myxopapillary ependymoma. (A) Sagittal T2-weighted image. (B) Axial T2-weighted image at the level of the L2 vertebra. (C) Axial T1-weighted image at the level of the L2 vertebra. (D) Fat-suppressed axial T1-weighted image after the administration of gadolinium at the level of the L2 vertebra.

and epidermoid cysts on MRI. A spinal teratoma is exceedingly rare, especially in occurrence elsewhere than the sacrococcygeal region and above the age of two years old.[100] An arachnoid cyst is a CSF-filled sac delineated by the arachnoid membrane that may be congenital or acquired and can grow because of a ventil-like mechanism, allowing CSF inflow and limited outflow. On MRI, their signal intensity is similar to CSF without contrast enhancement or diffusion restriction.[101]

Closure Defects of the Lumbosacral Spine on MRI

Most congenital diseases of the lumbosacral spine are embryologic closure defects or so-called spinal dys-

raphisms or neural tube defects. They result from problems in gastrulation, primary neurulation, or secondary neurulation, all leading to different anomalies.[102] Because of this, a wide range of anomalies and MRI scans can be acquired, from intrauterine to adult spinal MRI scans. The assessment of these MRI scans can best be done in a systematic manner. The assessment begins with defining whether the defect is open or closed, according to the Tortori-Donati classification.[103] Open dysraphism is then classified into myelomeningocele, myelocele, hemimyelomeningocele, or hemimyelocele. Closed dysraphism should be subsequently classified into dysraphisms with subcutaneous mass or without subcutaneous mass. Closed dysraphistic lesions with

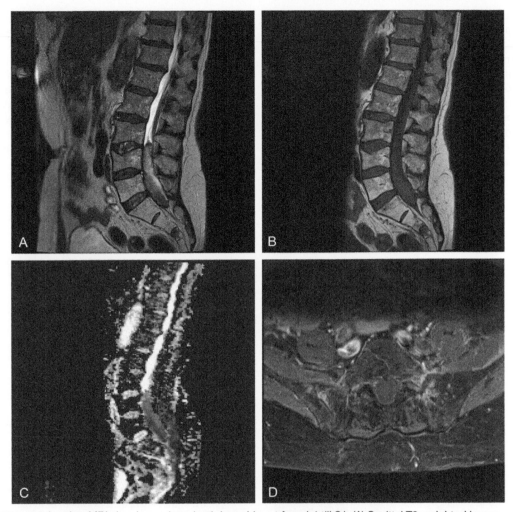

FIG. 22 Lumbar MRI showing an intradural dermoid cyst from L4 till S1. (A) Sagittal T2-weighted image
shows a relatively hyperintense lesion. (B) Sagittal T1-weighted image shows a hypointense lesion.
(C) Sagittal ADC image shows abnormal diffusion restriction. (D) Axial T1-weighted image after the
administration of gadolinium shows limited rim enhancement of the lesion.

subcutaneous mass include lipomas with dural defects, such as lipomyelomeningocele and lipomyelocele, terminal or nonterminal myelocystocele, and meningocele. Closed disraphistic lesions without subcutaneous mass are divided into simple or complex lesions. Simple lesions include intradural/filar lipoma, dorsal dermal sinus, tight filum terminale, and abnormally elongated spinal cord, which are often clinically translating into a tethered cord syndrome. Complex lesions include neurenteric cysts, split cord malformations (which should be divided into diplomyelia and diastematomyelia), dorsal enteric fistula, caudal agenesis, and segmental spinal dysgenesis. These lesions are rare and do not have specific quantitative or qualitative characteristics on MRI. We refer to specific textbooks on this topic.

Lumbosacral Vascular Malformations on MRI

Spinal vascular malformations include arteriovenous malformations, arteriovenous fistulas, and cavernomas. Diagnosis is frequently delayed as they are rare disorders and often mimic degenerative diseases of the spine. Digital subtraction angiography is often necessary for a proper diagnosis and in order to develop a treatment plan for these lesions. Because of their clinical presentation, MRI is often the first imaging available of these lesions. Therefore, recognition of vascular lesions on MRI is of the utmost importance.

Spinal arteriovenous malformations (SAVMs) are aberrant arteriovenous connections with an interposed nidus. On MRI, SAVM types cannot be properly distinguished or fully classified. They appear as a complex cluster of dilated and tortuous vessels, visible as mixed hyper- and hypointense tubular structures. Intensities are depending on flow velocity and direction and lesions are usually contrast enhancing. Venous congestive edema may be present in the spinal cord or conus and appears as a hyperintense signal on T2-weighted images and is accompanied by thickening of the spinal cord. There can be a trace of hemorrhages in the subarachnoid space or spinal cord. Fast MR angiography can be used to detect large single feeding vessels.[104, 105] Furthermore, exact location of the lesion and relationship with dura, spinal cord, and nerves should be described.

Spinal arteriovenous fistulas are also aberrant arteriovenous connections; however, they lack a nidus, instead presenting with a dural aberrant connection point between a radicular artery and radicular vein is present. Suggestive of a spinal arteriovenous fistula is a hyperintense signal change in the spinal cord and its thickening, as a result of venous congestion. Furthermore, ectatic intradural vascular structures adjacent to the spinal cord can be observed. A digital subtraction angiography is necessary to display the connection point[106, 107] (Fig. 23).

Spinal cavernomas can occur in the spinal cord and conus and therefore be visible on lumbosacral MRI. They are well-delineated lesions of varying sizes with a hypointense rim caused by their susceptibility artifact and hemosiderin deposits and a heterogeneous, often hyperintense core on T2-weighted images. The lesion has a raspberry- or mulberry-like appearance.[104] Spinal cavernomas are not visible on digital subtraction angiography.

CONCLUSION

Knowledge normal and pathological anatomical configuration and signal intensities characteristics on lumbar MRI helps the clinician in correctly diagnosing lumbar spinal pathology. However, clinical correlation with symptoms in the interpretation of lumbar MRI remains of utmost importance.

REFERENCES

1. Brinjikji W, Luetmer PH, Comstock B, et al. Systematic literature review of imaging features of spinal degeneration in asymptomatic populations. *AJNR Am J Neuroradiol.* 2015;36(4):811–816.
2. Chou R, Deyo RA, Jarvik JG. Appropriate use of lumbar imaging for evaluation of low back pain. *Radiol Clin North Am.* 2012;50(4):569–585.
3. Modic MT, Ross JS. Lumbar degenerative disk disease. *Radiology.* 2007;245(1):43–61.
4. Tien RD, Olson EM, Zee CS. Diseases of the lumbar spine: findings on fat-suppression MR imaging. *AJR Am J Roentgenol.* 1992;159(1):95–99.
5. Hannemann N, Bui-Mansfield LT. The "ABCDE" approach to the systematic assessment of lumbar spine MR examination. *Contemp Diagn Radiol.* 2018;41(24):1–7.
6. Been E, Kalichman L. Lumbar lordosis. *Spine J.* 2014;14(1):87–97.
7. Mauch F, Jung C, Huth J, Bauer G. Changes in the lumbar spine of athletes from supine to the true-standing position in magnetic resonance imaging. *Spine.* 2010;35(9):1002–1007.
8. Carrino JA, Campbell Jr PD, Lin DC, et al. Effect of spinal segment variants on numbering vertebral levels at lumbar MR imaging. *Radiology.* 2011;259(1):196–202.
9. Ucar D, Ucar BY, Cosar Y, et al. Retrospective cohort study of the prevalence of lumbosacral transitional vertebra in a wide and well-represented population. *Arthritis.* 2013;2013:461425.
10. Malanga GA, Cooke PM. Segmental anomaly leading to wrong level disc surgery in cauda equina syndrome. *Pain Physician.* 2004;7(1):107–110.
11. Castellvi AE, Goldstein LA, Chan D. Lumbosacral transitional vertebrae and their relationship with lumbar extradural defects. *Spine.* 1984;9(5):493–495.

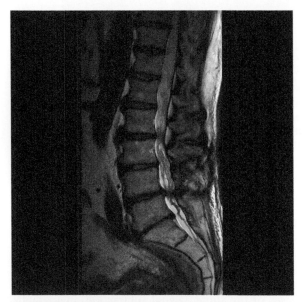

FIG. 23 T2-weighted image of a 77-year-old patient with a dural arteriovenous fistula. Note the hyperintense signal in the thickened spinal cord, as a sign of venous congestion. Furthermore, abnormal epidural veins are visible at the Th11-Th12 level.

12. Herrero CF, Garcia SB, Garcia LV, Aparecido Defino HL. Endplates changes related to age and vertebral segment. *Biomed Res Int.* 2014;2014:545017.

13. Moore RJ. The vertebral end-plate: what do we know? *Eur Spine J.* 2000;9(2):92–96.

14. Nouh MR, Eid AF. Magnetic resonance imaging of the spinal marrow: basic understanding of the normal marrow pattern and its variant. *World J Radiol.* 2015;7(12):448–458.

15. Małkiewicz A, Dziedzic M. Bone marrow reconversion-imaging of physiological changes in bone marrow. *Pol J Radiol.* 2012;77(4):45.

16. Adams A, Roche O, Mazumder A, Davagnanam I, Mankad K. Imaging of degenerative lumbar intervertebral discs; linking anatomy, pathology and imaging. *Postgrad Med J.* 2014;90(1067):511–519.

17. Andreisek G, Deyo RA, Jarvik JG, et al. Consensus conference on core radiological parameters to describe lumbar stenosis—an initiative for structured reporting. *Eur Radiol.* 2014;24(12):3224–3232.

18. Panjabi MM, White A. *Clinical Biomechanics of the Spine.* Lippincott Williams & Wilkins; 1990.

19. Nathoo N, Caris EC, Wiener JA, Mendel E. History of the vertebral venous plexus and the significant contributions of Breschet and Batson. *Neurosurgery.* 2011;69(5):1007–1014 [discussion 14].

20. Pearce JM. The craniospinal venous system. *Eur Neurol.* 2006;56(2):136–138.

21. Collie D, Brush J, Lammie G, et al. Imaging features of leptomeningeal metastases. *Clin Radiol.* 1999;54(11):765–771.

22. Deramo P, Agrawal V, Amos J, Patel N, Jefferson H. Does MRI of the thoracolumbar spine change management in blunt trauma patients with stable thoracolumbar spinal injuries without neurologic deficits? *World J Surg.* 2017;41(4):970–974.

23. Rajasekaran S, Vaccaro AR, Kanna RM, et al. The value of CT and MRI in the classification and surgical decision-making among spine surgeons in thoracolumbar spinal injuries. *Eur Spine J.* 2017;26(5):1463–1469.

24. Qureshi S, Dhall SS, Anderson PA, et al. Congress of neurological surgeons systematic review and evidence-based guidelines on the evaluation and treatment of patients with thoracolumbar spine trauma: radiological evaluation. *Neurosurgery.* 2019;84(1):E28–e31.

25. Mauch J, Carr C, Cloft H, Diehn F. Review of the imaging features of benign osteoporotic and malignant vertebral compression fractures. *Am J Neuroradiol.* 2018;39(9):1584–1592.

26. Zhou XJ, Leeds NE, McKinnon GC, Kumar AJ. Characterization of benign and metastatic vertebral compression fractures with quantitative diffusion MR imaging. *Am J Neuroradiol.* 2002;23(1):165–170.

27. Quinet RJ, Hadler NM, eds. *Diagnosis and Treatment of Backache. Seminars in Arthritis and Rheumatism.* Elsevier; 1979.

28. Bartels RH, Frenken CW. Lumbar spinal stenosis. *Ned Tijdschr Geneeskd.* 1993;137(11):529–532.

29. Verbiest H. A radicular syndrome from developmental narrowing of the lumbar vertebral canal. *J Bone Joint Surg.* 1954;36(2):230–237.

30. Yu LP, Qian WW, Yin GY, Ren YX, Hu ZY. MRI assessment of lumbar intervertebral disc degeneration with lumbar degenerative disease using the Pfirrmann grading systems. *PLoS One.* 2012;7(12), e48074.

31. Modic M, Steinberg P, Ross J, Masaryk T, Carter J. Degenerative disk disease: assessment of changes in vertebral body marrow with MR imaging. *Radiology.* 1988;166(1):193–199.

32. Zehra U, Bow C, Lotz JC, et al. Structural vertebral endplate nomenclature and etiology: a study by the ISSLS spinal phenotype focus group. *Eur Spine J.* 2018;27(1):2–12.

33. Zehra U, Cheung JPY, Bow C, Lu W, Samartzis D. Multidimensional vertebral endplate defects are associated with disc degeneration, modic changes, facet joint abnormalities, and pain. *J Orthop Res.* 2019;37(5):1080–1089.

34. Kokkonen SM, Kurunlahti M, Tervonen O, Ilkko E, Vanharanta H. Endplate degeneration observed on magnetic resonance imaging of the lumbar spine: correlation with pain provocation and disc changes observed on computed tomography diskography. *Spine (Phila Pa 1976).* 2002;27(20):2274–2278.

35. Chou D, Samartzis D, Bellabarba C, et al. Degenerative magnetic resonance imaging changes in patients with chronic low back pain: a systematic review. *Spine (Phila Pa 1976).* 2011;36(21 Suppl):S43–S53.

36. Splendiani A, Puglielli E, De Amicis R, Barile A, Masciocchi C, Gallucci M. Spontaneous resolution of lumbar disk herniation: predictive signs for prognostic evaluation. *Neuroradiology.* 2004;46(11):916–922.

37. Schizas C, Theumann N, Burn A, et al. Qualitative grading of severity of lumbar spinal stenosis based on the morphology of the dural sac on magnetic resonance images. *Spine.* 2010;35(21):1919–1924.

38. Abbati G, Bauer S, Winklhofer S, et al., eds. *MRI-based surgical planning for lumbar spinal stenosis. International Conference on Medical Image Computing and Computer-Assisted Intervention.* Springer; 2017.

39. Singh K, Samartzis D, Vaccaro AR, et al. Congenital lumbar spinal stenosis: a prospective, control-matched, cohort radiographic analysis. *Spine J.* 2005;5(6):615–622.

40. Wilmink JT. MR myelography in patients with lumbosacral radicular pain: diagnostic value and technique. *Neuroradiol J.* 2011;24(4):570–576.

41. Eberhardt K, Ganslandt O, Stadlbauer A. Functional and quantitative magnetic resonance myelography of symptomatic stenoses of the lumbar spine. *Neuroradiology.* 2014;56(12):1069–1078.

42. Sasaki K, Hasegawa K, Shimoda H, Keiji I, Homma T. Can recumbent magnetic resonance imaging replace myelography or computed tomography myelography for detecting lumbar spinal stenosis? *Eur J Orthop Surg Traumatol.* 2013;23(1):77–83.

43. Kuhn MJ, Youssef HT, Swan TL, Swenson LC. Lumbar epidural lipomatosis: the "Y" sign of thecal sac compression. *Comput Med Imaging Graph.* 1994;18(5):367–372.

44. Papavero L, Marques CJ, Lohmann J, Fitting T. Patient demographics and MRI-based measurements predict redundant nerve roots in lumbar spinal stenosis: a retrospective database cohort comparison. *BMC Musculoskelet Disord.* 2018;19(1):452.

45. Chen J, Wang J, Wang B, Xu H, Lin S, Zhang H. Postsurgical functional recovery, lumbar lordosis, and range of motion associated with MR-detectable redundant nerve roots in lumbar spinal stenosis. *Clin Neurol Neurosurg.* 2016;140:79–84.

46. Cong L, Zhu Y, Yan Q, Tu G. A meta-analysis on the clinical significance of redundant nerve roots in symptomatic lumbar spinal stenosis. *World Neurosurg.* 2017;105:95–101.

47. Marques CJ, Hillebrand H, Papavero L. The clinical significance of redundant nerve roots of the cauda equina in lumbar spinal stenosis patients: a systematic literature review and meta-analysis. *Clin Neurol Neurosurg.* 2018;174:40–47.

48. Cowley P. Neuroimaging of spinal canal stenosis. *Magn Reson Imaging Clin N Am.* 2016;24(3):523–539.

49. Wang G, Peng Z, Li J, Song Z, Wang P. Diagnostic performance of the nerve root sedimentation sign in lumbar spinal stenosis: a systematic review and meta-analysis. *Neuroradiology.* 2019;1–11.

50. Jarvik JG, Deyo RA. Diagnostic evaluation of low back pain with emphasis on imaging. *Ann Intern Med.* 2002;137(7):586–597.

51. Benzel E. Pseudoconcordance and the elephant in the room. *World Neurosurg.* 2020;133:xxiii–xxiv.

52. Prodi E, Grassi R, Iacobellis F, Cianfoni A. Imaging in spondylodiskitis. *Magn Reson Imaging Clin N Am.* 2016;24(3):581–600.

53. Raghavan M, Lazzeri E, Palestro CJ. Imaging of spondylodiscitis. *Semin Nucl Med.* 2018;48(2):131–147.

54. Stäbler A, Reiser MF. Imaging of spinal infection. *Radiol Clin.* 2001;39(1):115–135.

55. Kanna RM, Babu N, Kannan M, Shetty AP, Rajasekaran S. Diagnostic accuracy of whole spine magnetic resonance imaging in spinal tuberculosis validated through tissue studies. *Eur Spine J.* 2019;28(12):3003–3010.

56. Mittal S, Khalid M, Sabir AB, Khalid S. Comparison of magnetic resonance imaging findings between pathologically proven cases of atypical tubercular spine and tumour metastasis: a retrospective study in 40 patients. *Asian Spine J.* 2016;10(4):734–743.

57. Jacobs WB, Perrin RG. Evaluation and treatment of spinal metastases: an overview. *Neurosurg Focus.* 2001;11(6), e10.

58. Cole JS, Patchell RA. Metastatic epidural spinal cord compression. *Lancet Neurol.* 2008;7(5):459–466.

59. Klimo Jr P, Thompson CJ, Kestle JR, Schmidt MH. A meta-analysis of surgery versus conventional radiotherapy for the treatment of metastatic spinal epidural disease. *Neuro Oncol.* 2005;7(1):64–76.

60. Shah LM, Ross JS. Imaging of degenerative and infectious conditions of the spine. *Neurosurgery.* 2016;79(3):315–335.

61. Guillevin R, Vallee J-N, Lafitte F, Menuel C, Duverneuil N-M, Chiras J. Spine metastasis imaging: review of the literature. *J Neuroradiol.* 2007;34(5):311–321.

62. Schweitzer M, Levine C, Mitchell D, Gannon F, Gomella L. Bull's-eyes and halos: useful MR discriminators of osseous metastases. *Radiology.* 1993;188(1):249–252.

63. Charest-Morin R, Fisher CG, Sahgal A, et al. Primary bone tumor of the spine—an evolving field: what a general spine surgeon should know. *Global spine J.* 2019;9(1_suppl). 108S–16S.

64. Mechri M, Riahi H, Sboui I, Bouaziz M, Vanhoenacker F, Ladeb M. Imaging of malignant primitive tumors of the spine. *J Belg Soc Radiol.* 2018;102(1):56.

65. Jo VY, Fletcher CD. WHO classification of soft tissue tumours: an update based on the 2013 (4th) edition. *Pathology.* 2014;46(2):95–104.

66. Erlemann R. Imaging and differential diagnosis of primary bone tumors and tumor-like lesions of the spine. *Eur J Radiol.* 2006;58(1):48–67.

67. Ilaslan H, Sundaram M, Unni KK, Shives TC. Primary vertebral osteosarcoma: imaging findings. *Radiology.* 2004;230(3):697–702.

68. Yarmish G, Klein MJ, Landa J, Lefkowitz RA, Hwang S. Imaging characteristics of primary osteosarcoma: nonconventional subtypes. *Radiographics.* 2010;30(6):1653–1672.

69. Aoki J, Sone S, Fujioka F, et al. MR of enchondroma and chondrosarcoma: rings and arcs of Gd-DTPA enhancement. *J Comput Assist Tomogr.* 1991;15(6):1011–1016.

70. Campbell K, Shulman D, Janeway KA, DuBois SG. Comparison of epidemiology, clinical features, and outcomes of patients with reported ewing sarcoma and PNET over 40 years justifies current WHO classification and treatment approaches. *Sarcoma.* 2018;2018:1712964.

71. Rodallec MH, Feydy A, Larousserie F, et al. Diagnostic imaging of solitary tumors of the spine: what to do and say. *Radiographics.* 2008;28(4):1019–1041.

72. Christopher D, Fletcher JA, Krishnan U. *WHO classification of tumours of soft tissue and bone.* 4th ed. Lyon: International Agency for Research on Cancer; 2013:110–111.

73. Munk PL, Sallomi DF, Janzen DL, et al. Malignant fibrous histiocytoma of soft tissue imaging with emphasis on MRI. *J Comput Assist Tomogr.* 1998;22(5):819–826.

74. Lasocki A, Gaillard F, Harrison SJ. Multiple myeloma of the spine. *Neuroradiol J.* 2017;30(3):259–268.

75. Stäbler A, Baur A, Bartl R, Munker R, Lamerz R, Reiser M. Contrast enhancement and quantitative signal analysis in MR imaging of multiple myeloma: assessment of focal and diffuse growth patterns in marrow correlated with biopsies and survival rates. *AJR Am J Roentgenol.* 1996;167(4):1029–1036.

76. Smolders D, Wang X, Drevelengas A, Vanhoenacker F, De Schepper A. Value of MRI in the diagnosis of non-clival, non-sacral chordoma. *Skeletal Radiol.* 2003;32(6):343–350.

77. Cloran FJ, Pukenas BA, Loevner LA, Aquino C, Schuster J, Mohan S. Aggressive spinal haemangiomas: imaging correlates to clinical presentation with analysis of treatment algorithm and clinical outcomes. *Br J Radiol.* 2015;88(1055):20140771.

78. Montalti M, Amendola L. Solitary eosinophilic granuloma of the adult lumbar spine. *Eur Spine J.* 2012;21(Suppl 4):S441–S444.

79. Reddy P, Vannemreddy P, Nanda A. Eosinophilic granuloma of spine in adults: a case report and review of literature. *Spinal Cord.* 2000;38(12):766–768.

80. Iyer RS, Chapman T, Chew FS. Pediatric bone imaging: diagnostic imaging of osteoid osteoma. *Am J Roentgenol.* 2012;198(5):1039–1052.

81. Atesok KI, Alman BA, Schemitsch EH, Peyser A, Mankin H. Osteoid osteoma and osteoblastoma. *J Am Acad Orthop Surg.* 2011;19(11):678–689.

82. Zileli M, Çagli S, Basdemir G, Ersahin Y. Osteoid osteomas and osteoblastomas of the spine. *Neurosurg Focus.* 2003;15(5):1–7.

83. Lotfinia I, Vahedi P, Tubbs RS, Ghavame M, Meshkini A. Neurological manifestations, imaging characteristics, and surgical outcome of intraspinal osteochondroma. *J Neurosurg Spine.* 2010;12(5):474–489.

84. Sinelnikov A, Kale H. Osteochondromas of the spine. *Clin Radiol.* 2014;69(12):e584–e590.

85. Randall RL. Giant cell tumor of the sacrum. *Neurosurg Focus.* 2003;15(2), E13.

86. Shi LS, Li YQ, Wu WJ, Zhang ZK, Gao F, Latif M. Imaging appearance of giant cell tumour of the spine above the sacrum. *Br J Radiol.* 2015;88(1051):20140566.

87. Jansen J, Terwey B, Rama B, Markakis E. MRI diagnosis of aneurysmal bone cyst. *Neurosurg Rev.* 1990;13(2):161–166.

88. Sullivan RJ, Meyer JS, Dormans JP, Davidson RS. Diagnosing aneurysmal and unicameral bone cysts with magnetic resonance imaging. *Clin Orthop Relat Res.* 1999;366:186–190.

89. Zhai X, Zhou M, Chen H, et al. Differentiation between intraspinal schwannoma and meningioma by MR characteristics and clinic features. *Radiol Med.* 2019;124(6):510–521.

90. Iwata E, Shigematsu H, Yamamoto Y, et al. Preliminary algorithm for differential diagnosis between spinal meningioma and schwannoma using plain magnetic resonance imaging. *J Orthop Sci.* 2018;23(2):408–413.

91. Albayrak BS, Gorgulu A, Kose T. A case of intra-dural malignant peripheral nerve sheath tumor in thoracic spine associated with neurofibromatosis type 1. *J Neurooncol.* 2006;78(2):187–190.

92. Mauda-Havakuk M, Shofty B, Ben-Shachar S, Ben-Sira L, Constantini S, Bokstein F. Spinal and paraspinal plexiform neurofibromas in patients with neurofibromatosis type

93. Joseffer SS, Babu RP, Kleinman G. Plexiform neurofibroma of the cauda equina: case report. *Surg Neurol.* 2005;63(2):182–184 [discussion 4].

94. Wasa J, Nishida Y, Tsukushi S, et al. MRI features in the differentiation of malignant peripheral nerve sheath tumors and neurofibromas. *AJR Am J Roentgenol.* 2010;194(6):1568–1574.

95. Koeller KK, Shih RY. Intradural extramedullary spinal neoplasms: radiologic-pathologic correlation. *Radiographics.* 2019;39(2):468–490.

96. Honeyman SI, Warr W, Curran OE, Demetriades AK. Paraganglioma of the lumbar spine: a case report and literature review. *Neurochirurgie.* 2019;65(6):387–392.

97. Blaty D, Malos M, Palmrose T, McGirr S. Sporadic intradural extramedullary hemangioblastoma of the cauda equina: case report and literature review. *World Neurosurg.* 2018;109:436–441.

98. Baker KB, Moran CJ, Wippold FJ, et al. MR imaging of spinal hemangioblastoma. *Am J Roentgenol.* 2000;174(2):377–382.

99. Evans A, Stoodley N, Halpin S. Magnetic resonance imaging of intraspinal cystic lesions: a pictorial review. *Curr Probl Diagn Radiol.* 2002;31(3):79–94.

100. Pandey S, Sharma V, Shinde N, Ghosh A. Spinal intradural extramedullary mature cystic teratoma in an adult: a rare tumor with review of literature. *Asian J Neurosurg.* 2015;10(3):133.

101. Kukreja K, Manzano G, Ragheb J, Medina LS. Differentiation between pediatric spinal arachnoid and epidermoid-dermoid cysts: is diffusion-weighted MRI useful? *Pediatr Radiol.* 2007;37(6):556–560.

102. Reghunath A, Ghasi RG, Aggarwal A. Unveiling the tale of the tail: an illustration of spinal dysraphisms. *Neurosurg Rev.* 2019;1–18.

103. Tortori-Donati P, Rossi A, Biancheri R, Cama A. Congenital malformations of the spine and spinal cord. In: *Pediatric Neuroradiology.* Springer; 2005:1551–1608.

104. Krings T, Lasjaunias PL, Hans FJ, et al. Imaging in spinal vascular disease. *Neuroimaging Clin N Am.* 2007;17(1):57–72.

105. Doppman JL, Di Chiro G, Dwyer AJ, Frank JL, Oldfield EH. Magnetic resonance imaging of spinal arteriovenous malformations. *J Neurosurg.* 1987;66(6):830–834.

106. Wilbers J, Meijer FJ, Tuladhar A, de Vries J, van Dijk E, Boogaarts JD. Spinal dural arteriovenous fistula: frequently diagnosed late. *Ned Tijdschr Geneeskd.* 2013;157(12), A5909.

107. Jellema K, Tijssen C. Gijn Jv. Spinal dural arteriovenous fistulas: a congestive myelopathy that initially mimics a peripheral nerve disorder. *Brain.* 2006;129(12):3150–3164.

CHAPTER 15

Lumbosacral CT

ANDREW CHUNG • NASSIM LASHKARI • ELOISE STANTON •
OMAIR A. QURESHI • ZORICA BUSER • JEFFREY C. WANG
Department of Orthopaedic Surgery, Keck School of Medicine of the University of Southern
California, Los Angeles, CA, United States

LUMBOSACRAL ANATOMY

Osseous Anatomy

The lumbosacral spine consists of five lumbar (L1–L5) and five sacral vertebrae (S1–S5) and their associated intervertebral discs, nerves, muscles, ligaments, and blood vessels. Each vertebra consists of a vertebral body, vertebral arch, and seven processes. The vertebral bodies are responsible for absorbing most of the axial forces exerted on the vertebrae.[1] The vertebral arches and the dorsal part of the vertebral body along the vertebral column collectively form the spinal canal that houses the thecal sac. The arches contain pedicles on each side that predominantly blend into the superior articular process. From this, bony intersections arise the transverse processes, which are present bilaterally. Each vertebra has additional inferior processes. The superior and inferior processes articulate with the inferior and superior processes of the adjacent vertebrae, respectively, to create the facet joints. Approximately 20% of the axial load placed on the lumbosacral spine is transmitted through the facet joints. The seven processes of vertebrae serve as both origin and insertion points of the paraspinal muscles. They therefore are integral to the overall function of the spine, including its ability to move, bear-weight, and maintain proper alignment.[2]

The lumbar vertebrae have several unique properties that distinguish them from vertebrae of other vertebral levels. They have characteristically larger vertebral bodies, and shorter, thicker spinous processes. The larger bodies are a testament to the lumbar region's duty to bear a significant proportion of the weight of the upper limbs and trunk. Intervertebral discs are cartilaginous structures that provide additional cushioning between each vertebra. Stability is further conferred to the lumbar spine through the anterior and posterior longitudinal ligaments that run vertically on the ventral and dorsal aspects of the vertebral column, respectively.[3]

The five sacral vertebrae are fused together to form the sacrum, an upside-down triangular bone that resides at the base of the lumbar spine. With the exception of the L5-S1 intervertebral disc, due to ultimate fusion of the sacral vertebrae by adulthood, the sacral segments are not typically separated by intervertebral discs. The sacral promontory, the most anterior part of the sacrum, articulates with L5, forming part of the lumbosacral joint. In addition to the intrinsic stability imparted by the intervening intervertebral disc, this joint is further strengthened by the iliolumbar and lumbosacral ligaments.

The inferior portion of the sacrum articulates with the coccyx, which is another small triangular bone at the bottom of the spine that is thought, by many, to be a vestigial structure. Within the sacrum itself lies the continuation of the vertebral canal, the *sacral canal*, that terminates at an apex termed the *sacral hiatus*. While in the adult spine, the spinal cord typically ends at the level of L1-L2 as the *conus medullaris*, both dura mater and the filum terminale, which is a ligamentous condensation of pia mater, extends down from the conus through the sacral canal to the coccyx and serves as an anchor for the spinal cord.[4] Computed tomography (CT) has been found to be a primary imaging modality for demonstrating osteological pathology, including trauma, fractures, scoliosis, and in pre- and postoperative patients.[5]

Lumbosacral Intervertebral Discs

The intervertebral disc allows for flexibility of the spine while concomitantly conferring strength and shock absorptive ability. Intervertebral discs are composed of two main components: the *nucleus pulposus* centrally, and the *annulus fibrosus*, circumferentially. The nucleus pulposus has a gelatinous composition that allows for dissipation of force and protection against injury.[3] The annulus fibrosus is made of organized collagen I fibers that encircle and maintain the integrity of the inner nucleus pulposus. The nerve supply to the intervertebral disc is limited to only the outer annulus through the

Atlas of Spinal Imaging. https://doi.org/10.1016/B978-0-323-76111-6.00010-9

sinuvertebral nerve.[6,7] Attaching the disc to adjacent vertebrae are the cartilaginous endplates. These endplates serve two counteracting functions—to both be porous enough to allow for nutrient transport between disc cells, while remaining sufficiently sturdy to mitigate mechanical failure.[8] Pathological changes within the endplates including Schmorl nodes, calcification, fractures, and tears have clinically been correlated with disc degeneration and back pain.[8]

As humans age, the proteoglycan and collagen composition within the intervertebral disc are altered. Specifically, the pulposus loses its water content and ultimately becomes more fibrotic.[8] Consequently, the disc thins and then ultimately will calcify during the terminal stages of the degenerative process.[9–12] These changes ultimately impair mobility and increase the likelihood of onset of various disc-related pathologies that will be discussed in the later sections.[3] Pathologies such as degeneration of intervertebral discs and radiculopathy can be visualized and studied on CT and magnetic resonance imaging (MRI) with contrast enhancement.[13]

Anomalous Lumbosacral Anatomy

Anatomical variation seen in the lumbar and sacral region is partially due to sexual dimorphism and partially due to congenital defects that influence the movement and function of the vertebral column. The sacrum can vary slightly among males and females. Females usually have a shorter and wider sacrum and a less prominent sacral promontory that functions to help with easier delivery during childbirth.[4] Another anatomical variant seen in the lumbosacral region is the existence of lumbosacral transitional vertebrae. These can result from either of the following: (1) L5 fusing with the sacrum (sacralization), which yields six sacral vertebrae, and (2) S1 transitioning to a lumbar vertebra (lumbarization), resulting in only four sacral vertebrae. The lumbarized S1 vertebra typically has features similar to lumbar vertebrae. Either of these processes can occur partially or completely, unilaterally or bilaterally. These physiologic variations may impair the range of motion and weight-bearing abilities, which may contribute to spine pathology and lower back pain.[4,14] Due to its superior spatial resolution, CT may be the best imaging modality for characterization of lumbosacral transitional vertebra pathologies.[15]

Neurovasculature of the Lumbosacral Spine

The main blood supply to the lumbar vertebrae are the subcostal and lumbar arteries. The sacral vertebrae are supplied by the medial and bilateral sacral arteries. The red marrow of each vertebra's body receives a separate source of nutrients from vertebral canal branches from these main arteries. The spinal veins that run longitudinally along the vertebral canal form valveless venous plexuses. Blood flow direction is thus bidirectional and is contingent on pressure gradients.[2]

The nervous supply to both the sacral and lumbar vertebrae is from branches derived from the terminal spinal nerves. Meningeal branches of these spinal nerves innervate the lumbar and sacral vertebrae themselves. In the caudal spine, the spinal nerves increase in diameter, while the diameter of the intervertebral foramina decreases. This anatomical relationship contributes to certain pathologies of the lumbosacral spine to be discussed later.[2] By providing visualization of nerve roots, the cauda equina, and the spinal cord, CT myelography is useful in diagnosing these various pathologies.[15]

Lumbosacral Musculature

Both the lumbar and sacral vertebral regions serve as origin and attachment sites for numerous muscles. The erector spinae, interspinalis, intertransversarii, latissimus dorsi, rotatores, and serratus posterior inferior muscles all originate within the lumbar spine.[2] The piriformis muscle originates from the anterior surface of the sacrum. Furthermore, the coccygeus, the iliac muscles, gluteus maximus, multifidus lumborum, and erector spinae muscles all have various attachment site or sites of origin in the sacrum.[4] These paravertebral muscles atrophy with age through both degradation of skeletal muscle and infiltration of fat tissue.[16] These age-related changes increase the spine's susceptibility to pathology and may serve as an additional pain generator. Furthermore, they may be correlated to poorer outcomes following spine surgery.[17] CT scans can be used to assess muscular integrity via visualization of the functional cross-sectional area (FCSA) and fatty infiltration of atrophied paravertebral muscles.[18]

INDICATIONS FOR LUMBOSACRAL COMPUTED TOMOGRAPHY

Compared with plain radiography and magnetic resonance imaging (MRI), the ability of computed tomography (CT) to provide ultrafine spatial anatomic detail allows for optimal evaluation of bony anatomy and pathology. Furthermore, image reformatting and three-dimensional reconstructions allow the surgeon to better visualize spinal anatomy in the setting of difficult to visualize regions of the axial skeleton (e.g., sacrum) and when evaluating complex pathologies, e.g., severe spinal deformities, high-grade spondylolistheses, complex fractures, and neoplasms.

In light of these latter advantages, use of CT has become the gold standard for the initial evaluation of the traumatized lumbosacral spine and for evaluating bony fusion. Importantly, in the setting of neural compression, CT allows for better distinction between compression secondary to soft tissue versus bony pathology. Furthermore, CT is more sensitive than MRI and plain radiography when it comes to detecting pars defects and subtle pars fractures.

Finally, in patients with contraindications to MRI (the presence of certain pacemakers or defibrillators), CT myelogram is a useful surrogate to assess for soft tissue pathology. Specific benefits of CT are outlined in further detail later.

Stenosis Secondary to Bony Pathology

A comprehensive understanding of the pathologic condition being addressed is mandatory in the surgical planning process. In addition to ligamentous overgrowth and disc-related pathology, lumbar degenerative stenosis is often the consequence of hypertrophied or asymmetric facets or osteophytosis. These findings are often noted within the setting of adjacent segment degeneration (a purely radiographic finding) or adjacent segment disease (radiographic finding with clinical consequences) that oftentimes develops at levels adjacent to previous fusions. These rates may approach

36.1% in the lumbar spine and 25.6% in the cervical spine, at 10-year follow-up following arthrodesis.[19,20] In this setting, CT allows for the most accurate depiction of these latter bony structures. Distinguishing between primarily osseous versus soft tissue neural compression may be the deciding factor between the choices of surgical approach, maximizing the safety of the stenosis operation and optimizing success rates. Finally in conjunction with upright lateral plain radiographs, similar to supine MRI, supine CT may be useful in the diagnosis of dynamic stenosis that may occur in the setting of segmental instability (e.g., mobile spondylolisthesis). It has even been suggested that this latter method may be, in fact, superior to the more widely accepted standing flexion/extension lateral radiographs for the detection of segmental translation.

While a much more common cause of neural compression in the cervical spine, ossification of the posterior longitudinal ligament (OPLL) can also lead to neural compression in the cervical and lumbosacral spine (Fig. 1). The prevalence of OPLL in the United States has been reported to range from 0.1% to 0.7% with a mean age of the onset of 50 years.[21] MRI, while still useful to qualify neural compression in this setting, may be limited in characterizing the extent of ossified ligamentous tissue. In these instances, CT is indispensable for surgical planning[22] and characteristic CT features of OPLL have been described. For example, while initially described in the setting of cervical neural

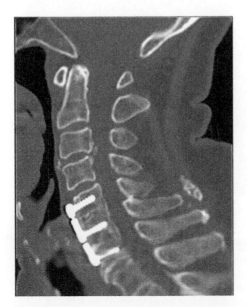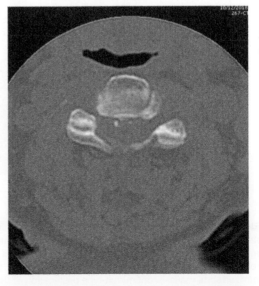

FIG. 1 Sagittal and axial computed tomography of the cervical spine demonstrating localized ossification of the posterior longitudinal ligament (OPLL) at the C3–4 disc space.

compression, the *double-layer sign* may be pathogno-monic for dural penetrance of the thecal sac by OPLL (Fig. 2). It is defined as the presence of a hypodense linear mass (representing a nonossified PLL) sandwiched between two hyperintense ossified rims.[23] When this is identified preoperatively, spinal surgeons should anticipate an increased likelihood for cerebrospinal fluid leak intra-operatively, if the surgical approach mandates a decompression at the affected level.

In general, OPLL can be divided into four types based on CT findings[21]:

(1) *Continuous*: OPLL spans multiple vertebral bodies in addition to crossing intervening disc spaces,
(2) *Segmental*: OPLL is limited to the vertebral body margins,
(3) *Mixed*: combination of the aforementioned,
(4) *Others*: OPLL may be primarily limited to the disc level.

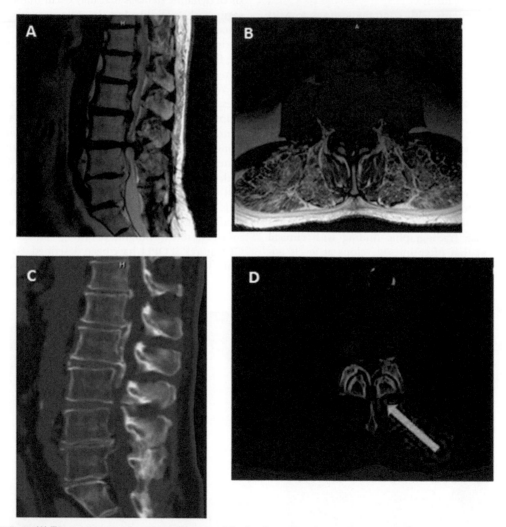

FIG. 2 (A) T2-weighted midsagittal MRI slice of the lumbar spine demonstrating significant multilevel stenosis secondary to spondylosis and a multisegment retrovertebral mass; (B) T2-weighted axial MRI image of the lumbar spine. Noted is severe central and subarticular stenosis secondary to circumferential compression; (C) Mid-sagittal CT image of the lumbar spine clearly delineates the etiology of the retrovertebral mass—continuous-type ossification of the posterior longitudinal ligament. Retrothecal ossification is also noted; (D) Axial CT image of the lumbar spine demonstrates ossified ligament flavum as the source of retrothecal compression.

While these latter classifications of OPLL may be useful prognosticators in the setting of myelopathy, no such correlations[24,25] that we are aware of have been described in the setting of lumbosacral OPLL.

Finally, there is a high correlation between OPLL and ossified ligamentum flavum,[22] the combination of which can potentially lead to circumferential neural compression. Again, a CT scan is invaluable in identifying these less common etiologies of stenosis and for planning the optimal surgical approach. Furthermore, as the risk of dural violation is potentially higher in these instances, this knowledge can be shared early on with patients during the preoperative planning process while discussing the risks and benefits of surgery.

Indications for CT Myelography

CT myelography combines the diagnostic benefits of CT with myelography. The addition of the myelogram allows for improved visualization of the neural elements (Fig. 3).[26] A myelogram is typically obtained by injecting noniodinated radiopaque contrast dye into the subarachnoid space via lumbar puncture. To obtain a CT myelogram, a traditional CT scan is then performed immediately following this.

The most common indications for CT myelography are: (1) the evaluation of neural compression when MRI is contraindicated (the presence of certain pacemakers or defibrillators) and (2) when osseous neural compression is suspected. When planning revision spinal surgery, CT myelograms can additionally prove useful, particularly in the setting of complex spinal deformity, or when substantial metal artifact on MRI interferes with accurate interpretation of imaging, i.e., if metal artifact reduction sequence [MARS] MRI is not readily available.

CT myelography may also be useful for the diagnosis of a postoperative cerebrospinal fluid leak (CSF) and the presence of a pseudomeningocele.[27] In the former, contrast extravasation outside of the thecal sac is diagnostic.

Finally, CT myelography can be as useful as an MRI for the diagnosis of arachnoiditis. Traditionally, three distinct patterns of arachnoiditis have been described based on MRI findings.[28]

(1) *Central adhesion of nerve roots*: nerves are clumped into one cord-like structure,

(2) *"Empty thecal sac" sign*: nerves are adherent to the meninges. With CT myelogram, only the high-intensity contrast agent is seen within the thecal sac. Nerves appear to be missing,

(3) *A nondistinct arachnoid mass within the thecal sac*: this is typically considered to signal the end stage of the inflammatory response. The arachnoid mater appears as a nonspecific mass-like structure that may result in a contrast block.

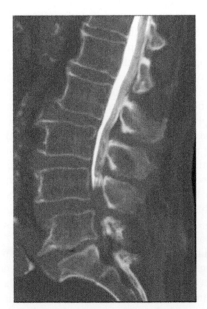 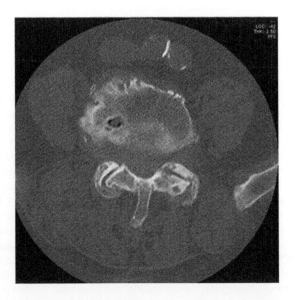

FIG. 3 Sagittal and axial CT myelogram demonstrating severe stenosis at the L4–5 level as evidenced by the contrast block at this level. The axial image clearly demonstrates the hypertrophic and dysmorphic facet joints that are contributing to canal stenosis.

Similar findings can be seen with CT myelography, although with perhaps less distinctive ability. Ultimately, however, radiographic findings do not appear to correlate with clinical symptomatology.[29]

Infection and Tumor

Metastases from primary pulmonary, renal, thyroid, breast, and prostatic malignancy are the most common tumors found in the spine. Primary tumors arising in the spine are rare. These include tumors of spinous structures and bone, which include intradural extramedullary tumors, intramedullary tumors, and extradural primary tumors such as chondrosarcoma, osteosarcoma, and chordoma.

Compared to plain radiographs, CT allows for improved visualization of bone mineralization and may subsequently allow for earlier detection of osseous lesions. CTs are particularly useful in the diagnosis of certain osteogenic tumors, such as osteoid osteomas or osteoblastomas, as they are not depicted with the use of plain radiography and have very characteristic appearances on CT. Consequently, CT has become the diagnostic test of choice for these latter pathologies.

Furthermore, as discussed prior, image reformatting options and three-dimensional reconstructions grant surgeons the ability to depict even minute discrepancies in bone mineralization that may allow for earlier diagnosis of tumors. Additionally, understanding whether or not a tumor is osteolytic or osteoblastic can help in both tumor diagnosis and surgical planning. Finally, while not as sensitive as MRI in this regard, CT may also allow for the identification of any concomitant soft tissue mass. Consequently, the acquisition of CT scans has become a staple of any preoperative plan that involves tumor resection.

While MRI remains the imaging modality of choice for the evaluation of spine infections, CT offers valuable diagnostic information and is an essential part of the preoperative workup. From a diagnostic standpoint, CT may help in the distinction between infection and tumor. For instance, infection generally results in vertebral body osteolysis, whereas tumor can be osteoblastic and may be more likely to involve the posterior elements.[30]

CT may additionally help in differentiating between pyogenic spondylitis and a granulomatous infection (e.g., tuberculosis or fungal infection). Granulomatous infections may exhibit radiographic traits similar to tumor such as pedicle invasion and associated soft tissue masses.[31] Paraspinal calcifications and vertebral fragmentation are unique features of tuberculous infections that may also be seen on CT.[32] Finally, in the setting of a concomitant neurologic deficit, CT myelogram can be obtained in patients with contraindications to undergoing MRI.

Lumbosacral Trauma

The spiral CT scan has become the standard for the initial radiologic evaluation of the polytraumatized patient. With the use of thin-section techniques and multiplanar reformatting, CT allows for a quick evaluation of the bony anatomy with high sensitivity in detecting fractures.[33] Furthermore, as routine acquisition of CT imaging of the chest, abdomen, and pelvis is performed in the traumatic setting, reformatting of the existing data to specifically evaluate the spine can often be included and enhanced based on the current CT scan. This ultimately decreases overall radiation exposure and evaluation times.

In general, CT remains the diagnostic study of choice for detecting posteriorly displaced fracture fragments that may result in spinal cord compression (i.e., burst fractures) and for the evaluation of bony involvement of the posterior osseous structures (Fig. 4). Misdiagnosis of burst from compression fractures can occur up to 25% of the time when relying solely on plain radiography.[34,35] It is important to note, however, that the diagnosis of posterior ligamentous injury, which is crucial to injury management, is best ascertained with the use of MRI.

Sacral fractures, particularly when accompanied by concomitant lumbar or pelvic fractures, can represent a substantial surgical challenge. Furthermore, with anomalous lumbosacral anatomy (i.e., lumbosacral transitional vertebrae and the so-called "dysmorphic" sacrum that may present in up to half of the adult population), the complexity of surgical fixation of these fractures may be exponentially increased. Sacral dysmorphism was initially characterized in the orthopedic trauma literature and encompasses any of the following seven radiographic findings: (1) collinearity of the upper sacrum with the cranial aspect of the iliac crests; (2) the presence of mammillary bodies in the alar region of the S1 segment; (3) larger, noncircular, misshapen upper sacral foramina best viewed on an pelvic outlet view; (4) residual disc between the S1 and S2 segments; (5) a steep alar slope that does not correspond well with the iliac cortical density on a lateral image; (6) tongue-in-groove-shaped sacroiliac articulation on an axial CT; and (7) anterior cortical indentation of the upper sacral segment on inlet imaging.[36,37] Preoperative CT with three-dimensional reconstructions is invaluable when characterizing the fracture pattern and for identifying any anomalous anatomy that may preclude safe execution of standard fixation approaches (e.g., sacroiliac or iliosacral screw fixation).[38] As will be discussed later, in these instances, the use of

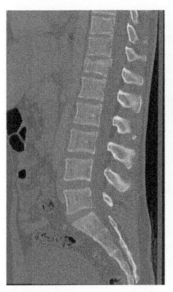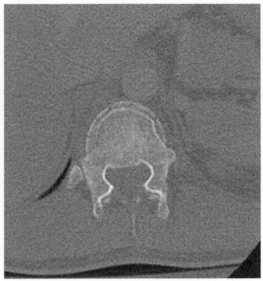

FIG. 4 Sagittal and axial computed tomography demonstrating a T12 burst fracture with mild retropulsion.

CT-based, computer-assisted navigation (CAN) can be of substantial benefit.

Sacroiliac Joint Pain

Sacroiliac joint pathology is a potential cause of low back pain that is becoming more widely recognized as of late (Fig. 5). While osteoarthritic change of the sac-roiliac joint may be appreciated on CT (i.e., joint space narrowing, subchondral sclerosis, cyst formation, and osteophytosis), to date, imaging findings on CT have not correlated with the presence of severity of patient symptomatology.[39,40]

Surgical Planning, Intra-Operative Surgical Navigation

In the case of complex fixed spinal deformities, CT serves as an invaluable adjunct to dynamic radio-graphs to ascertain the presence of any existing fusion masses (whether iatrogenic, congenital, etc.) that may necessitate more substantial corrective osteotomies. Furthermore, CT facilitates the identification of any unusual vertebral anatomy that may complicate the surgical approach. Three-dimensional reconstructions are particularly useful in these latter settings. Moreover, these imaging studies can then be utilized to create three-dimensional printed models of complex anat-omy that can aid in the preoperative planning process.

Similarly, in the revision surgical setting, fine-cut CT scans with sagittal and coronal reformatting can help to identify and qualify any existent fusion (interbody, intertransverse processes, or facets). Furthermore, any previous bony resections (laminectomy and laminot-omy defects), any iatrogenic fractures (pars and facets), and any adjacent-level spondylosis can all be identified with the use of CT.

For more routine cases, templating of screw trajec-tory, screw size, and interbody cage dimensions can all

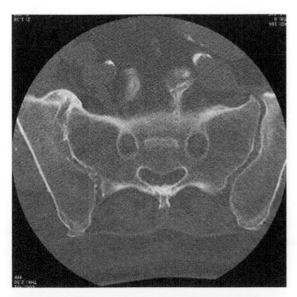

FIG. 5 Axial CT demonstrating right greater than left sacroiliac joint narrowing. Note autofusion of the left sacroiliac joint consistent with long-standing pathology.

be easily performed with the use of CT. However, it is important to first ensure that the measuring software being utilized is scaled appropriately.

Additionally, most computer-assisted intra-operative surgical navigation solutions are currently based off of CT scans. In the lumbosacral spine, computer-assisted navigation (CAN) can be utilized to place pedicle screws, pelvic screws (iliac, S2-alar), sacroiliac screws and can even assist with interbody placement. CAN has been shown to improve pedicle screw placement when compared to freehand or fluoroscopic techniques, and consequently, its use has become increasingly widespread. A recent review article found a 6% breach rate for navigated screws when compared to 15% for freehand screws.[41] Furthermore, placement of properly sized screws with optimal pedicle fill may improve overall construct biomechanics, which may prove invaluable in the setting of more complex spinal reconstructions and revision surgeries. Ultimately, the rate of secondary surgeries may consequently be reduced.[41]

More recently, CAN has been utilized to place iliosacral and sacroiliac screws with excellent results. This can be particularly useful in the setting of pelvic trauma where normal anatomy may be substantially distorted or in patients with anomalous anatomy.[42-44] While improved screw placement has not yet been shown to directly correlate with any clinically meaningful differences in the rates of associated complications,[45,46] as

CAN-use becomes increasingly widespread, it may indeed become standard of care. Finally, the use of CAN offers the additional benefits of decreased radiation exposure to the surgeon, operating room staff, and patients when compared to fluoroscopic-assisted surgery.[44]

Evaluation of Fusion

With reported rates of lumbar pseudoarthrosis of up to 56%, the ability to accurately identify pseudoarthrosis following lumbar spinal fusion is important.[47] While plain radiography is useful for routine tracking of fusion status, CT is well regarded as the gold standard imaging modality at ascertaining fusion status[47,48] with accuracy rates at predicting fusion of up to 96% with the use of fine-cut CT.[49] Currently, there is no universally accepted standardized criteria for assessing fusion status in the lumbosacral spine.

Indicators of fusion include bridging osseous trabeculations across the fused level with the lack of any radiolucency at the graft-bone interface (Fig. 6). Additionally, the presence of traversing bone between adjacent transverse processes or osseous integration of adjacent facets is indicative of fusion. Cage or device subsidence and the presence of haloing around pedicle screws and radiolucency around cage implants (typically 1 mm) are important markers of potential pseudoarthrosis.[48,50] However, it is important to differentiate screw loosening secondary to pseudoarthrosis

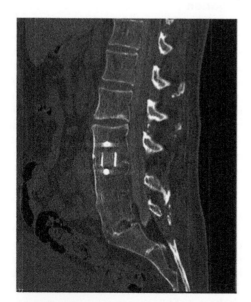 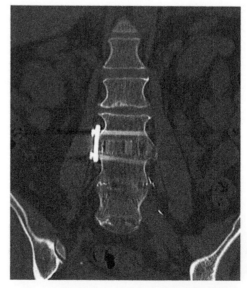

FIG. 6 Sagittal and axial computed tomography demonstrating a solid fusion mass across the L3 and L4 disc spaces. Note the column of solid bone between the two vertebrae with no evidence of peri-implant loosening or sclerosis.

from haloing secondary to infection or aseptic implant loosening.[51] Patient historical data, medical history, and laboratory data may help to exclude these latter less common, but nonetheless, important diagnoses. Furthermore, cystic changes around the endplate and a change in angulation between the pedicle screw axis and vertebral endplate on follow-up imaging studies may be indicative of screw loosening.[52]

Acquisition of Bone Mineral Density

Clinical CT studies performed for other indications in the abdomen, pelvis, or lumbar spine region contain unused quantitative information that can opportunistically assess vertebral bone mineral density (BMD). Although dual-energy X-ray absorptiometry (DXA) is the current standard for BMD assessment, studies comparing DXA to quantitative computed tomography (QCT) indicate that QCT of the spine is equal to or superior to DXA for the assessment of vertebral fracture risk.[53] CT attenuation, measured in Hounsfield units (HU), can be obtained from all clinical CT studies, thereby decreasing the need for additional radiation exposure or cost when evaluating BMD.[54,55] CT attenuation-derived T-scores are calculated and can be used to assess vertebral fracture risk or individuals at risk for metabolic bone disease. Recent studies have analyzed QCT T-scores to determine workup parameters for patients with osteoporosis; a QCT-derived T-score of − 3.0 is highly specific for osteoporosis.[54]

Case Example

A 60-year-old female with worsening symptoms of neurogenic claudication (Fig. 2). Axial MRI revealed significant central stenosis at L3–4. Midsagittal MRI demonstrates narrowing of the spinal canal diameter secondary to a nonspecific, diffuse retrovertebral mass. Axial CT imaging demonstrates calcification at L3–4 consistent with ossified ligamentum flavum. Mixed-type OPLL at upper lumbar levels is seen on midsagittal CT.

LIMITATIONS OF LUMBOSACRAL COMPUTED TOMOGRAPHY

Lumbosacral spinal pathology can commonly present as lower back pain. Pathologies presenting with lower back pain include known or suspected trauma, malignancy, infectious causes and inflammatory, autoimmune, and degenerative disease. The primary diagnostic imaging modalities used to evaluate the lumbosacral region in addition to CT include plain-film X-ray and magnetic resonance imaging (MRI).

It is estimated that spinal imaging studies reveal abnormalities in at least one-third of asymptomatic patients.[56] Implementation of an evidence-based, judicious, and selective approach to imaging of the lumbosacral region in clinical practice can contribute to a decrease in unnecessary cost, intervention, and patient exposure to harm.

Known advantages and limitations of the available imaging modalities have been well documented including the increase in ionizing radiation exposure when compared to plain radiography.[56] Additionally, in the presence of metal, X-ray attenuation may result in streak artifact during imaging reconstruction making visualization of pathology, difficult. Metals with lower attenuation coefficients such as plastic and titanium generate less artifact when compared to those with higher coefficients, such as stainless steel or cobalt chrome. However, this latter limitation may be a nonfactor in the future with a more widespread availability of dual-energy CTs.[31]

Indications for obtaining CT as well as other imaging in clinical practice are based primarily upon patient history, physical examination, suspected spinal pathology, and, if applicable, mechanism and type of injury. A brief overview of the use, advantages, and limitations of CT in comparison to X-ray and MRI for common lumbosacral spinal pathologies is presented later.

Trauma and Other Spinal Emergencies

Compared with plain radiography, CT is better able to visualize the complex anatomy of osseous structures. CT has been reported to have a sensitivity of 95% for the detection of lumbar fractures when compared to 86% by plain film.[57,58] In particular, CT is superior to plain radiography for the detection of fractures involving the posterior elements.[59–61] It is also the diagnostic study of choice for the assessment of sacral fractures. Traditional radiographs may only detect up to 30% of these fractures.[62] Numerous society guidelines including the American College of Radiology recommend that all adults and children older than 14 years of age undergo CT if they meet the criteria for spinal imaging.[63] However, while multiplanar CT is the clear initial diagnostic imaging modality of choice in the evaluation of lumbosacral trauma, there are some inherent limitations with its use.

In the presence of neurologic deficits or neurologic emergencies, such as acute cauda equina syndrome or conus medullaris syndrome, MRI is the diagnostic study of choice.[64–66] MRI is superior to CT for the evaluation of the posterior ligamentous complex (crucial for determining stability of the fracture), neural structures, and other surrounding soft tissue structures.[63,66] Of course, if a patient has a contraindication to MRI, CT can be used as an effective surrogate, particularly when combined with myelography.

Furthermore, plain radiography is readily available and an inexpensive imaging modality that allows for rapid assessment of the traumatized spine. In contrast to CT, weight-bearing and dynamic studies can be readily obtained with plain imaging. Also, due to much lower radiation dosages, the use of plain radiography should be first considered in the initial assessment and screening of spinal injury in children and adolescents.[67] From a radiation standpoint, a typical CT of the lumbosacral spine involves approximately 6 mSv of radiation exposure compared to approximately 1.5 mSv for plain radiographs.[68,69]

Inflammatory Disease

Seronegative spondyloarthropathies are common inflammatory diseases affecting the lumbosacral spine. These include ankylosing spondylosis (AS) and reactive arthritis. AS commonly affects the axial skeleton, including the sacroiliac joints, spinal apophyseal joints, and symphysis pubis. On the contrary, reactive arthritis presents with asymmetric oligoarthritis, conjunctivitis, and urethritis. Upright AP radiographs are generally sufficient to identify sacroiliitis and erosive changes in patients with suspected AS and should first be considered due to minimize patient radiation exposure.[70,71] In patients with equivocal radiographs, CT is more sensitive for the detection of structural changes and is best able to detect joint and enthesis erosion as well as fracture.[71] However, as CT is unable to provide diagnostic information on inflammation and has a poor ability to detect a soft tissue change, MRI tends to be superior in this regard.[71,72]

Infection

Spinal infections most commonly occur in the lumbar spine. The role of CT in infection is limited to the evaluation of bony destruction and localization of lesions for biopsy. CT is poorly sensitive in the detection of epidural abscesses when compared with MRI.[65,73,74] MRI with gadolinium contrast is the imaging modality of choice for all types of suspected spinal infection with sensitivity and specificity of more than 95%.[64,75]

Malignancy

In the setting of tumor, MRI with gadolinium remains the mainstay of diagnosis as it provides the clearest delineation of the spinal cord from surrounding structures and almost all intrinsic spinal cord tumors and metastases enhance with gadolinium.[76,77] However, as discussed prior, CT certainly has a role in the staging of the disease and when there is extensive bony involvement. Furthermore, needle biopsy under CT guidance is often useful when a diagnosis cannot be made based on imaging alone.[64]

Pediatrics and Other Special Populations

Conventional radiography remains the initial diagnostic imaging modality of choice in the pediatric patient presenting with lower back pain. Controversy exists in the literature regarding the best radiographic modality to use after plain radiographs. MRI is typically preferred as CT is associated with high amounts of radiation. A study by Shin et al.[78] that compared the effective dose of CT/PET in pediatric patients with malignancy found PET/MRI to have 1/5th equivalent of the effective dose of PET/CT. This same study found that the relative radiation dose from a single radiographic examination (0.04 mSv) was 27 times lower than the dose of a comparable CT. The use of CT in this population should be limited to the evaluation of high-energy injuries, polytrauma, workup of specific types of malignancy, monitoring healing from fracture, and when there is a high clinical suspicion of spinal injury in the setting of negative plain imaging.[67,79]

The use of imaging in pregnancy depends upon the imaging modalities available and indications for use. The American College of Obstetricians and Gynecologists recommend the use of MRI as a safer alternative to CT during pregnancy in cases in which both are equivalent in the setting of the diagnosis in question.[80] The use of CT should not be withheld if clinically indicated, but a thorough discussion of risks and benefits when the patient should take place.

Degenerative Diseases/Low Back Pain

MRI is minimally invasive, is highly sensitive and specific, and does not expose patients to ionizing radiation, and as such is considered the gold standard for the workup of suspected disc herniation.[65] Similarly, while CT scan can be useful for evaluating bony pathology, particularly for the purposes of surgical planning, MRI is the test of choice for the evaluation of stenosis.[65,81] For the diagnosis of spondylolysis, while CT is useful, single-photon emission CT (SPECT) and MRI are more sensitive in detecting early disease.[82] Further, MRI scans allow for better evaluation of any associated neural impingement. As mentioned throughout the chapter, CT and CT myelography can be used in those with contraindications to MRI (e.g., implanted cardiac devices).

CONCLUSION

Lumbosacral spinal pathologies are common and include trauma, malignancy, infection, and degenerative disease. Compared with plain radiography and MRI, CT provides ultrafine spatial anatomic detail that allows for optimal evaluation of bony anatomy and pathology. Furthermore, image reformatting and three-dimensional reconstructions allow the surgeon to better visualize spinal anatomy when evaluating complex anatomy and pathologies. Importantly, in the setting of neural compression, CT allows for better distinction between compression secondary to soft tissue versus bony pathology. In patients with contraindications to MRI (i.e., in the presence of certain pacemakers or defibrillators), CT myelogram is a useful surrogate to assess for soft tissue pathology. Ultimately, in many situations, a combination of imaging modalities may be necessary for the evaluation of the spine patient.

REFERENCES

1. DeSai C, Agarwal A. Neuroanatomy, spine. In: *StatPearls*. Treasure Island (FL): StatPearls Publishing; 2020. http://www.ncbi.nlm.nih.gov/books/NBK526133/. Accessed 19 March 2020.
2. Waxenbaum JA, Futterman B. Anatomy, back, lumbar vertebrae. In: *StatPearls*. Treasure Island (FL): StatPearls Publishing; 2020. http://www.ncbi.nlm.nih.gov/books/NBK459278/. Accessed 19 March 2020.
3. Waxenbaum JA, Futterman B. Anatomy, back, intervertebral discs. In: *StatPearls*. Treasure Island (FL): StatPearls Publishing; 2020. http://www.ncbi.nlm.nih.gov/books/NBK470583/. Accessed 19 March 2020.
4. Sattar MH, Guthrie ST. Anatomy, back, sacral vertebrae. In: *StatPearls*. Treasure Island (FL): StatPearls Publishing; 2020. http://www.ncbi.nlm.nih.gov/books/NBK551653/. Accessed 19 March 2020.
5. Balasubramanya R, Selvarajan SK. Lumbar spine imaging. In: *StatPearls*. StatPearls Publishing; 2020. http://www.ncbi.nlm.nih.gov/books/NBK553181/. Accessed 19 June 2020.
6. Jackson HC, Winkelmann RK, Bickel WH. Nerve endings in the human lumbar spinal column and related structures. *J Bone Joint Surg Am*. 1966;48(7):1272–1281.
7. Raj PP. Intervertebral disc: anatomy-physiology-pathophysiology-treatment. *Pain Pract*. 2008;8(1):18–44. https://doi.org/10.1111/j.1533-2500.2007.00171.x.
8. Lotz JC, Fields AJ, Liebenberg EC. The role of the vertebral end plate in low back pain. *Global Spine J*. 2013;3(3):153–164. https://doi.org/10.1055/s-0033-1347298.
9. Antoniou J, Goudsouzian NM, Heathfield TF, et al. The human lumbar endplate. Evidence of changes in biosynthesis and denaturation of the extracellular matrix with growth, maturation, aging, and degeneration. *Spine*. 1996;21(10):1153–1161. https://doi.org/10.1097/00007632-199605150-00006.
10. Roberts S, Menage J, Urban JP. Biochemical and structural properties of the cartilage end-plate and its relation to the intervertebral disc. *Spine*. 1989;14(2):166–174. https://doi.org/10.1097/00007632-198902000-00005.
11. Bernick S, Cailliet R. Vertebral end-plate changes with aging of human vertebrae. *Spine*. 1982;7(2):97–102. https://doi.org/10.1097/00007632-198203000-00002.
12. Bishop PB, Pearce RH. The proteoglycans of the cartilaginous end-plate of the human intervertebral disc change after maturity. *J Orthop Res*. 1993;11(3):324–331. https://doi.org/10.1002/jor.1100110303.
13. Haughton V. Medical imaging of intervertebral disc degeneration: current status of imaging. *Spine*. 2004;29(23):2751–2756. https://doi.org/10.1097/01.brs.0000148475.04738.73.
14. Konin GP, Walz DM. Lumbosacral transitional vertebrae: classification, imaging findings, and clinical relevance. *AJNR Am J Neuroradiol*. 2010;31(10):1778–1786. https://doi.org/10.3174/ajnr.A2036.
15. Tins B. Technical aspects of CT imaging of the spine. *Insights Imaging*. 2010;1(5–6):349–359. https://doi.org/10.1007/s13244-010-0047-2.
16. Dallaway A, Kite C, Griffen C, et al. Age-related degeneration of the lumbar paravertebral muscles: systematic review and three-level meta-regression. *Exp Gerontol*. 2020;133. https://doi.org/10.1016/j.exger.2020.110856, 110856.
17. Flexman AM, Street J, Charest-Morin R. The impact of frailty and sarcopenia on patient outcomes after complex spine surgery. *Curr Opin Anaesthesiol*. 2019;32(5):609–615. https://doi.org/10.1097/ACO.0000000000000759.
18. Hu Z-J, He J, Zhao F-D, Fang X-Q, Zhou L-N, Fan S-W. An assessment of the intra- and inter-reliability of the lumbar paraspinal muscle parameters using CT scan and magnetic resonance imaging. *Spine*. 2011;36(13):E868. https://doi.org/10.1097/BRS.0b013e3181ef6b51.
19. Ghiselli G, Wang JC, Bhatia NN, Hsu WK, Dawson EG. Adjacent segment degeneration in the lumbar spine. *J Bone Joint Surg Am*. 2004;86(7):1497–1503. https://doi.org/10.2106/00004623-200407000-00020.
20. Hilibrand AS, Carlson GD, Palumbo MA, Jones PK, Bohlman HH. Radiculopathy and myelopathy at segments adjacent to the site of a previous anterior cervical arthrodesis. *J Bone Joint Surg Am*. 1999;81(4):519–528. https://doi.org/10.2106/00004623-199904000-00009.
21. Kalb S, Martirosyan NL, Perez-Orribo L, Kalani MYS, Theodore N. Analysis of demographics, risk factors, clinical presentation, and surgical treatment modalities for the ossified posterior longitudinal ligament. *Neurosurg Focus*. 2011;30(3):E11. https://doi.org/10.3171/2010.12.FOCUS10265.
22. Epstein NE. Ossification of the yellow ligament and spondylosis and/or ossification of the posterior longitudinal ligament of the thoracic and lumbar spine. *J Spinal Disord*. 1999;12(3), 250–256.
23. Hida K, Iwasaki Y, Koyanagi I, Abe H. Bone window computed tomography for detection of dural defect associated

with cervical ossified posterior longitudinal ligament. *Neurol Med Chir (Tokyo).* 1997;37(2):173–175. discussion 175–176 https://doi.org/10.2176/nmc.37.173.

24. Mochizuki M, Aiba A, Hashimoto M, Fujiyoshi T, Yamazaki M. Cervical myelopathy in patients with ossification of the posterior longitudinal ligament. *J Neurosurg Spine.* 2009;10(2):122–128. https://doi.org/10.3171/2008.10. SPI08480.

25. Matsunaga S, Sakou T, Taketomi E, Komiya S. Clinical course of patients with ossification of the posterior longitudinal ligament: a minimum 10-year cohort study. *J Neurosurg.* 2004;100(3 Suppl Spine):245–248. https://doi.org/10.3171/spi.2004.100.3.0245.

26. Herkowitz HN, Garfin SR, Bell GR, Bumphrey F, Rothman RH. The use of computerized tomography in evaluating non-visualized vertebral levels caudad to a complete block on a lumbar myelogram. A review of thirty-two cases. *J Bone Joint Surg Am.* 1987;69(2):218–224.

27. Malhotra A, Kalra VB, Wu X, Grant R, Bronen RA, Abbed KM. Imaging of lumbar spinal surgery complications. *Insights Imaging.* 2015;6(6):579–590. https://doi.org/10.1007/s13244-015-0435-8.

28. Delamarter RB, Ross JS, Masaryk TJ, Modic MT, Bohlman HH. Diagnosis of lumbar arachnoiditis by magnetic resonance imaging. *Spine.* 1990;15(4):304–310. https://doi.org/10.1097/00007632-199004000-00011.

29. Petty PG, Hudgson P, Hare WS. Symptomatic lumbar spinal arachnoiditis: fact or fallacy? *J Clin Neurosci.* 2000;7(5):395–399. https://doi.org/10.1054/jocn.1999.0223.

30. Van Lom KJ, Kellerhouse LE, Pathria MN, et al. Infection versus tumor in the spine: criteria for distinction with CT. *Radiology.* 1988;166(3):851–855. https://doi.org/10.1148/radiology.166.3.3340783.

31. Brant-Zawadzki M, Burke VD, Jeffrey RB. CT in the evaluation of spine infection. *Spine.* 1983;8(4):358–364. https://doi.org/10.1097/00007632-198305000-00003.

32. De Backer AI, Mortelé KJ, Vanschoubroeck IJ, et al. Tuberculosis of the spine: CT and MR imaging features. *JBR-BTR.* 2005;88(2):92–97.

33. Inaba K, Munera F, McKenney M, et al. Visceral torso computed tomography for clearance of the thoracolumbar spine in trauma: a review of the literature. *J Trauma.* 2006;60(4):915–920. https://doi.org/10.1097/01.ta.0000196926.79065.6e.

34. Bagley LJ. Imaging of spinal trauma. *Radiol Clin N Am.* 2006;44(1):1–12. vii https://doi.org/10.1016/j.rcl.2005.08.004.

35. Bernstein MP, Young MG, Baxter AB. Imaging of spine trauma. *Radiol Clin N Am.* 2019;57(4):767–785. https://doi.org/10.1016/j.rcl.2019.02.007.

36. Gardner MJ, Morshed S, Nork SE, Ricci WM, Chip Routt ML. Quantification of the upper and second sacral segment safe zones in normal and dysmorphic sacra. *J Orthop Trauma.* 2010;24(10):622–629. https://doi.org/10.1097/BOT.0b013e3181cf0404.

37. Hwang JS, Reilly MC, Shaath MK, et al. Safe zone quantification of the third sacral segment in normal and

dysmorphic sacra. *J Orthop Trauma.* 2018;32(4):178–182. https://doi.org/10.1097/BOT.0000000000001100.

38. Miller AN, Routt MLC. Variations in sacral morphology and implications for iliosacral screw fixation. *J Am Acad Orthop Surg.* 2012;20(1):8–16. https://doi.org/10.5435/JAAOS-20-01-008.

39. Eno J-JT, Boone CR, Bellino MJ, Bishop JA. The prevalence of sacroiliac joint degeneration in asymptomatic adults. *J Bone Joint Surg Am.* 2015;97(11):932–936. https://doi.org/10.2106/JBJS.N.01101.

40. Elgafy H, Semaan HB, Ebraheim NA, Coombs RJ. Computed tomography findings in patients with sacroiliac pain. *Clin Orthop.* 2001;382:112–118. https://doi.org/10.1097/00003086-200101000-00017.

41. Luther N, Iorgulescu JB, Geannette C, et al. Comparison of navigated versus non-navigated pedicle screw placement in 260 patients and 1434 screws: screw accuracy, screw size, and the complexity of surgery. *J Spinal Disord Tech.* 2015;28(5):E298–E303. https://doi.org/10.1097/BSD.0b013e31828af33e.

42. Kraus MD, Krischak G, Keppler P, Gebhard FT, Schuetz UHW. Can computer-assisted surgery reduce the effective dose for spinal fusion and sacroiliac screw insertion? *Clin Orthop.* 2010;468(9):2419–2429. https://doi.org/10.1007/s11999-010-1393-6.

43. Ghisla S, Napoli F, Lehoczky G, et al. Posterior pelvic ring fractures: intraoperative 3D-CT guided navigation for accurate positioning of sacro-iliac screws. *Orthop Traumatol Surg Res.* 2018;104(7):1063–1067. https://doi.org/10.1016/j.otsr.2018.07.006.

44. Richter PH, Gebhard F, Dehner C, Scola A. Accuracy of computer-assisted iliosacral screw placement using a hybrid operating room. *Injury.* 2016;47(2):402–407. https://doi.org/10.1016/j.injury.2015.11.023.

45. Shin BJ, James AR, Njoku IU, Härtl R. Pedicle screw navigation: a systematic review and meta-analysis of perforation risk for computer-navigated versus freehand insertion. *J Neurosurg Spine.* 2012;17(2):113–122. https://doi.org/10.3171/2012.5.SPINE11399.

46. Verma R, Krishan S, Haendlmayer K, Mohsen A. Functional outcome of computer-assisted spinal pedicle screw placement: a systematic review and meta-analysis of 23 studies including 5,992 pedicle screws. *Eur Spine J.* 2010;19(3):370–375. https://doi.org/10.1007/s00586-009-1258-4.

47. Gruskay JA, Webb ML, Grauer JN. Methods of evaluating lumbar and cervical fusion. *Spine J.* 2014;14(3):531–539. https://doi.org/10.1016/j.spinee.2013.07.459.

48. Williams AL, Gornet MF, Burkus JK. CT evaluation of lumbar interbody fusion: current concepts. *AJNR Am J Neuroradiol.* 2005;26(8):2057–2066.

49. Carreon LY, Djurasovic M, Glassman SD, Sailer P. Diagnostic accuracy and reliability of fine-cut CT scans with reconstructions to determine the status of an instrumented posterolateral fusion with surgical exploration as reference standard. *Spine.* 2007;32(8):892–895. https://doi.org/10.1097/01.brs.0000259808.47104.dd.

50. Kanemura T, Matsumoto A, Ishikawa Y, et al. Radiographic changes in patients with pseudarthrosis after posterior

lumbar interbody arthrodesis using carbon interbody cages: a prospective five-year study. *J Bone Joint Surg Am.* 2014;96(10):e82. https://doi.org/10.2106/JBJS.L.01527.

51. Wimmer C, Gluch H. Aseptic loosening after CD instrumentation in the treatment of scoliosis: a report about eight cases. *J Spinal Disord.* 1998;11(5):440–443.

52. Aghayev E, Zullig N, Diel P, Dietrich D, Benneker LM. Development and validation of a quantitative method to assess pedicle screw loosening in posterior spine instrumentation on plain radiographs. *Eur Spine J.* 2014;23(3):689–694. https://doi.org/10.1007/s00586-013-3080-2.

53. Engelke K, Adams JE, Armbrecht G, et al. Clinical use of quantitative computed tomography and peripheral quantitative computed tomography in the management of osteoporosis in adults: the 2007 ISCD official positions. *J Clin Densitom.* 2008;11(1):123–162. https://doi.org/10.1016/j.jocd.2007.12.010.

54. Hendrickson NR, Pickhardt PJ, Del Rio AM, Rosas HG, Anderson PA. Bone mineral density T-scores derived from CT attenuation numbers (Hounsfield units): clinical utility and correlation with dual-energy X-ray absorptiometry. *Iowa Orthop J.* 2018;38:25–31. https://www.ncbi.nlm.nih.gov/pubmed/30104921.

55. Brett AD, Brown JK. Quantitative computed tomography and opportunistic bone density screening by dual use of computed tomography scans. *J Orthop Translat.* 2015;3(4):178–184. https://doi.org/10.1016/j.jot.2015.08.006.

56. Devlin VJ. *Spine Secrets Plus.* 2nd ed. Philadelphia, Pa: Elsevier/Mosby; 2012.

57. Diaz JJ, Cullinane DC, Altman DT, et al. Practice management guidelines for the screening of thoracolumbar spine fracture. *J Trauma.* 2007;63(3):709–718. https://doi.org/10.1097/TA.0b013e318142d2db.

58. Sheridan R, Peralta R, Rhea J, Ptak T, Novelline R. Reformatted visceral protocol helical computed tomographic scanning allows conventional radiographs of the thoracic and lumbar spine to be eliminated in the evaluation of blunt trauma patients. *J Trauma.* 2003;55(4):665–669. https://doi.org/10.1097/01.TA.0000048094.38625.B5.

59. Panda A, Das CJ, Baruah U. Imaging of vertebral fractures. *Indian J Endocrinol Metab.* 2014;18(3):295–303. https://doi.org/10.4103/2230-8210.131140.

60. McAfee PC, Yuan HA, Fredrickson BE, Lubicky JP. The value of computed tomography in thoracolumbar fractures. An analysis of one hundred consecutive cases and a new classification. *J Bone Joint Surg.* 1983;65(4):461–473.

61. Shah LM, Ross JS. Imaging of spine trauma. *Neurosurgery.* 2016;79(5):626–642. https://doi.org/10.1227/NEU.0000000000001336.

62. Mehta S, Auerbach J, Born C, Chin K. Sacral fractures. *J Am Acad Orthop Surg.* 2006;14(12):656–665. https://doi.org/10.5435/00124635-200611000-00009.

63. Jo A, Wilseck Z, Manganaro M, Ibrahim M. Essentials of spine trauma imaging: radiographs, CT, and MRI. *Semin Ultrasound CT MR.* 2018;39(6):532–550.

64. Skinner H. *Current Diagnosis and Treatment in Orthopedics.* 5th ed. New York: McGraw-Hill Professional Publishing; 2014. Revised.

65. Lavi ES, Pal A, Bleicher D, Kang K, Sidani C. MR imaging of the spine: urgent and emergent indications. *Semin Ultrasound CT MR.* 2018;39(6):551–569. https://doi.org/10.1053/j.sult.2018.10.006.

66. Goldberg AL, Kershah SM. Advances in imaging of vertebral and spinal cord injury. *J Spinal Cord Med.* 2010;33(2):105–116. https://doi.org/10.1080/10790268.2010.11689685.

67. Rodriguez DP, Poussaint TY, Rodriguez DP. Imaging of back pain in children. *AJNR Am J Neuroradiol.* 2010;31(5):787–802. https://doi.org/10.3174/ajnr.A1832.

68. Nguyen PK, Wu JC. Radiation exposure from imaging tests: is there an increased cancer risk? *Expert Rev Cardiovasc Ther.* 2011;9(2):177–183. https://doi.org/10.1586/erc.10.184.

69. Yu L. Radiation dose reduction in computed tomography: techniques and future perspective. *Imaging Med.* 2009;1(1):65–84. https://doi.org/10.2217/iim.09.5.

70. Devauchelle-Pensec V, D'Agostino M, Marion J, et al. Computed tomography scanning facilitates the diagnosis of sacroiliitis in patients with suspected spondylarthritis: results of a prospective multicenter French cohort study. *Arthritis Rheum.* 2012;64(5):1412–1419. https://doi.org/10.1002/art.33466.

71. Østergaard M, Lambert RG, Bianchi G. Imaging in ankylosing spondylitis. *Ther Adv Musculoskelet Dis.* 2012;4(4):301–311. https://doi.org/10.1177/1759720X11436240.

72. Weber U, Jurik A, Lambert R, Maksymowych W. Imaging in Spondyloarthritis: controversies in recognition of early disease. *Curr Rheumatol Rep.* 2016;18(9):1–12. https://doi.org/10.1007/s11926-016-0607-7.

73. Shah A, Ogink T, Nelson B, Harris B, Schwab H. Nonoperative management of spinal epidural abscess: development of a predictive algorithm for failure. *J Bone Joint Surg.* 2018;100(7):546–555. https://doi.org/10.2106/JBJS.17.00629.

74. Stratton A, Faris P, Thomas K. The prognostic accuracy of suggested predictors of failure of medical management in Patients with nontuberculous spinal epidural abscess. *Global Spine J.* 2018;8(3):279–285. https://doi.org/10.1177/2192568217719437.

75. Bond A, Manian FA. Spinal epidural abscess: a review with special emphasis on earlier diagnosis. *Biomed Res Int.* 2016;2016:6. https://doi.org/10.1155/2016/1614328.

76. Sevick RJ, Wallace CJ. MR imaging of neoplasms of the lumbar spine. *Magn Reson Imaging Clin N Am.* 1999;7(3):539–553 [ix].

77. Singh K, Samartzis D, Vaccaro A, Andersson G. Current concepts in the management of metastatic spinal disease. *J Bone Joint Surg.* 2006;88(4):434–442. https://doi.org/10.1302/0301-620X.88B4.17282.

78. Shin H, Myung-Joon K, Mi-Jung L. Comparison of effective radiation doses from X-ray, CT, and PET/CT in pediatric patients with neuroblastoma using a dose monitoring program. *Diagn Interv Radiol.* 2016;22(4):390–394. https://doi.org/10.5152/dir.2015.15221.

79. Kim P, Zhu X, Houseknecht E, Nickolaus D, Mahboubi S, Nance M. Effective radiation dose from radiologic studies in pediatric trauma patients. *World J Surg.* 2005;29(12):1557–1562. https://doi.org/10.1007/s00268-005-0106-x.

80. Committee Opinion No. 723 Summary: guidelines for diagnostic imaging during pregnancy and lactation. *Obstet Gynecol.* 2017;130(4):933–934. https://doi.org/10.1097/AOG.0000000000002350.

81. Bischoff RJ, Rodriguez RP, Gupta K, et al. A comparison of computed tomography-myelography, magnetic resonance imaging, and myelography in the diagnosis of herniated nucleus pulposus and spinal stenosis. *J Spinal Disord.* 1993;6(4):289–295. https://doi.org/10.1097/00002517-199306040-00002.

82. Bouras T, Korovessis P. Management of spondylolysis and low-grade spondylolisthesis in fine athletes. A comprehensive review. *Eur J Orthop Surg Traumatol.* 2015;25(S1):167–175. https://doi.org/10.1007/s00590-014-1560-7.

CHAPTER 16

Clinical Correlations to Specific Phenotypes and Measurements With Classification Systems: Lumbosacral Spine

ALEXANDER L. HORNUNG[a] • GARRETT K. HARADA[a] • ZAKARIAH K. SIYAJI[a,b] • HOWARD S. AN[a]
[a]Department of Orthopaedic Surgery, Rush University Medical Center, Chicago, IL, United States
[b]Department of Neurological Surgery, Rush University Medical Center, Chicago, IL, United States

INTRODUCTION

Over the past few decades, the management of lumbosacral spinal disease has become notoriously difficult, whereby complex biomechanics and heterogeneity in presenting conditions have challenged treating clinicians. In response, classification systems emerged, leading to expanded characterization of disease and improvements in treatment guidelines. Though the earliest classifications of the lumbosacral region were simply descriptive, advances in knowledge and technology have since led to systems resulting in measurable improvements in patient outcomes. Over time, the introduction of imaging techniques, such as plain radiographic films and tomography followed by CT, MRI, angiography, and myelography led to major advancements in taxonomic development.[1,2] These advancements led to the identification of various phenotypes or measurements that could be used to categorize lumbosacral disease and injury, assess boney anomalies, disc vitality, and alignment of the lumbosacral spine in relation to adjacent vertebrae, discs, and soft tissues. This chapter aims to highlight lumbosacral classifications with emphasis on measurement, phenotypic variation, and the clinical relevance of the various systems proposed.

CURRENT CLASSIFICATIONS
Alignment (Spinal Curvature)
Adult spinal deformity

Adult spinal deformity (ASD) has conventionally been defined as aberrant curvature or alignment of the spinal vertebrae.[3,4] While the vast majority of spinal deformity falls into the category of degenerative scoliosis, there are frequent incidences of ASD in patients with persistent adolescent idiopathic scoliosis.[3] As such, increased precedence is being placed on examining other, atypical deformities as novel research continues to unravel the complex, heterogeneous nature of the various disorders that fall within the diagnosis.[4] In 2006, the SRS and Schwab classifications were developed to address such issues and have subsequently been combined in routine clinical use.[5,6] The SRS-Schwab classification leverages full-spine (free-standing) radiographs to assess the hip joints and femoral heads in relation to a patient's underlying deformity.[3] In 2008, Kuntz described the CKIV Classification, which utilized some of the parameters in the SRS classification, such as thoracic kyphosis (TK) and lumbar lordosis (LL), but placed precedence on developing an age-dependent system that was further subcategorized by abnormal characteristics (location, severity, pattern) as well as overall global spinal alignment (Table 1).[7,8] Finally, in 2012, the SRS-Schwab classification was modified to include updated pelvic parameters, such as pelvic tilt (PT), pelvic incidence-lumbar lordosis (PI-LL) mismatch, and Cobb angle, as these factors had been previously correlated with clinical outcomes, such as disability, pain, and quality of life scores (Table 2).[6,8–12]

The currently used classification systems allow for an understanding of the impact of disease, mostly by leveraging radiographic findings, yet fail to accurately prognosticate the likelihood of complication rates. The most commonly utilized system is the SRS classification, and while it provides pertinent information regarding

TABLE 1
CKIV Classification of ASD

Patient age (year)

Infantile (0–2)

Juvenile (3–9)

Adolescent (10–18)

Adult (19–60)

Geriatric (> 60)

Spinal abnormality

Scoliotic, kyphotic, lordotic, mixed deformity curves

Major structural deformity curve standing deformity curve with greatest deviation from age-appropriate NUSA for 98.5% of the asymptomatic population

Scoliotic deformity curves

Scoliotic major structural deformity curve > age-appropriate NUSA for 98.5% of the population

Minor structural scoliotic curves remain > 25 degrees on side-bending radiographs

Scoliotic curves named for curve apex in spinal zones

Location (disc)

Occipitocervical: O-C2

Cervical: C2/C3 disc-C6/C7 disc

Cervicothoracic: C7-T1

Proximal thoracic: T1/T2 disc-T5

Main thoracic: T5/T6 disc-T11/T12 disc

Thoracolumbar: T12-L1

Lumbar: L1/L2 disc: L4/L5 disc

Lumbosacral: L5-S1

Kyphotic and lordotic deformity curves

Kyphotic major structural deformity curve > age-appropriate NUSA mean + 2.5 SD

Lordotic major structural deformity curve < age-appropriate NUSA mean – 2.5 SD

Minor structural kyphotic curves remain > adult NUSA mean + 1 SD on extension radiographs

Minor structural lordotic curves remain < adult NUSA mean – 1 SD on flexion radiographs

Kyphotic and lordotic curves named for Sagittal angle in spinal zones

Location (Vertebra)

Occipitocervical: O-C2

Cervical: C2-C7

Cervicothoracic: C6-T2

Proximal thoracic: T1-T5

Main thoracic: T4-T12

Thoracolumbar: T10-L2

Lumbar: L1-L5

Lumbosacral: L4-S1

Scoliokyphotic and scoliolordotic deformity curves

Structural scoliotic curve plus structural kyphotic curve in the same zone

Structural scoliotic curve plus structural lordotic curve in the same zone

Coronal imbalance

± Coronal imbalance, C7-S1 CVA (greater or less than age-appropriate NUSA mean ± 2.5 SD)

Sagittal imbalance

± Sagittal imbalance, C7-S1 SVA (greater or less than age-appropriate NUSA mean ± 2.5 SD)

Pelvic alignment, neutral

Coronal rotation PO > adult NUSA mean ± 2.5 SD

Sagittal rotation PT > or < adult NUSA mean ± 2.5 SD

NUSA, neutral upright spinal alignment.

TABLE 2
SRS Classification of Adult Spinal Deformity

Primary curve types

Single thoracic (ST)

Double thoracic (DT)

Double major (DM)

Triple major (TM)

Thoracolumbar (TL)

Lumbar "de novo"/idiopathic (L)

Primary sagittal plane deformity (SP)

Adult spinal deformity modifiers

Regional sagittal modifier (include only if outside normal range as listed)

(PT) Proximal thoracic (T2-T5): ≥+20 degrees

(MT) Main thoracic (T5-T12): ≥+50 degrees

(TL) Thoracolumbar (T10-L2): ≥+20 degrees

(L) Lumbar (T12-S1): ≥−40 degrees

Lumbar degenerative modifier (include only if present)

(DDD) 2 disc height and facet arthropathy based on X-ray include the lowest involved level between L1 and S1

TABLE 2 SRS Classification of Adult Spinal Deformity—cont'd
(LIS) Listhesis (rotational, lateral antero, retro) ≥ 3 mm includes the lowest level between L1 and L5
(JCT) Junctional L5-S1 curve ≥ 10 degrees (intersection angle superior endplates L5 and S1)
Global balance modifier (include only if imbalance present)
(SB) Sagittal C7 plumb ≥ 5 cm anterior or posterior to sacral promontory
(CB) Coronal C7 plumb ≥ 3 cm right or left of CSVL
SRS definition of regions
Thoracic: apex T2-T11-T12 disc
Thoracolumbar: apex T12-L1
Lumbar: apex L1-L2 disc-L4
Criteria for specific major curve types
Thoracic curves
• Curve ≥ 40 degrees
• Apical vertebral body lateral to C7 plumbline
• T1 rib or clavicle angle ≥ 10 degrees upper thoracic curves
Thoracolumbar and lumbar curves
• Curve ≥ 30 degrees
• Apical vertebral body lateral to CSVL
Primary sagittal plane deformity
• No major coronal curve
• One or more regional sagittal measurements (PT, MT, TL, L) outside

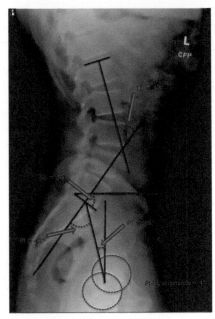

FIG. 1 Spinopelvic radiographic parameters. *LL*, lumbar lordosis; *PI*, pelvic incidence; *PT*, pelvic tilt; *SS*, sacral slope.

quality of life scores, though some recent evidence may suggest that differences up to 20 degrees may lead to acceptable outcomes as well.[9,13,16-20]

Recent literature indicates the need to reevaluate our current parameters to identify associations with perioperative complication rates in ASD patients.[9,13,16-20] While studies, such as Lafage et al., have described age-specific ASD classification systems, there still is ample opportunity to improve upon the current ASD schemes, as some researchers believe the patients' symptomology should have a larger role in their classification and treatment.[4,21] The current heterogeneity in the described classification systems at the time of the writing of this chapter further serves as evidence supporting the need for a more comprehensive system.

Facet Joints

Zygapophysial ("facet") joints are small articulations found along the entire length of the spine, providing stability and a restricted range of motion between adjacent vertebral segments. As such, with increasing age and cumulative biomechanical stress, the facet joints may undergo progressive degeneration and become a consistent source of back pain and disability.[22] Facet joints located in the lumbar spine are perhaps most

previously unconsidered factors (pelvic tilt, incidence, etc.) it fails to take into consideration other potentially relevant factors (comorbidities, treatment, alignment, and patient goals).[8,13] Perhaps the most commonly utilized system is the pelvic incidence/lumbar lordosis (PI-LL) mismatch calculation, which was described by the creators of the Schwab classification (Fig. 1). The PI-LL mismatch is a quick, simple calculation that is commonly applied for evaluation and preoperative planning. Furthermore, the PI-LL mismatch is a diagnostic marker in other pathologies, such as adjacent segment disease after lumbar fusion or pelvic dissociation.[14,15] A PI-LL mismatch < 10 degrees has traditionally been associated with improved postoperative health-related susceptible to such pathology, as corresponding vertebral segments and intervertebral discs experience greater flexibility, axial loads, and other concomitant degenerative changes.[23] Further, facet joint pathology has been notoriously difficult to identify through routine history and physical examination, as frequently the cause of pain, disability, or radicular symptoms is multifaceted and may require invasive diagnostic procedures to identify.[22,23] Such considerations have led to the development of numerous imaging-based classification systems, with hopes that specific facet phenotypes may best correlate with presenting symptoms and help identify which patients will respond appropriately to specific interventions.[24-26]

Lumbar facet arthropathy

Lumbar facet arthropathy (LFA) is a form of osteoarthritis that occurs in the lumbar zygapophysial joints.[27,28] LFA is often portrayed as a result of degenerative processes, such as excessive loading or abnormal movement patterns, but may occur as a result of trauma as well. Generally speaking, LFA occurs as the synovium in the facet joint begins to fail, leading to erosions, decreased disc space, and subchondral osteosclerosis.[25] LFA presents most commonly at L4-L5, though all levels of the lumbar vertebral column may be involved, and often results in complaints of chronic low back pain or radiculopathy due to spinal cord compression.[22] Three classification systems are currently utilized to describe lumbar facet arthropathy (Tables 3–5).

Despite expansive efforts concerning LFA classification schema development, there is no current consensus on any of these classifications. A study by

TABLE 4
Weishaupt et al. Classification

Grade	Criteria
0	Normal facet joint space (2 ± 4 mm width)
1	Narrowing of the facet joint space (< 2 mm) and/or small osteophytes and/or mild hypertrophy of the articular processes
2	Narrowing of the facet joint space and/or moderate osteophytes and/or moderate hypertrophy of the articular process and/or mild subarticular bone erosions
3	Narrowing of the facet joint space and/or large osteophytes and/or severe hypertrophy of the articular process and/or severe subarticular bone erosions and/or subchondral cysts

TABLE 5
Pathria et al. Classification

Grade	Description
1	Normal; no degeneration
2	Mild; joint space narrowing or mild osteophyte
3	Moderate; sclerosis or moderate osteophyte
4	Severe; marked osteophyte or subchondral cysts

TABLE 3
Grogan et al. Classification

Grade	Description
1	Uniformly thick cartilage which covers the articular surface plus well-defined cartilage over articular processes
2	Cartilage covers the entire articular surface with evidence of irregular regions or erosion, interspace is irregular or noncrescentic
3	Cartilage incompletely covers the articular surfaces with underlying bone exposed
4	Cartilage is absent from the articular surface (may have trace amounts). Voids are evident with low MRI signals within the interspace

Kettler et al. in 2006, which set kappa or ICC at > 0.40 (moderate agreement), was carried out to determine which system to recommend statistically for clinical use. Their efforts yielded two classifications that met their recommendation standards, namely the Pathria and Weishaupt systems.[25] Additionally, they included the Grogan system, which is also utilized in clinical care, despite the that the classification did not meet study standards.[25,27] As a whole, the agreement set on this study is low compared to the research community's standards. The heterogeneity in classification systems as well as the lack of agreement at the time of the writing of this chapter necessitates further evaluation. Examination of which of the aforementioned systems correlates "better" with patient symptoms or clinical outcomes could be completed in a comparative analysis similar to that described by Kettler et al. in 2006.[25,29]

Vertebral Endplate

Endplate degeneration

Modic changes (MC) are currently defined as signal changes in vertebral subchondral bone marrow present on magnetic resonance.[30] The sentinel study by M.T. Modic et al., first described Modic changes in 1989 using T1-weighted sagittal MRI.[31] These changes have been strongly associated with degenerative spinal pathologies, specifically degenerative disc disease.[30,32,33] Type 1 MC has been correlated with low back pain (LBP) in numerous studies although its role in the pathogenies of LBP is under scrutiny.[34] To date, three main types of MC have been delineated (Fig. 2).[35]

Currently, only Modic type 1 has been associated with low back pain in study populations, despite recent evidence the Modic type 2 changes may be more prevalent in individuals with greater fat mass.[34] According to a study by Mitra et al., Modic changes represent a pathologic progression from acute (Modic type 1) to other chronic forms with Modic type 2 resulting in improvement of the patients' symptoms.[36,37] Overall, most hypotheses about the pathogenesis and role of Modic changes in degeneration are speculative, despite the classification's widespread use in the research community. Continued analysis of the role of type 3 changes in spinal pathologies, with specific attention to the progression of degenerative etiologies, is necessary to elucidate the relationship with patient symptoms. Furthermore, it is important to note that recent studies have proposed a combined classification system that utilizes not only Modic changes, but Pfirrmann grading, high-intensity zones, and loss of disc height as well.[38] Continued analysis of algorithmic approaches that leverage multiple classical scoring systems may provide better prognostic utility when evaluating the spine for degeneration.[38–40]

Schmorl's nodes

Schmorl's nodes (SN) are a subclassification of herniation that results in the nucleus pulpous (NP) being pushed through the cartilage and endplate.[41,42] In most cases, SN are asymptomatic findings on imaging modalities but may become painful over time.[43,44] Despite numerous postulates as to the pathogenesis of SN (autoimmunity, trauma, degeneration, etc.), no single theory is currently accepted.[43–45] Previous studies indicated SN is associated with the degeneration of the vertebral discs. With the wide variability of reported prevalence

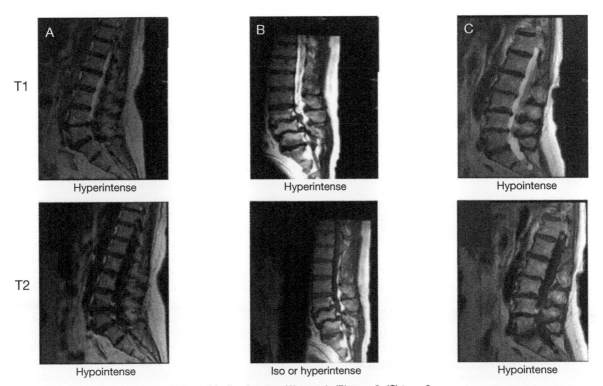

FIG. 2 Modic changes (A) type 1; (B) type 2; (C) type 3.

data, 3.8%–76%, precedence has been placed not only on examining the different etiologies of SN but on classifying it as well.[45] Currently, at least one study has proposed a classification system. The classification is broken into five categories based on the contour, morphology, and typology of the lesion.[45]

Despite continued research, such as that by Mok et al. which described the association between SN and disc degeneration, the clinical relevance of SN remains uncertain as the explanatory mechanism or pathogenesis to lower back pain has not been fully elucidated.[43,45,46] Additionally, conflicting evidence about the progression of SN to disc degenerative symptomology exists, making prognostication inherently difficult.[46] The initial results of the classification system described by Samartzis et al are promising with an excellent intraobserver (kappa = 0.88) and good interobserver reliability (mean kappa = 0.79).[45] Despite the initial findings, it is important to note that the intraobserver reliability was calculated with a small observer sample size ($n = 2$) and is a logical starting place for future analysis.[45] Additionally, further studies investigating the prognostic utility and reliability of the aforementioned system as well as mechanistic evaluations of the pathophysiology of SN is necessary.

Intervertebral Discs
Annular fissure
Annular fissures are defined as a disruption in at least one layer of the annulus fibrous.[47] Annular fissures occur not only between the annular fibers but from the vertebral column as well.[48] Despite the typical asymptomatic nature of annular fissures, some may progress to simple annular fissures without herniation or herniated nucleus pulposus with radiculopathy depending on the severity and extent of the insult.[41,47] Currently, fissures are classified by their involvement, location, and continuity (Table 6).[41,48,49]

TABLE 6 Raj et al. Classification	
Grade	**Description**
0	No visible tears, normal nucleus
1	Tears are less than one-third of the distance through the annulus fibrosus
2	Tears extend further toward the disc edge, there is no presence of bulging, compression, or gross deformity
3	Tears have completely disrupted the disc and are encroaching on PLL

The current classification for annular fissures, despite its descriptive value, fails in regard to prognostic usefulness.[50] Despite the commonality of annular fissures, we cannot currently reliably identify them on MRI as well as grade or classify them based on clinical symptoms.[50] Currently, multiple studies have explored the presence of high-intensity zones (HIZ) as a means of elucidating the existence or complexity of annular fissures, even though they can occur as a result of alternative pathological processes.[51,52] Preliminary analysis indicates that the signal intensity on T2-weighted images has correlated with annular fissures, whereas the presence of intensity on a T1-weighted image appears to suggest different pathophysiology.[53] Systematizing annular fissure MRI findings into a classification system has been suggested, but as of the writing of this chapter it has not been fabricated. It is the current recommendation of experts in the field to develop large-scale studies assessing the role of HIZ in annular fissure while cultivating a standardized classification system that utilizes the pathophysiologic progression of annular fissures.[50]

Disc degeneration
Disc degeneration is one of the most common spine-related presentations.[25,33,41] Degeneration is currently considered to be related to aggravating factors, such as surgery, metabolic injury, or trauma which leads to deteriorating processes (chondrocyte proliferation, cell death, dehydration, etc.) over time.[43,45,54,55] As a result of degeneration, the spine may become more susceptible to injury and progress to unfavorable symptomologies such as developing chronic low back pain.[25,41,55] The most commonly utilized classification systems for degeneration, Pfirrmann grades and Thompson Classification, will be examined in the subsequent sections.

Pfirrmann grading. In 2001, Pfirrmann et al. created a scoring system for disc degeneration based on T2-weighted magnetic resonance findings.[56] Specifically, the score aims to provide standardized nomenclature for describing disc abnormalities among spinal surgeons. The Pfirrmann classification system utilizes an algorithmic approach leveraging four criteria for describing disc degeneration, specifically structure, signal intensity, height, and the ability to distinguish the nucleus from the annulus.[56,57] The scores are classified as one of the five grades depending on MRI findings such as disc height, intensity, and the distinction between anatomical landmarks (Fig. 3).

The strengths of the Pfirrmann system lie in its simplicity, completeness, and proven research utility. Despite demonstrated reliability, specifically, intrarater, of Pfirrmann grading the classification falls short as

Grade	Structure	Signal intensity (T2)	Vertebral disc height	Reference
I	Bright, homogenous	Hyperintense	Normal	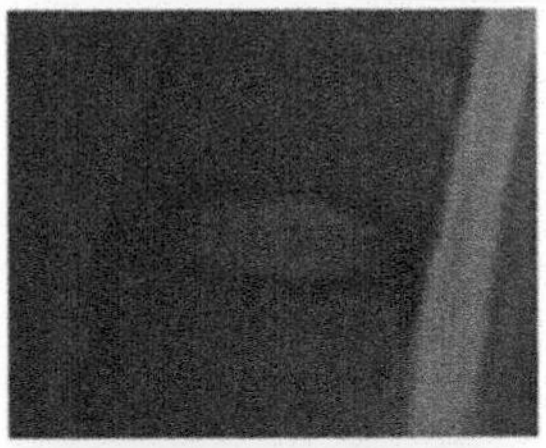
II	Heterogeneous; horizontal banding may be present	Hyperintense	Normal	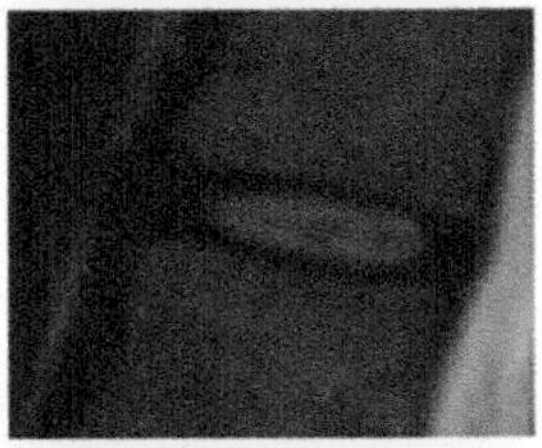
III	Grey, heterogeneous;	Transitional	Slightly decreased	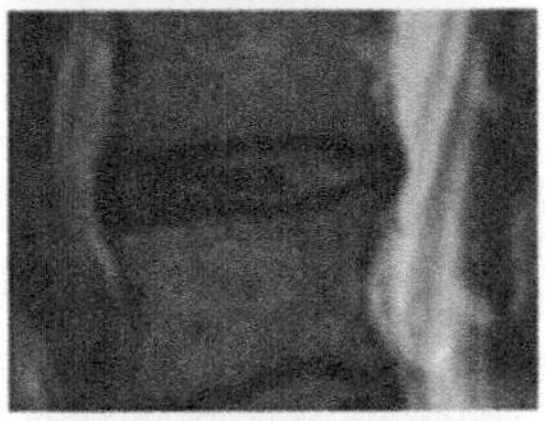
IV	Grey or black, heterogeneous	Slightly hypointense	Slightly to moderately decreased	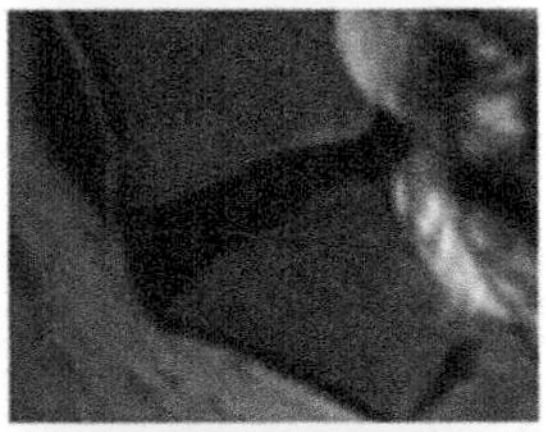
V	Black, heterogeneous	Hypointense	Severely decreased or collapsed	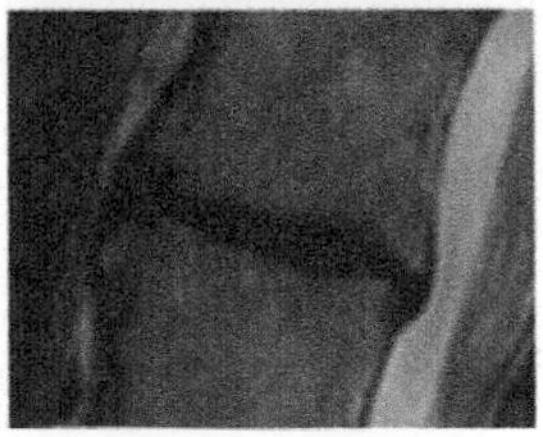

FIG. 3 Pfirrmann classification system.

multiple limitations of the system have been considered.[39] First, Pfirrmann grading has been described as being subjective.[58] As such, some studies have found that the Pfirrmann system only provides acceptable agreement among different observers, which calls its communicational consistency into question.[59] Furthermore, the Pfirrmann grading system has been under recent scrutiny for the lack of interobserver reliability, particularly when comparing disc degeneration between the elderly and younger patients.[39] Additionally, some argue that the 5-level system should be abandoned in favor of an 8-level system that expands grade C to 2 grades (3 and 4) and Grade D to 3 grades (5, 6, and 7).[57] This allows clinicians to more accurately take into account the effect of age on the degeneration of the spine.[57] Finally, advancements in biomechanical and magnetic resonance imaging technologies, such as glycosaminoglycan chemical exchange saturation, micro-nano structural, and 9.4T

TABLE 7
Jensen Classification

Grade	Nucleus	Annulus	Endplate	Vertebral Body
1	Bulging gel	Discrete fibrous laminae	Hyaline, uniform thickness	Rounded margins
2	Peripheral white fibrous tissue	Mucinous material between laminae	Irregular thickness	Pointed margins
3	Consolidated fibrous tissue	Extensive mucinous infiltration; loss of annular-nuclear demarcation	Focal defects in cartilage	Small chondrophytes or osteophytes at margins
4	Horizontal clefts parallel to endplate	Focal disruptions	Fibrocartilage extending from subchondral bone; irregularity and focal sclerosis in subchondral bone	Osteophytes < 2 mm
5	Clefts extended through nucleus and annulus		Diffuse sclerosis	Osteophytes > 2 mm

MRI, have let experts speculate that each could improve upon the currently utilized Pfirrmann system.[40,60,61] Of note, decreased variability in scoring severity with the adoption of these technologies has been postulated.[60,61]

Thompson classification. In 1990, Thompson et al. develop a gross morphological classification scheme for the lumbar intervertebral disc. The grading system separates midsagittal sections into five succinct categories (Table 7) of degeneration.[62]

While not as clinically useful as its counterpart, namely the Pfirrmann system, the Thompson classification exhibits an excellent intraobserver agreement (87%–91%) with an adequate to good interobserver agreement (61%–88%).[62] Despite being in use today, the clinical utility of the Thompson classification has fallen under scrutiny. The inherent limitations of the Thompson system, namely that it requires in vitro disc samples, curtail the system's widespread usage, limiting it to mostly the academic realm.[25]

Disc herniation

Disc herniation is described as a part of the disc nucleus that has slipped, ruptured, or bulged into the spinal canal.[47,63] Herniation is often the result of increased loading or pressure on the vertebral column which leads to degeneration over time, though sudden insults may also lead to herniation.[47,64] As the disc protrudes, patients may experience radicular symptoms, including pain, numbness/tingling, or weakness.[64] To date, multiple studies have examined individuals with herniations through multiple modalities (e.g., autopsies, computerized tomography (CT), magnetic resonance imaging (MRI), etc.).[65,66] There are currently three

main classification systems to describe disc herniations, as outlined in Tables 8–10 and Fig. 4.

TABLE 8
Jensen

Type	Description
Normal	Normal disc pathology
Bulge	Symmetric circumferential extension of the disc beyond interspace
Protrusion	Focal extension of the disc beyond interspace
Extrusion	The base of disc material is smaller than any other disc material dimension

TABLE 9
CTF Classification

Morphology
Protrusion
Extrusion
Intravertebral
Containment
Continuity
Relation with PLL complex
Volume
Composition
Location

TABLE 10
Hao Classification

(A)

	Features	Score
Clinical manifestation (CM)		
Pain		
	Slight lower limb(s) pain, tolerable without analgesics for > 6 weeks	1
	Heavy lower limb(s) pain, tolerable with analgesics for > 6 weeks	2
	Severe lower limb(s) pain, intolerable with analgesics for > 6 weeks	3
Nervous function		
	Slight involvement of nerves (numbness in any nerve between L4-S1)	1
	Involvement of nerves (strength decreasing 1–2 grade in digital extensor L4-S1)	2
	Muscle strength decreasing ≥ 3 grade, plus dysfunction of the sphincter (foot-drop or uroschesis)	3
Straight Let Raising Test (SLRT)		
	≥ +70 degrees	1
	+30–50	2
	≤ +30 degrees	3
Imaging findings		
CT or MRI cross-section		
Central		
	1. Protrusion of spinal sagittal diameter < 30%	1
	2. Protrusion of spinal sagittal diameter 30%–50%	2
	3. Protrusion of spinal sagittal diameter > 50%	3
Paramedian		
	1. lateral recess stenosis by protrusion < 30%	1
	2. lateral recess stenosis by protrusion 30%–50%	2
	3. lateral recess stenosis by protrusion > 50%	3
Foraminal		
	1. Intervertebral foramen stenosis by protrusion < 30%	1
	2. Intervertebral foramen stenosis by protrusion 30%–50%	2
	3. Intervertebral foramen stenosis by protrusion > 50%	3

(B)
6-SCORE V-TYPE CRITERIA

Type		Points
I		2
II		3
III		4
A	CM score of 3 and image finding score of 1	
B	CM score of 2 and image finding score of 2	
C	CM score of 1 and image finding score of 3	
IV		5
V		6

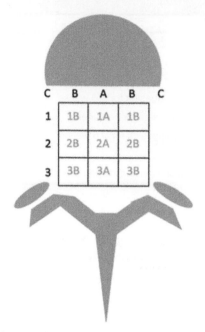

FIG. 4 Grading of herniations using the MSU schematic involves a two-character scoring system, location (A–C) as well as severity (1–3). For example, a score of 1C indicates the herniation is lateral to the established gridlines and does not extend into zone 2.

Currently, the Jensen and CTF classification system is the most commonly utilized system for describing lumbar disc pathology.[67] Researchers and physicians dispute the clinical relevance of these systems.[67-69] In an attempt to revitalize the classification of disc herniations, two separate research teams developed their own original systems. While the MSU system offers great interobserver reliability, as high as 98%, it is not without its faults.[68] Recent criticism of the system cites oversimplicity in the system, which led the authors to question the classification's clinical relevance.[67,69] The Hao system currently leverages a 6-score V-type system that can be used to score and evaluate future patients.[69] Due to the novelty of the study, little follow-up, aside from the initially reported 98% interexaminer reliability, has been initiated.[70] As a whole, the current heterogeneity in classification systems amplifies the need for further evaluation to determine clinical correlations.

Trauma and fracture classifications

Lumbosacral fractures are complex and exhibit heterogeneous nature as a result of the multiple ways they may be sustained.[71] Over the years, numerous classification systems have been developed and subsequently discarded. In light of novel imaging modalities, increased efforts have been made to develop a singular, original classification system that not only organizes lumbosacral fractures but allows for consistent treatment across providers.[72,73] To date, despite the best efforts by experts, no such system exists. This had led to the use of multiple classification schemes, which are explored in the following sections.

Brief history of the classification of lumbosacral fractures. The exploration and development of lumbosacral fracture classification systems has been a long, arduous journey. The advent of these classification systems can be traced back to the mid-1900s when Boehler described five categories of spinal fractures.[74] While the system leveraged physiologically relevant information, namely the type of injury (compression, flexion, extension, etc.), it was ultimately served as a starting for other early classification systems, such as Watson-Jones (1938) and Nicoll (1949).[75,76] While each of these systems utilized different techniques to explain fracture subtleties, spinal solidity, and anatomy respectively, they both placed precedence on the ligamental stability in their schemes.[71,73]

Fracture classification was reinvigorated in 1963 with the advent of the Holdsworth classification. Drawing on the previously described models, specifically the role of the posterior spinous ligament in the Watson-Jones model and bony anatomy in the Nicoll model, Holdsworth proposed a two-column theory that placed precedence on the biomechanical stress or trauma of each injury subtype, thereby integrating all three of the previously proposed systems. An attempt to reexamine Holdsworth scheme, focused specifically on the anterior column, was carried out by Kelly and Whiteside in 1968.[77] Despite the limited sample ($n = 11$), the classification paved the way for subsequent classifications, namely Denis and McAfee.[71,73]

While each of the aforementioned classification systems served as the chief schema in their respective times, all were eventually replaced in favor of novel mechanistic considerations or a more objective measurement provided by the advancement in imaging modalities.[73] It is important to note that despite the use of newer imaging modalities, some more recent classification systems, namely the McAfee, Ferguson-Allen, and McCormack Classification (Load Sharing Classification), were eventually replaced as pathophysiology implications were elucidated.[71,73,78-80]

Roy-Camille classification. In 1984, Roy-Camille proposed a classification system for sacral fractures, placing attention on U-shaped injury patterns.[81] The system categorizes the fractures into three types based on the location of the cranial or rostral portion.[73] Injury types 1 and 2 describe degeneration or trauma as a result of flexion whereas type III predominately indicates extension injuries (Table 11).[81]

Denis classification. Mechanical implications were again postulated in 1983 with the proposal of the Denis classification system.[82] Unlike any previously described classification, the Denis system leveraged a three-column theory: anterior, middle, and posterior. In light of a radiographic study of 412 patients, Denis not only outlined four groups of fractures (compression, burst, seat-belt, and fracture-dislocations) but was able to describe them based on column location as well (Table 12).[82]

TABLE 11
Roy-Camille Classification

Type	Description
1	Simple focal kyphosis of the upper sacral segments
2	Anterior displacement and kyphosis, with impaction
3	Posterior displacement and lordosis with override

TABLE 12
Denis Classification

Section A	Section B
Anterior column	**Type A**
Anterior longitudinal ligament	Fracture of both endplates without kyphosis
Anterior two-thirds of the body	Mechanism of injury: pure axial load
Anterior two-thirds of the disc	Predilection site: low lumbar region
Middle column	**Type B**
Posterior one-third of the vertebral body	Fracture of the superior endplate (CT may also demonstrate a sagittal split of the lower endplate)
Posterior one-third of the intervertebral disc (annulus fibrosus)	Most frequent burst fracture
Posterior longitudinal ligament	Mechanism of injury: axial load and flexion
Posterior column	Predilection site: thoracolumbar junction
Everything posterior to the PLL	**Type C**
	Fracture of the inferior endplate
	Mechanism of injury: probably axial load and flexion
	No particular site pattern could be identified
	Type D
	Burst rotation fracture
	Burst fracture with comminution of the vertebral body, large central defect on CT, loss of posterior height, an increase of the interpedicular distance, vertical fracture of the lamina, bone retropulsed into the spinal canal
	Mechanism of injury: axial load and rotation
	Predilection site: mid lumbar region
	Type E
	Burst lateral flexion fracture
	The fractured posterior wall of the vertebral body with fragment extrusion toward the side of the flexion
	Mechanism of injury: axial load and lateral flexion

Magerl AO. Described in 1994 by Magerl et al., this scheme again utilizes a mechanistic approach to spinal fracture evaluation.[83] Unlike the Denis classification system, the Magerl AO categorizes injuries into 3 types, encompassing 53 models.[71] The strength of the Magerl AO study was its sample size as 1445 patients were examined in the constructive process of this classification scheme.[73] Leveraging simple physics parameters, such as force vectors, with the appearance of the bone provided a comprehensive description of spinal injury (Table 13).[71,73]

Thoracolumbar Injury Classification and Scoring System (TLICS). Drawing on the efforts of Magerl et al., the Thoracolumbar Injury Classification and Scoring System (2002) aimed not only to universalize the process of classifying fracture injuries but to simplify it as well.[84–86] Unlike the Magerl AO, the TLICS evaluates neurological status, posterior ligamentous complex integrity, and provides descriptive morphology of the injury. Additionally, this classification utilizes a scoring system that provides an algorithmic approach, much like the Spinal Instability Neoplastic Score (SINS), for evaluating the necessity of surgical treatment.[87] It is also important to note that a similar system was developed for sacral injuries as well (Table 14).

AOSpine classification(s). Despite the advent of the TLICS, there was still no widespread (i.e., international) implementation of a single classification system for spinal fractures, specifically those in the lumbar and sacral spines.[88] For this reason, the AO Spine Classification Group was developed for not only the lumbar system but the sacral classification as well (Table 15). Central to these newly developed systems was the addition of neurological parameters as well as supplementary modifiers, like concomitant injuries or comorbidities.[89,90]

TABLE 13
Magerl AO Classification

A: Compression injuries	B: Distraction injuries	C: Torsion injuries
A1: Impaction fractures	B1: Predominantly transligamentous flexion-distraction injury	C1: Rotation-compression injury
A1.1: Endplate impaction	B1.1: With transverse disc disruption	C1.1: Impaction
A1.2: Wedge impaction	B1.1.1: Flexion subluxation	C1.2: Split
A1.3: Vertebral body collapse	B1.1.2: Anterior dislocation	C1.3: Burst
A2: Split fractures	B1.1.3: Either 1.1 or 1.2 + a fracture of the articular processes	C2: Rotation-distraction injury
A2.1: Frontal	B1.2: With type A vertebral body fracture	C2.1: With transligamentous flexion-distraction
A2.2: Sagittal	B2: Predominantly osseous flexion-distraction injury	C2.2: With transosseous flexion-distraction
A2.3: Pincer	B2.1: Transverse bi column fracture	C2.3: With hyperextension-distraction
A3: Burst fractures	B2.2: Posterior osseous disruption with transverse disc disruption	C3: Rotational shear injury
A3.1: Incomplete burst	1: Through the pedicles	
A3.2: Burst split	2: Through the interarticular portions (flexion spondylolysis)	
A3.3: Complete burst	B2.3: With type A vertebral body fracture	
1: Pincer	1: Through the pedicles	
2: Flexion	2: Through the isthmus	
3: Axial	B3: Anterior disruption through the disc	
	B3.1: Hyperextension-subluxation	
	B3.2: Hyperextension-spondylolysis	
	B3.3: Posterior dislocation	

TABLE 14
TLICS Scoring

Section A	
Parameter	**Points**
Morphology	
Compression fracture	1
Burst fracture	2
Translational/rotational	3
Distraction	4
Neurologic involvement	
Intact	0
Nerve root	2
Cord, conus medullaris	
Incomplete	3
Complete	2
Cauda equina	3
Posterior ligamentous complex	
Intact	0
Injury suspected/indeterminate	2
Injured	3

Section B	
Management Strategy	**Points**
Nonoperative	0–3
Nonoperative or operative	4
Operative	≥ 5

These additions lead the researchers to adopt a novel system that they felt would provide physicians with ample information to classify the pathology and prepare treatment plans.[90]

Isler classification. In the 1990s, Isler proposed classifications for lumbosacral fractures near the articulation sites.[91,92] The classification utilizes a simple three typological scheme describing the directionality of the fracture indicating what subsequent structures may have been impacted (Table 16).[73]

Significance. Currently, the most widely utilized classifications differ by anatomical location. For lumbar fractures, the Denis and Magerl AO systems are frequently employed, though some studies report that the Magerl

AO is not totally useful clinically as it provides too much information to be applicable for everyday clinical decision-making.[87] On the other hand, sacral fractures also use the Denis classification and commonly leverage the Roy-Camille, Isler, and the AO sacral systems as well depending on fracture orientation. Generally speaking, the fault of fracture classifications is that they are either too simple or too cumbersome to use clinically.[87,90] Additionally, fracture schemes fail to provide sufficient repeatability. As a whole, the current state of fracture classification systems illustrates the importance of generating simple, useful, and repeatable assessments for prognostication. Furthermore, the newer classifications, namely the AOSpine classifications by region, have not been subjected to the validation and scrutiny of the previously proposed systems though preliminary evidence of the reliability has been promising.[93] Further analysis of the newest classification is warranted.[93,94]

Other Pathologies and Spinal Instability
Spondylolistheses
Spondylolisthesis is defined as a shift, movement, or translation of a vertebral body relative to adjacent levels.[41] Spondylolistheses can occur in the anterior, posterior, or lateral planes and arise from a variety of etiologies (namely, degeneration or overuse).[47,95] Spondylolisthesis may warrant further radiographic or CT assessment depending on patient complaints to determine stability, stenosis, and degree of compression (if present).[96] Although surgery may ultimately be necessary for patients with symptomatic spondylolisthesis, treatment recommendations remain controversial.[97] Spondylolisthesis is broken into two distinctions: degenerative and isthmic. Currently, there is a considerable overlap between classification systems for spondylolisthesis. It is important to note that only one classification system, the Wiltse-Newman, describes the etiology of spondylolisthesis and categorizes the severity of isthmic spondylolisthesis (Tables 17–22).[98]

Notwithstanding its widespread use, ultimately the Meyerding classification's utility for lumbar spondylolisthesis is minimal. The lack of clinical utility is the result of an inability to further classify lumbar spondylolisthesis between grades I and II as well as modify the scores with factors associated with commonly measured clinical outcomes, such as disc height, pelvic incidence, or other spinopelvic parameters.[97,99] Both of the SDSG classifications were created to describe high-grade and lumbosacral spondylolisthesis, respectively.[100–102]

As a result of the shortcomings of the previous systems, two novel classification systems were developed in 2014: the Clinical and Radiographic Degenerative

TABLE 15
AOSpine Thoracolumbar Injury Classification System

A: Compression injuries	Neurological status
Type A injuries involve the anterior portion of the vertebral column with an intact posterior tension band (the group of muscles, ligaments and processes/pedicles that maintain the integrity of the vertebral column).	N0: Neurologically intact
A0: No or clinically insignificant fractures of the spinous or transverse processes	N1: Transient deficit
A1: Wedge compression injuries	N2: Radiculopathy
A2: Split or pincer-type injuries	N3: Incomplete spinal cord injury or CE syndrome
A3: Also known as incomplete burst injuries	N4: Complete spinal cord injury
A4: Complete burst injuries	NX: Unknown neurological status
B: Distraction injuries	**Modifiers**
Type B injuries involve the anterior or posterior tension band.	M1: Unknown tension band injury status
B1: Chance fractures	M2: Comorbidities
B2: Posterior tension band disruption injuries	
B3: Hyperextension injuries	
C: Translation injuries	
Type C injuries involve displacement in any direction. No subtypes are present as there are numerous possibilities of dislocating fractures.	

TABLE 16
Isler Classification

Type I	Fracture occurs lateral to the L5/S1 facet
Type II	Fractures line involves the L5/S1 facet
Type III	Fracture line extends medially to the L5/S1 facet

TABLE 17
Meyerding Classification

Grade I	$\leq 25\%$
Grade II	25%–50%
Grade III	50%–75%
Grade IV	75%–100%
Grade V	> 100%

TABLE 18
SDSG—Spondylolisthesis Classification

Low grade (< 50% slippage)	
Type 1	PI < 45
Type 2	PI $45 < x < 60$
Type 3	PI > 60
High grade (> 50% slippage)	
Type 4	Balanced pelvis
Type 5	Retroversed pelvis, balanced column
Type 6	Retroversed pelvis, unbalanced column

Spondylolisthesis (CARDS) system and French classification for lumbar degenerative spondylolisthesis (French).[1,103] Both systems have shown initial promise and have their respective strengths. The CARDS system has been hailed for its simplicity, clinical utility, and reliability despite not taking into account spinopelvic measurements.[99,103] On the other hand, the French system leverages a more comprehensive approach, similar to the adult spinal deformity classification purposed by Schwab et al., allowing for more detail to be used in patient assessment.[11,104] To date, only a single study has examined the studies against each other.[103] Before the adoption of one system over the other, further

TABLE 19
SDSG Revised Classification

Grade	Sacropelvic Balance	Spinopelvic Balance	Type
Low-grade	Normal pelvic incidence	–	1
	High pelvic incidence	–	2
High-grade	Balanced	–	3
	Unbalanced	Balanced	4
		Unbalanced	5

TABLE 20
CARDS Classification

Type	Description
A	Advanced disc space collapse without kyphosis
B	Disc height partially preserved, translation < 5 mm
C	Disc height partially preserved, translation > 5 mm
D	Kyphotic alignment

TABLE 21
French Classification

Type	Description
1	SVA < 4 cm, SL > 5, LL > PI
2	SVA < 4 cm, SL = 5, LL > PI
3	SVA < 4 cm, LL < PI, PT < 25
4	SVA < 4 cm, LL < PI, PT > 25
5	SVA > 4 cm

SVA, sagittal vertical axis; *SL*, segmental lordosis; *LL*, lumbar lordosis

TABLE 22
Wiltse-Newman Classification

Type I	Dysplastic	A congenital defect in pars
Type II	Isthmic	
	A	Pars fatigue fracture
	B	Pars elongation due to multiple healed stress fracture
	C	Pars acute fracture
Type III	Degenerative	Facet instability without a pars fracture
Type IV	Traumatic	Acute posterior arch fracture other than pars
Type V	Neoplastic	Pathologic destruction of pars

iterations are necessary to determine the clinical significance of each system.

Finally, despite the development of two novel classification systems, the Mac-Thiong and Marchetti-Bartolozzi, for recategorizing isthmic spondylolistheses, the Wilste-Newman is still the most commonly utilized isthmic spondylolisthesis schema. Currently, analysis of the use of magnetic resonance imaging (MRI) and single-photon emission computed tomography (SPECT) as a means of classifying spondylolitic lesions have been documented. These studies are preliminary and have only been done for adolescents.[105-107] Future validation and logistical insights are required before their widespread adoption into the orthopedic spinal community.

Diffuse idiopathic skeletal hyperostosis

Diffuse idiopathic skeletal hyperostosis (DISH) is explained as a proliferation of ossific, or calcific, processes in the spine.[108-110] DISH is mostly described in individuals over the age of 50 and typically occurs in the thoracic spine but has been identified in the lumbar segment as well.[111-114] The condition often results in pain and immobility due not only to the progression of joint space stenosis but an enlargement of the epiphysis as well.[108,110] Currently, the Resnick and Niwayama and the Utsinger criteria are the most widely utilized accepted classifications (Tables 23 and 24).[115,116]

A review by Kuperus et al. in 2017 highlights the current state of DISH classification systems.[117] Currently, there remains discordance regarding the various classifications set forth as over 20 sets of classifications have been set forth. Whether it be the location, the number of affected vertebra, or thickness, the underpinnings of each study seem to be based on each author's opinion on the pathological progression of DISH.[117] Recent literature highlights the shape and location, namely the involvement of the anterior or posterior longitudinal ligament, paired with the Resnick criteria as a means of further classifying DISH.[117] Moreover, a scoring system utilizing imagining modalities scoring the amount of ossification as well as the involvement of extraspinal

TABLE 23
Resnick and Niwayama

Criteria	Description
1	Calcification and ossification along the anterolateral aspect of ≥ 4 contiguous vertebral bodies with/without associated localized excrescences at the intervening body-disc junctions
2	Relative preservation of disc height in the involved segment with absence of extensive radiographic changes of DDD including the vacuum phenomena and vertebral body marginal sclerosis
3	Absence of apophyseal joint ankylosis and SI joint erosion, sclerosis, or intraarticular osseous fusion

TABLE 24
Utsinger

Criteria	Description
1	Continuous ossification along the anterolateral aspect of ≥ 4 contiguous vertebral bodies
2	Continuous ossification along the anterolateral aspect of ≥ 2 contiguous vertebral bodies
3	Symmetrical and peripheral enthesopathy involving the posterior heel, superior patella, or olecranon. The new bone has a well-defined cortical margin

locations was also proposed by Mata et al.[118] The Mata classification was further modified to a progressive sextet by Yaniv et al.[119] Additionally, recent literature documents the characteristic DISH computed tomography findings have been initiated.[120,121] A study by Leibushor et al. was one of the first to utilize the applied CT findings, namely intraarticular ankylosis (a common finding in DISH patients) to the already established Resnick classification criteria.[120] Future investigation into the evolution and pathophysiology of DISH as well as novel imagining modalities not only allows for the development of a DISH classification that meets the needs of the orthopedic spine community but also will allow for the development of novel, prospective analyses to truly cement the postulated system's significance in the clinical realm.

Spinal instability

Spinal instability is described as an abnormal increase in the lumbar range of motion.[122] The causes of instability range from trauma to congenital defects, utilizing a variety of techniques to determine the stability of the spine. Of note, lumbar flexion-extension radiographs are commonly used to examine the integrity of spondylolisthetic segments with > 2–4 mm of translation or 7–20 rotation considered abnormal on functional radiographs.[123–125] Finally, fluoroscopic video assessment of the sagittal plane, cross-sectional size, and activation of the paraspinal muscle, as well as flexion relaxation studies, have also been utilized to examine lumbar stability.[126–128]

SINS. Despite the heterogeneity in the pathogenesis of lumbar instability, the only current standardized scoring system for instability is defined for neoplastic processes.[27,122] In 2010, the Spinal Instability Neoplastic Score (SINS) was developed to ensure consistent communication across physicians from a variety of specialties, but have prognostic surgical value as well.[122,129] While only 5 points are attributed to the lumbosacral spine in regard to the location in the overall SINS score, it nonetheless has been used to describe neoplastic lumbar instability and its accompanying symptoms.[129–132] The tool assesses six variables and provides a score for each component (Table 25).[122] These scores can be easily added and applied to the three predetermined thresholds that serve to guide the enacting surgeon's decision-making process on a per-patient basis.[70,133]

While multiple studies have indicated interobserver agreement as well as high sensitivity (95.7%) and specificity (79.5%), the clinical significance of SINS is not without scrutiny.[122,134–136] Despite the recommendation of referral for patients with SINS ≥ 7 and surgery for those with scores ≥ 13, the threshold values are currently under consideration. Two studies proposed alternative thresholds to those presently recommended in an attempt to address poorer outcomes, namely severe adverse effects (SAEs) and those related to no surgical interventions.[70,133,137,138] Additionally, the relatively novel nature of this scoring system has not allowed sufficient time for large enough studies to elucidate any correlations with SINS score and clinical outcomes.[135] Of the studies that have been conducted on the prognostic value of the scoring system, the vast majority of evidence has been rated as low to very low.[70,133] Furthermore, according to recent literature, the value of the SINs score as a prognostic tool may have been initially

TABLE 25
Spine Instability Neoplastic Score (SINS)

Location	Points
Junctional (O-C2; C7-T2; T11-L1; L5-S1)	3
Mobile spine (C3-6; L2-4)	2
Semirigid (T3-10)	1
Rigid (S2-S5)	0
Mechanical pain	
Yes	3
No	2
Pain free lesion	1
Bone lesion quality	
Lytic	2
Mixed	1
Blastic	0
Spine alignment	
Subluxation/translation present	4
Deformity (kyphosis/scoliosis)	2
Normal	0
Vertebral body collapse	
> 50% collapse	3
< 50% collapse	2
No collapse with > 50% body involved	1
None of the above	0
Involvement of posterior element	
Bilateral	3
Unilateral	1
None of the above	0

TABLE 26
White and Panjabi Classification

Element	Points
Anterior elements nonfunctioning or destroyed	2
Posterior elements nonfunctioning or destroyed	2
Radiograph	4
Flexion-extension	
Sagittal plane translation > 4.5 mm of 15%	2
Sagittal plane rotation (in degrees)	
15 at L1-L2, L2-L3 and L3-L4	2
20 at L4-5	2
25 at L5-S1	2
Resting	
Sagittal plane displacement > 4.5 mm of 15%	2
Relative sagittal plane angulation > 22 (degrees)	2
Cauda equina damage	3
Dangerous loading anticipated	1

Notwithstanding its long clinical utility, the White Panjabi system is not without its shortcomings. Lack of agreement and ambiguity of definitions are the most commonly cited downsides of the system. Additionally, heterogeneity in imaging techniques may alter the measurement portion of the system. Further determination of set definitions, such as what constitutes a "dangerous load," is necessary to fully exploit this scoring system's clinical potential.[142]

Bertolotti's syndrome
Bertolotti's syndrome was first described in 1917 by Mario Bertolotti.[143] Bertolotti's syndrome, also known as lumbosacral transitional vertebra, is an abnormal partial or total fusion of the transverse process at L5-S1.[144] While this anatomical variant is often diagnosed in young adults, there is evidence to indicate that its presence may be underdiagnosed and pain may arise later in life due to the heterogeneity of the disorder (Table 27).[144,145]

Despite the increasing evidence that Bertolotti's syndrome may be more prevalent in the population than initially anticipated, anywhere from 4.6% to 35.6%, the application of the Castellvi classification has been called into question, specifically for nontypical anatomy.[145-147] Additionally, Bertolotti's syndrome

overstated as the system does not take into account all of the factors that may affect spinal stability, thereby leaving out relevant information for decision information and outcome analysis.[70,133,139] Future studies are necessary to further examine the utility of the SINS score for lumbosacral instability in daily clinical practice.

White Panjabi. Proposed in the 1970s, the White and Panjabi method leverages a multifaceted system that combines radiographic findings and physical examination with the biomechanical stress anticipated for a patient, to determine spinal instability.[140,141] A score ≥ 5 indicated instability of the spine (Table 26).[142]

TABLE 27
Castellvi Classification
Type I: Enlarged and dysplastic transverse process (≥ 19 mm)
(a) Unilateral
(b) Bilateral
Type II: Pseudo-articulation of the transverse process and sacrum with incomplete sacralization or lumbarization; plus enlargement of transverse process with pseudarthrosis
(a) Unilateral
(b) Bilateral
Type III: Transverse process fuses with the sacrum, complete lumbarization or sacralization, enlarged transverse process with complete fusion
(a) Unilateral
(b) Bilateral
Type IV: Combination of type III on one side and type IIa on the contralateral side

does not necessarily correlate with symptoms of low back pain.[148,149] Multiple studies have postulated that while the Castellvi classification provides a simplistic approach to categorizing Bertolotti's syndrome in normal anatomy nothing substitutes an accurate description of anatomical variants. The clinical significance of Bertolotti's syndrome remains unknown despite its correlation with lower back pain as further investigation is necessary. Moreover, while numbering lumbosacral vertebrae may be beneficial for future surgery for other ailments, specifically concerning instrumentation placement, there is no current indication for surgical intervention.[149]

CONCLUSION

Given the abundance of lumbar spine injuries, constant attempts to generalize similar imaging findings have been iterated. An understanding of the genesis of these various classification schemes is invaluable as it not only directs future research but allows for elucidation into each of their significance clinically. Ideally, classification schemes should convey utility to their users simplistically and reliably. While there are many systems outlined here which have not yet been subjected to the scrutiny of their predecessors, it is important to reiterate that there are many that provide clear utility in clinical decision-making and research. The dynamic

nature of the classification system lends itself quite easily to the realization that many novel developments are on the horizon ahead.

REFERENCES

1. Hesselink JR. Spine imaging: history, achievements, remaining frontiers. *AJR Am J Roentgenol.* 1988;150:1223–1229.
2. Hoeffner EG, Mukherji SK, Srinivasan A, et al. Neuroradiology back to the future: spine imaging. *AJNR Am J Neuroradiol.* 2012;33:999–1006.
3. Diebo BG, Shah NV, Boachie-Adjei O, et al. Adult spinal deformity. *Lancet.* 2019;394:160–172.
4. Naresh-Babu J, Viswanadha AK, Ito M, et al. What should an ideal adult spinal deformity classification system consist of?: Review of the factors affecting outcomes of adult spinal deformity management. *Asian Spine J.* 2019;13:694–703.
5. Lowe T, Berven SH, Schwab FJ, et al. The SRS classification for adult spinal deformity: building on the King/Moe and Lenke classification systems. *Spine (Phila Pa 1976).* 2006;31:S119–S125.
6. Schwab F, Farcy JP, Bridwell K, et al. A clinical impact classification of scoliosis in the adult. *Spine (Phila Pa 1976).* 2006;31:2109–2114.
7. Kuntz IV C, Shaffrey CI, Ondra SL, et al. Spinal deformity: a new classification derived from neutral upright spinal alignment measurements in asymptomatic juvenile, adolescent, adult, and geriatric individuals. *Neurosurgery.* 2008;63:25–39.
8. Dagdia L, Kokabu T, Ito M. Classification of adult spinal deformity: review of current concepts and future directions. *Spine Surg Relat Res.* 2019;3:17–26.
9. Glassman SD, Bridwell K, Dimar JR, et al. The impact of positive sagittal balance in adult spinal deformity. *Spine (Phila Pa 1976).* 2005;30:2024–2029.
10. Schwab F, Lafage V, Farcy JP, et al. Surgical rates and operative outcome analysis in thoracolumbar and lumbar major adult scoliosis: application of the new adult deformity classification. *Spine (Phila Pa 1976).* 2007;32:2723–2730.
11. Schwab F, Ungar B, Blondel B, et al. Scoliosis Research Society-Schwab adult spinal deformity classification: a validation study. *Spine (Phila Pa 1976).* 2012;37:1077–1082.
12. Berjano P, Langella F, Ismael MF, et al. Successful correction of sagittal imbalance can be calculated on the basis of pelvic incidence and age. *Eur Spine J.* 2014;23(suppl 6):587–596.
13. Lafage R, Schwab F, Challier V, et al. Defining spino-pelvic alignment thresholds: should operative goals in adult spinal deformity surgery account for age? *Spine (Phila Pa 1976).* 2016;41:62–68.
14. Rothenfluh DA, Mueller DA, Rothenfluh E, et al. Pelvic incidence-lumbar lordosis mismatch predisposes to

adjacent segment disease after lumbar spinal fusion. *Eur Spine J.* 2015;24:1251–1258.

15. Hart RA, Badra MI, Madala A, et al. Use of pelvic incidence as a guide to reduction of H-type spino-pelvic dissociation injuries. *J Orthop Trauma.* 2007;21:369–374.

16. Takemoto M, Boissière L, Vital J-M, et al. Are sagittal spinopelvic radiographic parameters significantly associated with quality of life of adult spinal deformity patients? Multivariate linear regression analyses for pre-operative and short-term post-operative health-related quality of life. *Eur Spine J.* 2017;26:2176–2186.

17. Bess S, Line B, Fu K-M, et al. The health impact of symptomatic adult spinal deformity: comparison of deformity types to united states population norms and chronic diseases. *Spine (Phila Pa 1976).* 2016;41:224–233.

18. Presciutti SM, Louie PK, Khan JM, et al. Sagittal spinopelvic malalignment in degenerative scoliosis patients: isolated correction of symptomatic levels and clinical decision-making. *Scoliosis Spinal Disord.* 2018;13:28.

19. Zhang H-C, Zhang Z-F, Wang Z-H, et al. Optimal pelvic incidence minus lumbar lordosis mismatch after long posterior instrumentation and fusion for adult degenerative scoliosis. *Orthop Surg.* 2017;9:304–310.

20. Merrill RK, Kim JS, Leven DM, et al. Beyond pelvic incidence–lumbar lordosis mismatch: the importance of assessing the entire spine to achieve global sagittal alignment. *Global Spine J.* 2017;7:536–542.

21. Lafage R, Schwab F, Glassman S, et al. Age-adjusted alignment goals have the potential to reduce PJK. *Spine (Phila Pa 1976).* 2017;42:1275–1282.

22. Perolat R, Kastler A, Nicot B, et al. Facet joint syndrome: from diagnosis to interventional management. *Insights Imaging.* 2018;9:773–789.

23. Manchikanti L, Kaye AD, Boswell MV, et al. A systematic review and best evidence synthesis of effectiveness of therapeutic facet joint interventions in managing chronic spinal pain. *Pain Physician.* 2015;48.

24. Little JW, Grieve TJ, Cramer GD, et al. Grading osteoarthritic changes of the zygapophyseal joints from radiographs: a reliability study. *J Manipulative Physiol Ther.* 2015;38:344–351.

25. Kettler A, Wilke HJ. Review of existing grading systems for cervical or lumbar disc and facet joint degeneration. *Eur Spine J.* 2006;15:705–718.

26. Kellgren JH, Lawrence JS. Radiological assessment of osteo-arthrosis. *Ann Rheum Dis.* 1957;16:494–502.

27. Gellhorn AC, Katz JN, Suri P. Osteoarthritis of the spine: the facet joints. *Nat Rev Rheumatol.* 2013;9:216–224.

28. Binder DS, Nampiaparampil DE. The provocative lumbar facet joint. *Curr Rev Musculoskelet Med.* 2009;2:15–24.

29. Zhou X, Liu Y, Zhou S, et al. The correlation between radiographic and pathologic grading of lumbar facet joint degeneration. *BMC Med Imaging.* 2016;16:27.

30. Albert HB, Kjaer P, Jensen TS, et al. Modic changes, possible causes and relation to low back pain. *Med Hypotheses.* 2008;70:361–368.

31. Modic MT, Ross JS, Masaryk TJ. Imaging of degenerative disease of the cervical spine. *Clin Orthop Relat Res.* 1989;109–120.

32. Rahme R, Moussa R. The Modic vertebral endplate and marrow changes: pathologic significance and relation to low back pain and segmental instability of the lumbar spine. *AJNR Am J Neuroradiol.* 2008;29:838–842.

33. Roudsari B, Jarvik JG. Lumbar spine MRI for low back pain: indications and yield. *AJR Am J Roentgenol.* 2010;195:550–559.

34. Teichtahl AJ, Urquhart DM, Wang Y, et al. Modic changes in the lumbar spine and their association with body composition, fat distribution and intervertebral disc height - a 3.0 T-MRI study. *BMC Musculoskelet Disord.* 2016;17:92.

35. Järvinen J, Karppinen J, Niinimäki J, et al. Association between changes in lumbar Modic changes and low back symptoms over a two-year period. *BMC Musculoskelet Disord.* 2015;16:98.

36. Mitra D, Cassar-Pullicino VN, McCall IW. Longitudinal study of vertebral type-1 end-plate changes on MR of the lumbar spine. *Eur Radiol.* 2004;14:1574–1581.

37. Chen Y, Yang H, Zhang L, et al. Analyzing the influence of Modic changes on patients with lower back pain undergoing conservative treatment. *Pain Res Manag.* 2019;2019:8185316.

38. Riesenburger RI, Safain MG, Ogbuji R, et al. A novel classification system of lumbar disc degeneration. *J Clin Neurosci.* 2015;22:346–351.

39. Rim DC. Quantitative Pfirrmann disc degeneration grading system to overcome the limitation of Pfirrmann disc degeneration grade. *Korean J Spine.* 2016;13:1–8.

40. Sher I, Daly C, Oehme D, et al. Novel application of the Pfirrmann disc degeneration grading system to 9.4T MRI: higher reliability compared to 3T MRI. *Spine (Phila Pa 1976).* 2019;44:E766–E773.

41. Ract I, Meadeb JM, Mercy G, et al. A review of the value of MRI signs in low back pain. *Diagn Interv Imaging.* 2015;96:239–249.

42. Schmorl G. Die gesunde und kranke Wirbelsaule im Rontgenbild. In: *Pathologisch-anatomische Untersuchungen;* 1952.

43. Mok FP, Samartzis D, Karppinen J, et al. ISSLS prize winner: prevalence, determinants, and association of Schmorl nodes of the lumbar spine with disc degeneration: a population-based study of 2449 individuals. *Spine (Phila Pa 1976).* 2010;35:1944–1952.

44. Kyere KA, Than KD, Wang AC, et al. Schmorl's nodes. *Eur Spine J.* 2012;21:2115–2121.

45. Samartzis D, Mok FPS, Karppinen J, et al. Classification of Schmorl's nodes of the lumbar spine and association with disc degeneration: a large-scale population-based MRI study. *Osteoarthr Cartil.* 2016;24:1753–1760.

46. Rustenburg CME, Faraj SSA, Ket JCF, et al. Prognostic factors in the progression of intervertebral disc degeneration: Which patient should be targeted with regenerative therapies? *JOR Spine.* 2019;2, e1063.

47. Kushchayev SV, Glushko T, Jarraya M, et al. ABCs of the degenerative spine. *Insights Imaging*. 2018;9:253–274.
48. Tenny S, Gillis CC. Annular disc tear. In: *StatPearls*; 2020.
49. Raj PP. Intervertebral disc: anatomy-physiology-pathophysiology-treatment. *Pain Pract*. 2008;8:18–44.
50. Teraguchi M, Samartzis D, Hashizume H, et al. Classification of high intensity zones of the lumbar spine and their association with other spinal MRI phenotypes: the Wakayama Spine Study. *PLoS One*. 2016;11, e0160111.
51. Schellhas KP, Pollei SR, Gundry CR, et al. Lumbar disc high-intensity zone. Correlation of magnetic resonance imaging and discography. *Spine (Phila Pa 1976)*. 1996;21:79–86.
52. Peng B, Hou S, Wu W, et al. The pathogenesis and clinical significance of a high-intensity zone (HIZ) of lumbar intervertebral disc on MR imaging in the patient with discogenic low back pain. *Eur Spine J*. 2006;15:583–587.
53. Suthar P, Patel R, Mehta C, et al. MRI evaluation of lumbar disc degenerative disease. *J Clin Diagn Res*. 2015;9:Tc04–Tc09.
54. Fardon DF. Nomenclature and classification of lumbar disc pathology. *Spine (Phila Pa 1976)*. 2001;26:461–462.
55. Fardon DF, Williams AL, Dohring EJ, et al. Lumbar disc nomenclature: version 2.0: recommendations of the combined task forces of the North American Spine Society, the American Society of Spine Radiology, and the American Society of Neuroradiology. *Spine (Phila Pa 1976)*. 2014;39:E1448–E1465.
56. Pfirrmann CW, Metzdorf A, Zanetti M, et al. Magnetic resonance classification of lumbar intervertebral disc degeneration. *Spine (Phila Pa 1976)*. 2001;26:1873–1878.
57. Griffith JF, Wang YX, Antonio GE, et al. Modified Pfirrmann grading system for lumbar intervertebral disc degeneration. *Spine (Phila Pa 1976)*. 2007;32:E708–E712.
58. Hebelka H, Lagerstrand K, Brisby H, et al. The importance of level stratification for quantitative MR studies of lumbar intervertebral discs: a cross-sectional analysis in 101 healthy adults. *Eur Spine J*. 2019;28:2153–2161.
59. Urrutia J, Besa P, Campos M, et al. The Pfirrmann classification of lumbar intervertebral disc degeneration: an independent inter- and intra-observer agreement assessment. *Eur Spine J*. 2016;25:2728–2733.
60. Schleich C, Muller-Lutz A, Zimmermann L, et al. Biochemical imaging of cervical intervertebral discs with glycosaminoglycan chemical exchange saturation transfer magnetic resonance imaging: feasibility and initial results. *Skelet Radiol*. 2016;45:79–85.
61. Togao O, Hiwatashi A, Wada T, et al. A qualitative and quantitative correlation study of lumbar intervertebral disc degeneration using glycosaminoglycan chemical exchange saturation transfer, Pfirrmann grade, and T1-rho. *AJNR Am J Neuroradiol*. 2018;39:1369–1375.
62. Thompson JP, Pearce RH, Schechter MT, et al. Preliminary evaluation of a scheme for grading the gross morphology of the human intervertebral disc. *Spine (Phila Pa 1976)*. 1990;15:411–415.
63. Benzakour T, Igoumenou V, Mavrogenis AF, et al. Current concepts for lumbar disc herniation. *Int Orthop*. 2019;43:841–851.
64. Kreiner DS, Hwang SW, Easa JE, et al. An evidence-based clinical guideline for the diagnosis and treatment of lumbar disc herniation with radiculopathy. *Spine J*. 2014;14:180–191.
65. Jensen MC, Brant-Zawadzki MN, Obuchowski N, et al. Magnetic resonance imaging of the lumbar spine in people without back pain. *N Engl J Med*. 1994;331:69–73.
66. Lurie JD, Tosteson AN, Tosteson TD, et al. Reliability of magnetic resonance imaging readings for lumbar disc herniation in the Spine Patient Outcomes Research Trial (SPORT). *Spine (Phila Pa 1976)*. 2008;33:991–998.
67. Li XK, Wu ZG, Ding T, et al. Revisiting the nomenclature and grading schemes for disc degeneration: issues to be solved. *Spine J*. 2015;15:2594–2595.
68. Mysliwiec LW, Cholewicki J, Winkelpleck MD, et al. MSU classification for herniated lumbar discs on MRI: toward developing objective criteria for surgical selection. *Eur Spine J*. 2010;19:1087–1093.
69. Hao DJ, Duan K, Liu TJ, et al. Development and clinical application of grading and classification criteria of lumbar disc herniation. *Medicine (Baltimore)*. 2017;96, e8676.
70. Versteeg AL, van der Velden JM, Verkooijen HM, et al. The effect of introducing the Spinal Instability Neoplastic Score in routine clinical practice for patients with spinal metastases. *Oncologist*. 2016;21:95–101.
71. Aebi M. Classification of thoracolumbar fractures and dislocations. *Eur Spine J*. 2010;19(suppl 1):S2–S7.
72. Ghobrial GM, Jallo J. Thoracolumbar spine trauma: review of the evidence. *J Neurosurg Sci*. 2013;57:115–122.
73. Azam MQ, Sadat-Ali M. The concept of evolution of thoracolumbar fracture classifications helps in surgical decisions. *Asian Spine J*. 2015;9:984–994.
74. Böhler L. *Die Technik der Knochenbruchbehandlung im Frieden und im Kriege*; 1943.
75. Watson-Jones R. The results of postural reduction of fractures of the spine. *J Bone Joint Surg Am*. 1938;20:567–586.
76. Nicoll EA. Fractures of the dorso-lumbar spine. *J Bone Joint Surg Br*. 1949;31:376–394.
77. Kelly RP, Whitesides Jr TE. Treatment of lumbodorsal fracture-dislocations. *Ann Surg*. 1968;167:705–717.
78. McAfee PC, Yuan HA, Fredrickson BE, et al. The value of computed tomography in thoracolumbar fractures. An analysis of one hundred consecutive cases and a new classification. *J Bone Joint Surg Ser A*. 1983;65:461–473.
79. Ferguson RL, Allen Jr BL. A mechanistic classification of thoracolumbar spine fractures. *Clin Orthop Relat Res*. 1984;189:77–88.
80. McCormack T, Karaikovic E, Gaines RW. The load sharing classification of spine fractures. *Spine*. 1994;19:1741–1744.
81. Roy-Camille R, Saillant G, Gagna G, et al. Transverse fracture of the upper sacrum. Suicidal jumper's fracture. *Spine (Phila Pa 1976)*. 1985;10:838–845.

82. Denis F. The three column spine and its significance in the classification of acute thoracolumbar spinal injuries. *Spine*. 1983;8:817–831.

83. Magerl F, Aebi M, Gertzbein SD, et al. A comprehensive classification of thoracic and lumbar injuries. *Eur Spine J*. 1994;3:184–201.

84. Lee JY, Vaccaro AR, Lim MR, et al. Thoracolumbar injury classification and severity score: a new paradigm for the treatment of thoracolumbar spine trauma. *J Orthop Sci*. 2005;10:671–675.

85. Sethi MK, Schoenfeld AJ, Bono CM, et al. The evolution of thoracolumbar injury classification systems. *Spine J*. 2009;9:780–788.

86. Sethi RK, Yanamadala V, Shah SA, et al. Improving complex pediatric and adult spine care while embracing the value equation. *Spine Deform*. 2019;7:228–235.

87. Divi SN, Schroeder GD, Oner FC, et al. AOSpine-Spine Trauma Classification system: the value of modifiers: a narrative review with commentary on evolving descriptive principles. *Global Spine J*. 2019;9:77s–88s.

88. Reinhold M, Audigé L, Schnake KJ, et al. AO spine injury classification system: a revision proposal for the thoracic and lumbar spine. *Eur Spine J*. 2013;22:2184–2201.

89. Vaccaro AR, Oner C, Kepler CK, et al. AOSpine thoracolumbar spine injury classification system: fracture description, neurological status, and key modifiers. *Spine (Phila Pa 1976)*. 2013;38:2028–2037.

90. Schroeder GD, Kurd MF, Kepler CK, et al. The development of a universally accepted sacral fracture classification: a survey of AOSpine and AOTrauma members. *Global Spine J*. 2016;6:686–694.

91. Isler B, Ganz R. Classification of pelvic girdle injuries. *Unfallchirurg*. 1990;93:289–302.

92. Isler B, Ganz R. Classification of pelvic ring injuries. *Injury*. 1996;27(suppl 1):3–12.

93. Mo AZ, Miller PE, Glotzbecker MP, et al. The reliability of the AOSpine Thoracolumbar Classification System in children: results of a multicenter study. *J Pediatr Orthop*. 2020. https://doi.org/10.1097/bpo.0000000000001521. Epub ahead of print.

94. Gibbs WN, Doshi A. Sacral fractures and sacroplasty. *Neuroimaging Clin N Am*. 2019;29:515–527.

95. Niggemann P, Kuchta J, Grosskurth D, et al. Spondylolysis and isthmic spondylolisthesis: impact of vertebral hypoplasia on the use of the Meyerding classification. *Br J Radiol*. 2012;85:358–362.

96. Matz PG, Meagher RJ, Lamer T, et al. Guideline summary review: an evidence-based clinical guideline for the diagnosis and treatment of degenerative lumbar spondylolisthesis. *Spine J*. 2016;16:439–448.

97. Evans N, McCarthy M. Management of symptomatic degenerative low-grade lumbar spondylolisthesis. *EFORT Open Rev*. 2018;3:620–631.

98. Wiltse LL, Newman PH, Macnab I. Classification of spondylolisis and spondylolisthesis. *Clin Orthop Relat Res*. 1976;23–29.

99. Kepler CK, Hilibrand AS, Sayadipour A, et al. Clinical and radiographic degenerative spondylolisthesis (CARDS) classification. *Spine J*. 2015;15:1804–1811.

100. DeWald CJ, Vartabedian JE, Rodts MF, et al. Evaluation and management of high-grade spondylolisthesis in adults. *Spine (Phila Pa 1976)*. 2005;30:S49–S59.

101. Mac-Thiong JM, Duong L, Parent S, et al. Reliability of the Spinal Deformity Study Group classification of lumbosacral spondylolisthesis. *Spine (Phila Pa 1976)*. 2012;37:E95–102.

102. Labelle H, Mac-Thiong JM, Roussouly P. Spino-pelvic sagittal balance of spondylolisthesis: a review and classification. *Eur Spine J*. 2011;20(suppl 5):641–646.

103. Kong C, Sun X, Ding J, et al. Comparison of the French and CARDS classifications for lumbar degenerative spondylolisthesis: reliability and validity. *BMC Musculoskelet Disord*. 2019;20:382.

104. Gille O, Bouloussa H, Mazas S, et al. A new classification system for degenerative spondylolisthesis of the lumbar spine. *Eur Spine J*. 2017;26:3096–3105.

105. Herman MJ, Pizzutillo PD. Spondylolysis and spondylolisthesis in the child and adolescent: a new classification. *Clin Orthop Relat Res*. 2005;46–54.

106. Arima H, Suzuki Y, Togawa D, et al. Low-intensity pulsed ultrasound is effective for progressive-stage lumbar spondylolysis with MRI high-signal change. *Eur Spine J*. 2017;26:3122–3128.

107. Dhouib A, Tabard-Fougere A, Hanquinet S, et al. Diagnostic accuracy of MR imaging for direct visualization of lumbar pars defect in children and young adults: a systematic review and meta-analysis. *Eur Spine J*. 2018;27:1058–1066.

108. Olivieri I, D'Angelo S, Palazzi C, et al. Diffuse idiopathic skeletal hyperostosis: differentiation from ankylosing spondylitis. *Curr Rheumatol Rep*. 2009;11:321–328.

109. Mader R, Sarzi-Puttini P, Atzeni F, et al. Extraspinal manifestations of diffuse idiopathic skeletal hyperostosis. *Rheumatology (Oxford)*. 2009;48:1478–1481.

110. Mader R, Baraliakos X, Eshed I, et al. Imaging of diffuse idiopathic skeletal hyperostosis (DISH). *RMD Open*. 2020;6. https://doi.org/10.1136/rmdopen-2019-001151. Epub ahead of print.

111. Otsuki B, Fujibayashi S, Takemoto M, et al. Diffuse idiopathic skeletal hyperostosis (DISH) is a risk factor for further surgery in short-segment lumbar interbody fusion. *Eur Spine J*. 2015;24:2514–2519.

112. Otsuki B, Fujibayashi S, Tanida S, et al. Outcomes of lumbar decompression surgery in patients with diffuse idiopathic skeletal hyperostosis (DISH). *J Orthop Sci*. 2019;24:957–962.

113. Mader R, Buskila D, Verlaan JJ, et al. Developing new classification criteria for diffuse idiopathic skeletal hyperostosis: back to square one. *Rheumatology (Oxford)*. 2013;52:326–330.

114. Mader R, Verlaan JJ, Buskila D. Diffuse idiopathic skeletal hyperostosis: clinical features and pathogenic mechanisms. *Nat Rev Rheumatol*. 2013;9:741–750.

115. Resnick D, Niwayama G. Radiographic and pathologic features of spinal involvement in diffuse idiopathic skeletal hyperostosis (DISH). *Radiology*. 1976;119:559–568.

116. Utsinger PD. Diffuse idiopathic skeletal hyperostosis. *Clin Rheum Dis*. 1985;11:325–351.

117. Kuperus JS, de Gendt EEA, Oner FC, et al. Classification criteria for diffuse idiopathic skeletal hyperostosis: a lack of consensus. *Rheumatology (Oxford)*. 2017;56:1123–1134.

118. Mata S, Chhem RK, Fortin PR, et al. Comprehensive radiographic evaluation of diffuse idiopathic skeletal hyperostosis: development and interrater reliability of a scoring system. *Semin Arthritis Rheum*. 1998;28:88–96.

119. Yaniv G, Bader S, Lidar M, et al. The natural course of bridging osteophyte formation in diffuse idiopathic skeletal hyperostosis: retrospective analysis of consecutive CT examinations over 10 years. *Rheumatology (Oxford)*. 2014;53:1951–1957.

120. Leibushor N, Slonimsky E, Aharoni D, et al. CT abnormalities in the sacroiliac joints of patients with diffuse idiopathic skeletal hyperostosis. *AJR Am J Roentgenol*. 2017;208:834–837.

121. Oudkerk SF, de Jong PA, Attrach M, et al. Diagnosis of diffuse idiopathic skeletal hyperostosis with chest computed tomography: inter-observer agreement. *Eur Radiol*. 2017;27:188–194.

122. Fourney DR, Frangou EM, Ryken TC, et al. Spinal instability neoplastic score: an analysis of reliability and validity from the spine oncology study group. *J Clin Oncol*. 2011;29:3072–3077.

123. Hayes MA, Howard TC, Gruel CR, et al. Roentgenographic evaluation of lumbar spine flexion-extension in asymptomatic individuals. *Spine (Phila Pa 1976)*. 1989;14:327–331.

124. White III AA, Panjabi MM. The basic kinematics of the human spine. A review of past and current knowledge. *Spine (Phila Pa 1976)*. 1978;3:12–20.

125. Kanayama M, Abumi K, Kaneda K, et al. Phase lag of the intersegmental motion in flexion-extension of the lumbar and lumbosacral spine. An in vivo study. *Spine (Phila Pa 1976)*. 1996;21:1416–1422.

126. McGill SM, Kippers V. Transfer of loads between lumbar tissues during the flexion-relaxation phenomenon. *Spine (Phila Pa 1976)*. 1994;19:2190–2196.

127. Teyhen DS, Flynn TW, Bovik AC, et al. A new technique for digital fluoroscopic video assessment of sagittal plane lumbar spine motion. *Spine (Phila Pa 1976)*. 2005;30:E406–E413.

128. Sanchez-Zuriaga D, Lopez-Pascual J, Garrido-Jaen D, et al. A comparison of lumbopelvic motion patterns and erector spinae behavior between asymptomatic subjects and patients with recurrent low back pain during pain-free periods. *J Manipulative Physiol Ther*. 2015;38:130–137.

129. Fisher CG, Schouten R, Versteeg AL, et al. Reliability of the Spinal Instability Neoplastic Score (SINS) among radiation oncologists: an assessment of instability secondary to spinal metastases. *Radiat Oncol*. 2014;9:69.

130. Filis AK, Aghayev KV, Doulgeris JJ, et al. Spinal neoplastic instability: biomechanics and current management options. *Cancer Control*. 2014;21:144–150.

131. Arana E, Kovacs FM, Royuela A, et al. Spine Instability Neoplastic Score: agreement across different medical and surgical specialties. *Spine J*. 2016;16:591–599.

132. Campos M, Urrutia J, Zamora T, et al. The Spine Instability Neoplastic Score: an independent reliability and reproducibility analysis. *Spine J*. 2014;14:1466–1469.

133. Versteeg AL, Verlaan JJ, Sahgal A, et al. The Spinal Instability Neoplastic Score: impact on oncologic decision-making. *Spine (Phila Pa 1976)*. 2016;41(suppl 20):S231–S237.

134. Fox S, Spiess M, Hnenny L, et al. Spinal Instability Neoplastic Score (SINS): reliability among spine fellows and resident physicians in orthopedic surgery and neurosurgery. *Global Spine J*. 2017;7:744–748.

135. Dosani M, Lucas S, Wong J, et al. Impact of the Spinal Instability Neoplastic Score on surgical referral patterns and outcomes. *Curr Oncol*. 2018;25:53–58.

136. Dakson A, Leck E, Brandman DM, et al. The clinical utility of the Spinal Instability Neoplastic Score (SINS) system in spinal epidural metastases: a retrospective study. *Spinal Cord*. 2020. https://doi.org/10.1038/s41393-020-0432-8. Epub ahead of print.

137. Lam TC, Uno H, Krishnan M, et al. Adverse outcomes after palliative radiation therapy for uncomplicated spine metastases: role of spinal instability and single-fraction radiation therapy. *Int J Radiat Oncol Biol Phys*. 2015;93:373–381.

138. Shi DD, Hertan LM, Lam TC, et al. Assessing the utility of the Spinal Instability Neoplastic Score (SINS) to predict fracture after conventional radiation therapy (RT) for spinal metastases. *Pract Radiat Oncol*. 2018;8:e285–e294.

139. Xu C, Yin M, Sun Z, et al. An independent inter-observer reliability and intra-observer reproducibility evaluation of SINS scoring and Kostuik classification systems for spinal tumor. *World Neurosurg*. 2020. https://doi.org/10.1016/j.wneu.2020.02.038. Epub ahead of print.

140. Panjabi MM, White III AA. Basic biomechanics of the spine. *Neurosurgery*. 1980;7:76–93.

141. White A, Panjabi MM. *Clinical Biomechanics of the Spine*. Philadelphia, PA: Lippincott; 1990.

142. Kim CW, Perry A, Garfin SR. Spinal instability: the orthopedic approach. *Semin Musculoskelet Radiol*. 2005;9:77–87.

143. Bertolotti M. Contributo alla conoscenze dei vizi di differenzazione regionale del racide con speciale riguardo alla assimilazione sacrale della V. lombare. *Radiol Med*. 1917;4:113–144.

144. Jancuska JM, Spivak JM, Bendo JA. A review of symptomatic lumbosacral transitional vertebrae: Bertolotti's syndrome. *Int J Spine Surg*. 2015;9:42.

145. Alonzo F, Cobar A, Cahueque M, et al. Bertolotti's syndrome: an underdiagnosed cause for lower back pain. *J Surg Case Rep*. 2018;2018, rjy276.

146. Castellvi AE, Goldstein LA, Chan DP. Lumbosacral transitional vertebrae and their relationship with lumbar extradural defects. *Spine (Phila Pa 1976)*. 1984;9:493–495.

147. Bron JL, van Royen BJ, Wuisman PI. The clinical significance of lumbosacral transitional anomalies. *Acta Orthop Belg*. 2007;73:687–695.

148. Konin GP, Walz DM. Lumbosacral transitional vertebrae: classification, imaging findings, and clinical relevance. *AJNR Am J Neuroradiol*. 2010;31:1778–1786.

149. Matson DM, Maccormick LM, Sembrano JN, et al. Sacral dysmorphism and lumbosacral transitional vertebrae (LSTV) review. *Int J Spine Surg*. 2020;14:14–19.

150. Gille O, Challier V, Parent H, et al, The French Society of Spine Surgery (SFCR). Degenerative lumbar spondylolisthesis. Cohort of 670 patients, and proposal of a new classification. *Orthop Traumatol Surg Res*. 2014;100(6):S311–S315. https://doi.org/10.1016/j.otsr.2014.07.006.

CHAPTER 17

Future Trends in Spinal Imaging

ZAKARIAH K. SIYAJI[a] • FAYYAZUL HASSAN[a] • GARRETT K. HARADA[a] • MORGAN B. GIERS[b] • HOWARD S. AN[a] • DINO SAMARTZIS[a] • PHILIP K. LOUIE[c]
[a]Department of Orthopaedic Surgery, Rush University Medical Center, Chicago, IL, United States, [b]School of Chemical, Biological and Environmental Engineering, Oregon State University, Corvallis, OR, United States, [c]Department of Neurosurgery, Virginia Mason Medical Center, Seattle, WA, United states

INTRODUCTION

Imaging methods of the spine have greatly expanded since the advent of X-rays for the use of plain radiographs (c.1895), providing anatomical clarity for diagnosis and treatment of the cervical, thoracic, lumbar, and sacral vertebrae. The complex anatomy of the vertebrae and irregular contours and geometry of the spinal elements have influenced the rapid development of more precise imaging modalities. Various advancements to two- and three-dimensional (i.e., 2D, 3D, respectively) imaging through plain radiographs, computed tomography (CT), magnetic resonance imaging (MRI), ultrasound, and EOS imaging along with multiple dimensional views of the spine are continuously optimized. Future developments in imaging may improve the assessment of pedicle screw placement and image definition, reduce radiation, provide quantitative information about disc and other soft tissue composition, and provide autonomous spinal mapping using artificial intelligence (AI).

FUTURE OF PLAIN RADIOGRAPHS

Plain radiographs utilize a heterogeneous emission of X-rays projected in the direction of a detector, ultimately curating an image established through components of the intervening objects, including composition as well as density. Plain radiographs may see improvements by providing image intensification, digital detectors, and radiosensitive screen amplifications. Although plain radiographs demonstrate a substantial degree of reliability, computed tomography (CT) has become the primary choice in imaging spinal injuries while obtaining similar measurements to plain radiographs.[1] Many may transpose their diagnostic care toward CT imaging over plain radiographs. Computed tomography utilizes a computerized X-ray imaging method in which a beam of X-rays is directed at the patient and rapidly circumvolved around the patient to develop cross-sectional images of the patient's body. Plain radiographs are increasingly replaced by contemporary imaging methods, including, but not limited to, intraoperative CT (ICT), 3D imaging, and the newfound application of AI and augmented reality (AR). Several reasons exist for the gradual phasing out of plain radiographs. Foremost are the limitations on types of features visible in the image. Such limitations are evident when soft tissue, high image resolution, and 3D characteristics are desired. For example, identification of bone loss on plain radiographs is typically not appreciable until over 30%–40% loss has occurred.[2] Furthermore, these limitations persist when detecting pedicle screws with a "safe" misguided freehand placement. Instead, CT technology boasts a higher accuracy and, therefore, a better-suited imaging technique for the confirmation of suspected incorrect screw positioning.[3] Plain radiographs have also proven inadequate in terms of cervical spine assessment following blunt trauma due to poor visibility of the entire cervical spine. An accompanying CT scan is often required to assay the cervical spine accurately, eliminating the need for a plain radiograph.[4] These circumstances have indicated the urgency to adopt alternative and more modern methods in spinal imaging.

FUTURE OF COMPUTED TOMOGRAPHY

The use of CT imaging in the United States has significantly increased in the past two decades, although its growth has slowed in recent years.[5,6] Additionally, pediatric CT usage has seen a significant decrease due to concerns for excessive radiation exposure.[6] The increase in adult CT usage has brought about concerns about the health risks associated with radiation exposure.[5,6] Regardless, CT remains an often-used tool for adult patients to obtain detailed images of the spine and, in some cases, even offers reduced radiation doses compared to some standard techniques.

Fluoroscopy and CT are standard techniques for surgical navigation.[7] Computed tomography has been shown to expose physicians to less radiation than fluoroscopy; however, radiation exposure for patients was higher.[7] Intraoperative CT systems have improved accuracy and success in spine surgery.[7-12] Comparative studies with fluoroscopic-based techniques have repeatedly found intraoperative CT imaging to have superior accuracy and less radiation exposure for the surgeon.[7-11] Additionally, modifications to amperage, scan, and scout length radiation exposure for patients can also be reduced compared to standard CT imaging.[11] However, a novel technique using a detachable pedicle marker and probe combined with pulsed fluoroscopy has been shown to considerably reduce radiation exposure for both patients and physicians while maintaining comparable accuracy to standard fluoroscopy and intraoperative CT imaging.[3]

Co-registration or image fusion of CT images with preoperative MRI can enhance navigation for spinal procedures.[13] A problem with attempting to fuse MRI with CT arises from patient positioning changing between the different imaging procedures.[13] The study by Hille et al.[14] utilized a multisegmented approach for image registration to account for this issue. The fusion of MRI with CT using this multisegmented approach may provide the greatest benefit to spinal metastases being targeted by radiofrequency ablations. The multisegmented approach takes significantly less time for registration compared to the landmark-based directive (an average of 24 s per vertebra vs an average of 8 min per vertebra), illustrating that this technique can be integrated practically into the clinical workflow.[14]

A case study of two patients analyzed the usage of co-registered intraoperative CT and MRI for the resection of intradural spinal tumors.[13] For one of the patients, additional preoperative diffusion tensor imaging (DTI) was also co-registered with the other imaging modalities. In each case, the co-registration of intraoperative CT with MRI and DTI enhanced navigation during tumor removal. The study reported that the addition of DTI with intraoperative CT helped with the localization of the tumor and allowed for about 90% removal, which would have been unlikely without the co-registration of DTI.[13]

Machine learning applications for spinal imaging are continually evolving. A team of medical researchers at Pusan National University Hospital in Busan, Korea, developed a machine learning model to predict osteoporosis from Hounsfield units of lumbar CT images.[15] Machine learning models for the identification and classification of vertebral fractures from CT images have also been developed.[16,17] Deep learning has also been utilized for the automatic segmentation of lumbosacral nerves from CT images to aid in the 3D reconstruction of targeted areas for the viability assessment of transforaminal steroid injection.[17] Compared to manual segmentation, the deep learning model saves considerable time.[17] There are additional models being developed. Machine learning for spinal imaging will be an area of rapid growth in the upcoming years.

FUTURE OF MAGNETIC RESONANCE IMAGING

Magnetic resonance imaging provides high-resolution multiplanar images of vertebral and soft tissue anatomy without posing any risks associated with radiation exposure, proving to be the diagnostic procedure of choice for most spinal pathologies. This imaging modality offers relatively high sensitivity and specificity for the assessment of infections, tumors, disc degeneration, pathologic fractures, and disc herniations. However, MRI is relatively expensive and has a variable degree of utility in obese, claustrophobic, and pacemaker-dependent patients.

Sodium, T1-rho, UTE, and gagCEST MRI

Standard proton MRI lacks the ability to provide direct markers for tissue viability.[18] Sodium MRI takes advantage of sodium-potassium pumps and other biochemical mechanisms maintaining transmembrane sodium gradients by quantifying intracellular and extracellular sodium levels to better identify tissue viability.[18] However, the detection of sodium signals is challenging and requires high field strengths to obtain images of the same resolution as standard MRI.[18] Due to the many constraints, sodium MRI is considered clinically infeasible for routine use.[18] However, many methodological advances are beginning to bring sodium MRI to a level where it can be used in practical clinical settings.[18]

To address the limited signal intensities in cortical bone, ultrashort echo time (UTE) sequences were developed to elicit hyperintense signals of cartilage (e.g., the cartilaginous endplate) and osseous structures.[19] Other methodologies have also used echo time with varying degrees of success. These include short tau inversion recovery protocols, allowing the suppression of adipose tissue.[20]

Magnetic resonance imaging techniques are continuously being developed, involving additional applications that manipulate magnetic field directionality. For example, T1-rho MRI is a technique developed for use in cartilage imaging and takes advantage of directionality manipulation, but has been utilized readily to detect proteoglycan content of the disc to facilitate early identification of degenerative disc changes.[21] With a similar line of thinking in assessing early-stage disc degeneration, Kim et al.[22] aimed to assess the feasibility of quantifying glycosaminoglycan chemical exchange saturation transfer (gagCEST) values in human intervertebral discs using a 3T MRI scanner.[22] The study proved that in in vivo gagCEST, quantification in human lumbar intervertebral discs is feasible at 3T in combination with successful B_0 inhomogeneity correction without significant hardware modifications.[22] However, the clinical applications, in particular in the context of spine surgery, of gagCEST, along with T1-rho MRI are constantly being evaluated and validation on a large scale is needed.

The proliferation of MRI innovations has proven instrumental in the field of spine surgery, allowing increased diagnostic yields for various pathologies. Several studies have demonstrated that quantitative MRI can differentiate between signals in herniated discs and annular tears when compared with discs lacking gross abnormalities.[23-25] Similarly, Li et al.[26] demonstrated the potential of sodium MRI in identifying the structure of the knee and its association with cartilage degeneration. Such techniques may be applied to the intervertebral discs and their association with low back pain. More recently, evidence surrounding other sequences has gained additional clinical utility.[26] For example, UTE MRI has led to the description by Pang et al.[27] of the "UTE Disc Sign," a finding represented by a hyperintense or hypointense band across a degenerative disc associated with chronic low back pain and disability.[27] These findings not only highlight the utility of these added sequences but also suggest MRI's potential to contribute to refined phenotyping of patients, identifying the pain generating source and potentially predicting outcomes after spine surgery.

Synthetic MRI

Synthetic magnetic resonance imaging (MRI) provides an alternative advantage by producing multiple synthetic contrasts from a single sequence. This technique

has been mainly used for brain diseases; however, a recent study evaluated its feasibility in spinal imaging. According to Vargas et al.,[28] synthetic images of acceptable quality were acquired in 53% less time than those of conventional MRI.[28] Essentially, this decrease in diagnostic time is crucial in retrieving quantitative measurements of the spine much more quickly than current methods. Historically, the spinal cord has presented challenges for MR imaging due to the various differentiated tissue types characterizing spinal fluid, bone, and air. This renders conventional MRI techniques occasionally unable to differentiate between the spinal cord and other tissues accurately. To address this issue, a study by Tsagkas et al.[29] utilized an averaged magnetization inversion recovery acquisitions (AMIRA) sequence to segment the spinal cord from gray matter and white matter. The group found the AMIRA sequence to be a more time-efficient, accurate, and reproducible MR imaging approach within the spinal cord.[29] In a separate article,[30] the group focused on the automatic detection of lumbar vertebrae in MRI imaging. A novel detection algorithm based on deep learning was utilized to produce an accuracy of 98.6% and a precision of 98.9% in detecting vertebras. These results indicated that a lumbar detection network supported by deep learning can be trained to detect its target without annotated MRI images successfully. This can help increase the degree of clinical efficiency when evaluating spinal MRIs.

FUTURE OF EOS BIPLANAR X-RAY

The EOS imaging system operates by performing two simultaneous X-rays of the patient from the anteroposterior and lateral views. These 2D images are utilized to reconstruct a 3D model of the spine. Another significant benefit is the reduced radiation dose compared to traditional X-rays and other imaging methods. These benefits make EOS imaging an enticing alternative to other 3D imaging methods. However, since the 3D image is a reconstruction produced from X-rays, the 3D reconstruction does not provide information on soft tissues. Additionally, the 3D model requires manual reconstruction by a radiologist.[31]

EOS boasts high interobserver reproducibility and intraobserver repeatability in its applications for scoliosis and sagittal balance.[31] These involve measurements from the 2D X-rays as well as the 3D reconstruction of the spine. The reproducibility and repeatability of apical vertebral orientation measurements from the EOS 3D spine reconstruction and 3D CT scans showed no statistically significant difference.[31] However, it is essential to note that patient positioning can affect EOS measurements as the apparatus requires patients to be standing upright and facing a particular direction. The patient can be improperly positioned up to ± 10 degrees and still result in acceptable images.[31]

EOS has also been shown to be more accurate for vertebral osteoporosis than dual-energy X-ray absorptiometry. For axial spondyloarthritis, EOS was comparable to conventional radiography. However, the EOS imaging system was not an excellent alternative to MRI for analyzing disc degeneration and other soft tissues. As expected, MRI had greater image visibility and better detection of soft tissue pathology.[31]

X-ray and CT angiography are both typically utilized to garner bone information; however, each comes with its limitations. X-ray provides only 2D images, while CT risks a significant radiation dose. As an alternative, the EOS system provides a method to produce 3D models of the spine with low radiation exposure. As previously mentioned, the 3D image must be manually reconstructed. This requires the radiologist to manually mark the vertebral bodies' positions, which can take more than an hour, limiting the number of patients that can be imaged daily. This limitation can be overcome using convolution neural networks. By applying a convolution neural network to the acquired X-rays, the 3D reconstruction can be automated and performed much more quickly, allowing for more patients to be imaged each day.[32]

FUTURE OF ULTRASOUND IMAGING

Ultrasound imaging employs high-frequency sound waves to image internal organs. Ultrasound can be noninvasive by operating the transducer on the skin. In other cases, invasive ultrasound, such as endoscopic or transvaginal ultrasound, can be performed to obtain better images of the organs of interest. Compared to other imaging modalities, the risk posed to patients by ultrasound is low since it has no ionizing radiation. The few risks involve heating of tissue and cavitation. Due to this overall low risk, ultrasound is an attractive technology to aid in surgical and diagnostic applications for spinal diseases.

Anesthetic Application

Neuraxial anesthesia is widely applied as a means of pain control for surgical procedures as well as labor.[33-35] Neuraxial anesthesia is typically applied using palpation and surface landmarks as guidance for needle injection.[33-35] This tends to be a complicated procedure, especially in cases of obesity or prior spinal injury. Errors in injection anesthesia can lead to

complications, including permanent neurological damage.[33] Preoperative and intraoperative use of ultrasound can guide the injection, thus reducing these risks. Intraoperative use is even more challenging, requiring the anesthetist to handle the transducer and needle simultaneously.[34] Due to these barriers, the adoption of ultrasound-guided neuraxial anesthesia has been limited.[35]

One novel approach is to use software that automatically marks spinal landmarks as the ultrasound is being performed and then utilizes the marks to triangulate the site and trajectory of the injection.[17] This approach had an excellent first-attempt success rate for neuraxial anesthesia compared to the traditional palpation-based method.[33] Real-time ultrasound guidance can be of better advice as the anesthetist can directly observe the needle during injection. A preliminary study using a paramedian transverse approach with real-time ultrasound guidance found a high first-attempt success rate.[34] There is yet another approach to identify the injection site using machine learning automatically. A support vector machine model was built and trained to identify the injection site based on the classification of the bone/interspinous region.[35]

Intraoperative Ultrasound

Intraoperative ultrasound (IoUS) in spinal surgery has a long history dating back to 1951. However, ultrasound did not immediately become widely used for spinal procedures. It was not until the 1980s, where many applications of IoUS for spinal surgery were reported. In the present, IoUS for spinal surgery enjoys significant usage across many spinal pathologies.[36]

Pedicle screws for the lumbar spine's stability during fusion or other spinal procedures are generally considered a safe procedure. Still, there remains a risk of screws being malpositioned (with rates reported to be around 10%–15%), leading to potential neurovascular complications and the need for surgical revision.[37] A study analyzed the use of intraosseous ultrasound to determine accurate pedicle screw placement.[37] The ultrasound technique was compared to postoperative CT scanning. The correct interpretation of the ultrasound images by three investigators occurred in 99% of cases with no false negatives.[37] Additionally, one investigator had no prior experience in interpreting intraosseous ultrasound images, thus showing that this technique can be adopted with a low learning curve.[37]

IoUS can aid in visualization during spinal surgery, reducing complications and injuries, and improving success rates.[38,39] IoUS can be used to observe lumbar spinal surgery, blood vessels and other organs on the approach path and can confirm if they have been adequately displaced.[38] The study performed by Nojiri et al.[38] was able to visualize the organs for all the patients with no organ injury or massive bleeding. Overall, the research shows the utility of IoUS for real-time visualization of blood vessels and organs during surgery, which can help prevent serious injury.

In another case involving the surgery of intradural spinal tumors, IoUS was used to visualize the tumors. IoUS helped determine if laminectomy was sufficient, needed extension, and learning the best myelotomy to be performed. Lastly, IoUS was then used to determine if the total excision of the tumor was achieved. In 7 patients out of 69, laminectomies needed to be extended, and in only 1 case, subtotal excision was observed and needed additional resection.[39] Thus, IoUS can be of great use to determine the extent of excision and incisions required. Furthermore, it can be used to ascertain the success of the surgery and, in cases of incomplete success, lead to an immediate remedy.

Diagnostic Application

The use of ultrasound for diagnostic purposes cannot be understated. Frequent diagnostic imaging can expose patients and physicians to harmful radiation from X-ray. Ultrasound is an imaging modality without ionizing radiation and would thus eliminate this risk if it could be adequately substituted for select diagnostic procedures. Additionally, ultrasound is more accessible to populations in remote or low socioeconomic regions.

Scoliosis evaluation involves the measurement of the Cobb angle obtained from radiographs. This diagnostic evaluation is considered the gold standard but comes with the risks of high exposure to radiation.[40,41] Several other imaging modalities have been proposed to reduce radiation exposure, but these methods do not eliminate exposure or provide the same level of visualization.[40,41]

Three-dimensional ultrasound provides an avenue to remove ionizing radiation with excellent visualization altogether. One such ultrasound system developed for scoliosis assessment, Scolioscan, was studied for its reliability and validity for identifying adolescent idiopathic scoliosis.[40] A similar study also analyzed Scolioscan for the best ultrasound angle between the use of the spinous processes and the transverse processes as landmarks for consistent and accurate measurement curve severity.[41] In both studies, Scolioscan was compared to the traditional Cobb angle measurement using radiographs. Both studies observed high reliability as well as an excellent correlation of the ultrasound angles with

the Cobb angles.[40,41] The latter study also found no significant difference in the reliability of validity between the ultrasound angles.[41] Ultimately, this demonstrates the use of ultrasound as a diagnostic modality that can reduce patient exposure to radiation.

The diagnostic use of ultrasound can also aid in treatment procedures. The magnetically controlled growing rod (MCGR) system was developed to treat early-onset scoliosis, compared to a traditional growing rod system where the rod needs to be lengthened periodically via invasive surgery. Alternatively, MCGR requires no surgery and rod lengthening can be performed more frequently.[42] However, this also results in increased amounts of radiation as the spine would need to be imaged by radiography before and after lengthening.[42] To combat this limitation, ultrasound has been employed to assist in rod lengthening with the use of plain radiographs. A prospective study imaged patients using ultrasound to find and lengthen the rods.[42] The new procedure was found to be comfortable and practical to implement. Due to the limitations of ultrasound imaging itself, neither the assessment of complications in the implants themselves nor the assessment of fusion blocks at the proximal and distal fixation points is possible.[42] Hence, periodic radiographs are still required. However, with this method, the number of radiographs can be reduced while allowing frequent lengthening, thereby reducing the risk of complications from radiation, in particular in the young where radiation-induced bone and soft tissue sarcomas may occur.[42]

Decreasing radiation exposure

Radiation is known as the emission of energy and can be either electromagnetic or particulate. Electromagnetic radiation utilizes photons that consist of energy, but without mass or charge. Conversely, particulate radiation contains particles that have mass and energy, but not necessarily an electric charge. Concerns regarding radiation have been well documented and noted previously above. Unfortunately, surgeons and surgical staff must endure the potential for radiation exposure during minimally invasive spine surgeries due to the heightened necessity for intraoperative imaging in these procedures. As concerns over physician and patient radiation exposure increase (due to a rise in minimally invasive spine surgeries requiring such techniques[43]), the importance of decreasing radiation has been prioritized. This goal has been deemed feasible in particular spine-related surgical procedures, resulting in reduced radiation exposure to patients and no adverse postoperative effects.[44] As the focus toward successful surgeries with reduced radiation becomes increasingly prevalent, numerous methods emerge to assist in making it a reality, including ultra-low-radiation imaging (ULRI) with image enhancement. ULRI is a technique that is just as it sounds, an imaging source that emits radiation but in minimal doses. Image enhancement refers to the process of altering digital images to make results sufficient for proper analysis. ULRI coordinated with image enhancement allows for substantial radiation reduction in minimally invasive procedures while maintaining adequate visualization during surgery and remaining in accordance with procedure safety.[45] Image enhancement software, such as NuVasive's *LessRay*, allows surgeons to scale down their dependence on radiation-inducing imaging during procedures. The concept of image enhancement software utilizes full-dose preoperative fluoroscopic images as a reference to form a conglomerated image of the necessary spinal levels, ultimately reducing radiation emissions by approximately 75%.[46] Parallel to ULRI with image enhancement, computer-assisted image-guided spinal navigation (such as ICT) also paves the way for diminished radiation exposure to surgeons. An ICT scanner allows surgeons to utilize the benefits of CT scans during procedures, enabling surgeons to sync preexisting scans with current ones. Ultimately, this supports surgeons in efficiently executing critical decisions in the operating room. The use of ICT in alliance with spinal navigation yields results similar to using traditional fluoroscopy with the supplemental contribution of reduced radiation.[47] Additionally, the utilization of ICT reduces radiation exposure in patients. This is in addition to the benefits of enhanced patient safety from the reduced rate of screw positioning.[11]

Alongside ICT and ULRI with enhanced imaging, the use of pulsed fluoroscopy (PF) paired with detachable pedicle marker and probe (DPMP) has emerged as a technique to decrease radiation. Pulsed fluoroscopy is identified as a tool utilizing a combination of pulse frequency and dose to reduce radiation exposure to patients while simultaneously enhancing image quality. Pulsed fluoroscopy and DPMP have allowed for decreased radiation exposure to both the surgical team and patients, all while maintaining accuracy during the procedure.[3] The reduced radiation approach should be the new standard in the future of spine imaging upon the enlightenment of the proficiency and feasibility of reduced radiation in minimally invasive surgeries.

ASSESSING INTERVERTEBRAL DISC METABOLISM AND TRANSPORT FOR PRECISION SPINE CARE

The intervertebral disc is the largest avascular structure in the human body, requiring disc cells to be uniquely suited to survival in a harsh environment, including a low nutrient supply of glucose and oxygen and high metabolite concentration of lactic acid, leading to low pH.[48] Despite the suitability of IVD cells for this environment, changes in disc structure and subsequent small changes in nutrient supply can threaten the survival of endogenous IVD cells as well as transplanted cells. As the cells die, due to a mixture of nutrient limitations, biomechanical problems, and signaling cascades, the ability of the disc to remodel its extracellular matrix (ECM) declines and the disc degenerates. All discs undergo some structural changes with age, including reorganization of ECM components and calcification of the disc endplate, an important part of the disc nutrient supply.[48] Capillaries are lost, and contact with the marrow cavities decreases.[48] Additionally, the ECM changes in the annulus fibrosus (AF) and nucleus pulposus (NP) also cause decreased diffusion in those regions.[49-51] Mature disc cells use glucose and produce lactic acid.[52] Although they do not require much oxygen to live,[53] cell activity and ECM synthesis are reduced at low concentrations.

Fundamental studies of the disc often focus on regenerative medicine. Disc regeneration strategies focus on targeting molecular pathways of ECM degeneration. This could theoretically be accomplished by supplementing anabolic factors (usually by adding cells), increasing production of anabolic factors (by growth factors), or decreasing production of catabolic factors (through growth factor or cytokine therapy). One major challenge to these approaches is their reliance on increasing cell activity or density in a nutrient-starved environment. In order to make these regenerative treatments successful, there will likely need to be an imaging approach to determine the nutrient capacity for each disc being considered for a biological therapy.

There are several imaging methods that are being used to study disc metabolism and transport phenomena. Magnetic resonance imaging can be used to study water diffusion in the disc in vivo using diffusion-weighted imaging (DWI) and apparent diffusion coefficient (ADC) mapping.[54] In a study of 100 patients' MRIs, ADC maps of NPs in 435 discs showed diffusion coefficients varied by up to 75% among discs with the same Pfirrmann grade.[49] Recently, DTI studies have investigated diffusion in the disc and detected pathological changes at early stages of cartilage degeneration.[55-58] There have been a few excellent studies that have answered disc transport phenomena-related questions using medical imaging of small-molecule surrogates in the disc.[59,60]

Ratio of R1p dispersion and -OH chemical exchange saturation transfer (RROC) imaging is sensitive to pH changes in ex vivo porcine discs without being confounded by variation in GAG concentration.[61] Endogenous glucose changes are apparent on T1ρ-weighted dynamic glucose-enhanced (DGE) MRI.[62] Glucose changes could also theoretically be determined using [^{18}F]2-fluoro-2-deoxy-D-glucose (^{18}F-FGD) positron emission tomography.[63,64] Finally, magnetic resonance spectroscopy has been demonstrated to quantify metabolites, specifically lactate and proteoglycans, and has been applied to aid surgeons in identifying painful discs for surgical intervention.[9]

APPLICATIONS OF ARTIFICIAL INTELLIGENCE

Artificial intelligence (AI) is an overarching field that contains subjects, such as machine learning (ML) and deep learning (DL). Machine learning is a statistical method that absorbs data and their results to train a computer algorithm, which may later perform predictions on unseen data, while deep learning has a layered structure that creates an artificial neural network. This artificial neural network has autonomy, which allows it to learn the complexity further, performing intelligent decisions on its own. The applications of AI in spinal imaging are continuously studied and endlessly evolving although the full extent of their applications has yet to be applied. It is well known that the potential of AI may allow for enhancements to existing techniques and modalities of spine care. Machine learning and deep learning, in conjunction with current technologies, augment traditional approaches further to enhance the scope of a clinician's accuracy, further optimizing pre-, post-, and perioperative treatment. The applications of AI present itself through 3D construction of the spine, enhanced image resolution, improvements to perioperative navigation techniques, and postoperative patient satisfaction outcome predictions.

Three-Dimensional Construction of the Spine

Analyzing MRI and CT images, machine learning identifies spinal markers, creating augmented simulations as well as printable structures, which exhibit an enhanced view of the patient's spine. Three-dimensional rendering of anatomical structures through image stitching software communicates in conjunction with artificial intelligence to outline necessary anatomy. This novel pairing improves upon stand-alone imaging, sharing insight into both visual and physical aspects of the spine. In a study concerning 3D printing in orthopedic case preparation, it was found that the use of the generated anatomical models significantly

increased surgical precision while decreasing intraoperative bleeding, surgical time, and, consequently, the amount of anesthesia required.[65] Further, machine learning may serve in concert with augmented reality for minimally invasive surgical navigation systems through 3D modeling in augmented space. In preparation for pedicle screw instrumentation, the augmented reality surgical navigation (ARSN) was anointed as a replacement to the fluoroscopy-guided minimally invasive method. Although it was found that both offered similar navigation efficiency, the ARSN system did not involve radiation. This potential presents surgeons with the opportunity to perform spine-related operations in a protective lead garment-free environment.[62]

Deep Learning for Lesion Detection and Classification

Deep learning is a subset within machine learning that is designed to automatically and adaptively learn the priority features from data through the backward calculation of weights in a layered structure; this process is known as backpropagation. The method commences with the final layer, traversing in reverse until the initial layer. This approach enhances decision making, filtering, and classifying data into cohorts that would allow the algorithm to make intelligent decisions with improved accuracy compared to the manual feature engineering that ML requires. Computer vision algorithms are DL algorithms, which are applied through a convolutional neural network (CNN) to classify images. The CNN does so using the layered DL structure to differentiate characteristics that would distinguish it from other models. It is believed that CNN algorithms may offer enhancements to traditional diagnostic methods of oncological spinal tumors on MRI. In the case where spinal schwannoma and meningioma were identified on T1- and T2-weighted MRI, diagnosis by both radiologists and the CNN was found to have performed at levels comparable to that of experienced radiologists.[66] Consequently, this has opened avenues to further applications within the scope of spinal oncology for optimized assistance in diagnosis and identification of complex anatomical structures, an issue that ML algorithms often failed to address. Further, the CNN algorithm may be implemented to identify relevant spinal anatomy and degenerative conditions.

The *Spine Explorer* is a deep learning-based software that automates spinal mapping of vertebral bodies and their intervertebral discs for quantification and analysis of the relative cervical, thoracic, and lumbosacral anatomy. The *Spine Explorer* was designed to identify degenerative spine conditions for improved speed and precision of data collection.[67] In turn, this standardizes methods that may enhance the quality of research concerning degenerative spinal condition while offering additions to the clinician's armamentarium of diagnostic tools. Much like the case where spinal tumors were differentiated, neural networks may also possess the ability to grade spinal stenosis in patients suffering from pain, numbness, or weakness in the arms or legs.[68] This is possible through the layered structure of the CNN, which maps the spinal canal and cord. Inevitably, deep learning and convoluted neural networks serve to augment the clinician's intuition and the precision of their diagnosis for optimal patient satisfaction outcomes.

CONCLUSIONS

Improved image quality, decreased radiation exposure, faster imaging and analysis, improved reliability, and intraoperative use have been guiding factors in the evolution of spinal imaging. Less reliance on plain radiographs while exploring new technologies, such as ML reconstructions or using standard tools in novel ways, such as intraoperative ultrasound, has decreased radiation risk while improving surgical techniques. Intraoperative CT provides surgeons with great guidance in real time to assist in navigating challenging anatomy. Magnetic resonance imaging has long been an expensive and time-consuming imaging technology. New MRI techniques being developed improve both image acquisition time and diagnostic information that can be obtained. Novel imaging can further assess metabolism and transport of materials into and out of the disc, allowing for refined patient selection/stratification that can also inform dose and approach for regenerative biologics of the disc as well as facilitate precision spine care. Machine learning is at the forefront of impressive automatic classification, reconstruction, and analysis of spinal features. The quick automatic analysis provided by machine learning can intraoperatively assist navigation during surgery. These developments in spinal imaging are reducing intra- and postoperative complications for both patients and physicians, leading to overall superior satisfaction and outcomes, as well as identifying the source of the pain for operative planning, managing patient expectations, and improved patient outcomes. The utility between advances in imaging coupled with the unraveling and implications of AI and ML approaches toward imaging and predictive modeling will continue to expand in the years to come and usher in a new age of precision spine care.

REFERENCES

1. Abdel MP, Bodemer WS, Anderson PA. Supine thoracolumbar sagittal spine alignment: comparing computerized tomography and plain radiographs. *Spine.* 2012;37:340–345.
2. Berquist TH. Imaging of the postoperative spine. *Radiol Clin N Am.* 2006;44:407–418. https://doi.org/10.1016/j.rcl.2006.01.002.
3. Marco RAW, Curry MC, Mujezinovic F, Linton J. Decreased radiation exposure using pulsed fluoroscopy and a detachable pedicle marker and probe to place pedicle screws: a comparison to current fluoroscopy techniques and CT navigation. *Spine Deform.* 2020;8:405–411. https://doi.org/10.1007/s43390-020-00086-5.
4. Lee B-S, Jo B-K, Bin S-I, Kim J-M, Lee C-R, Kwon Y-H. Hinge fractures are underestimated on plain radiographs after open wedge proximal tibial osteotomy: evaluation by computed tomography. *Am J Sports Med.* 2019;47:1370–1375.
5. Gale SC, Gracias VH, Reilly PM, Schwab CW. The inefficiency of plain radiography to evaluate the cervical spine after blunt trauma. *J Trauma.* 2005;59:1121–1125.
6. Hess EP, Haas LR, Shah ND, Stroebel RJ, Denham CR, Swensen SJ. Trends in computed tomography utilization rates: a longitudinal practice-based study. *J Patient Saf.* 2014;10:52–58.
7. Dietrich TJ, Peterson CK, Zeimpekis KG, Bensler S, Sutter R, Pfirrmann CWA. Fluoroscopy-guided versus CT-guided lumbar steroid injections: comparison of radiation exposure and outcomes. *Radiology.* 2019;290:752–759.
8. Wen B-T, Chen Z-Q, Sun C-G, et al. Three-dimensional navigation (O-arm) versus fluoroscopy in the treatment of thoracic spinal stenosis with ultrasonic bone curette: a retrospective comparative study. *Medicine.* 2019;98:e15647.
9. Yu JYH, Fridley J, Gokaslan Z, Telfeian A, Oyelese AA. Minimally invasive thoracolumbar corpectomy and stabilization for unstable burst fractures using intraoperative computed tomography and computer-assisted spinal navigation. *World Neurosurg.* 2019;122:e1266–e1274.
10. Scheufler K-M, Cyron D, Dohmen H, Eckardt A. Less invasive surgical correction of adult degenerative scoliosis, part I: technique and radiographic results. *Neurosurgery.* 2010;67:696–710.
11. Scarone P, Vincenzo G, Distefano D, et al. Use of the airo mobile intraoperative CT system versus the O-arm for transpedicular screw fixation in the thoracic and lumbar spine: a retrospective cohort study of 263 patients. *J Neurosurg Spine.* 2018;29:397–406.
12. Carl B, Bopp M, Pojskic M, Voellger B, Nimsky C. Standard navigation versus intraoperative computed tomography navigation in upper cervical spine trauma. *Int J Comput Assist Radiol Surg.* 2019;14:169–182.
13. Scullen T, Riffle J, Koga S, Kalyvas J. Novel technique of coregistered intraoperative computed tomography and preoperative magnetic resonance imaging and diffusion tensor imaging navigation in spinal cord tumor resection. *Ochsner J.* 2019;19:43–48.

14. Hille G, Saalfeld S, Serowy S, Tönnies K. Multi-segmental spine image registration supporting image-guided interventions of spinal metastases. *Comput Biol Med.* 2018;102:16–20.

15. Nam KH, Seo I, Kim DH, Lee JI, Choi BK, Han IH. Machine learning model to predict osteoporotic spine with hounsfield units on lumbar computed tomography. *J Korean Neurosurg Soc.* 2019;62:442–449.

16. Muehlematter UJ, Mannil M, Becker AS, et al. Vertebral body insufficiency fractures: detection of vertebrae at risk on standard CT images using texture analysis and machine learning. *Eur Radiol.* 2019;29:2207–2217.

17. Burns JE, Yao J, Summers RM. Vertebral body compression fractures and bone density: automated detection and classification on CT images. *Radiology.* 2017;284:788–797.

18. Madelin G, Lee J-S, Regatte RR, Jerschow A. Sodium MRI: methods and applications. *Prog Nucl Magn Reson Spectrosc.* 2014;79:14–47.

19. Bae WC, Chen PC, Chung CB, Masuda K, D'Lima D, Du J. Quantitative ultrashort echo time (UTE) MRI of human cortical bone: correlation with porosity and biomechanical properties. *J Bone Miner Res.* 2012;27:848–857.

20. O'Connell MJ, Hargaden G, Powell T, Eustace SJ. Whole-body turbo short tau inversion recovery MR imaging using a moving tabletop. *AJR Am J Roentgenol.* 2002;179:866–868.

21. Regatte RR, Akella SVS, Borthakur A, Kneeland JB, Reddy R. In vivo proton MR three-dimensional T1ρ mapping of human articular cartilage: initial experience. *Radiology.* 2003;229:269–274.

22. Kim M, Chan Q, Anthony M-P, Cheung KMC, Samartzis D, Khong P-L. Assessment of glycosaminoglycan distribution in human lumbar intervertebral discs using chemical exchange saturation transfer at 3 T: feasibility and initial experience. *NMR Biomed.* 2011;24:1137–1144. https://doi.org/10.1002/nbm.1671.

23. Cui Y-Z, Yang X-H, Liu P-F, Wang B, Chen W-J. Preliminary study on diagnosis of lumbar disc degeneration with magnetic resonance T1ρ, T2 mapping and DWI quantitative detection technologies. *Eur Rev Med Pharmacol Sci.* 2016;20:3344–3350.

24. Chokan K, Murakami H, Endo H, et al. Evaluation of water retention in lumbar intervertebral disks before and after exercise stress with T2 mapping. *Spine.* 2016;41:E430–E436.

25. Trattnig S, Stelzeneder D, Goed S, et al. Lumbar intervertebral disc abnormalities: comparison of quantitative T2 mapping with conventional MR at 3.0 T. *Eur Radiol.* 2010;20:2715–2722.

26. Li X, Majumdar S. Quantitative MRI of articular cartilage and its clinical applications. *J Magn Reson Imaging.* 2013;38:991–1008.

27. Pang H, Bow C, Cheung JPY, et al. The UTE disc sign on MRI: a novel imaging biomarker associated with degenerative spine changes, low back pain, and disability. *Spine.* 2018;43:503–511.

28. Vargas MI, Drake-Pérez M, Delattre BMA, Boto J, Lovblad K-O, Boudabous S. Feasibility of a synthetic MR imaging sequence for spine imaging. *AJNR Am J Neuroradiol.* 2018;39:1756–1763.

29. Tsagkas C, Horvath A, Altermatt A, et al. Automatic spinal cord gray matter quantification: a novel approach. *AJNR Am J Neuroradiol.* 2019;40:1592–1600.

30. Zhou Y, Liu Y, Chen Q, Gu G, Sui X. Automatic lumbar MRI detection and identification based on deep learning. *J Digit Imaging.* 2019;32:513–520.

31. Melhem E, Assi A, El Rachkidi R, Ghanem I. EOS® biplanar X-ray imaging: concept, developments, benefits, and limitations. *J Child Orthop.* 2016;10:1–14.

32. Chen C-C, Fang Y-H. Using bi-planar X-ray images to reconstruct the spine structure by the convolution neural network. In: *Future Trends in Biomedical and Health Informatics and Cybersecurity in Medical Devices.* Springer International Publishing; 2020:80–85.

33. Oh TT, Ikhsan M, Tan KK, et al. A novel approach to neuraxial anesthesia: application of an automated ultrasound spinal landmark identification. *BMC Anesthesiol.* 2019;19:57.

34. Liu Y, Qian W, Ke X-J, Mei W. Real-time ultrasound-guided spinal anesthesia using a new paramedian transverse approach. *Curr Med Sci.* 2018;38:910–913.

35. Yu S, Tan KK, Sng BL, Li S, Sia ATH. Lumbar ultrasound image feature extraction and classification with support vector machine. *Ultrasound Med Biol.* 2015;41:2677–2689.

36. Ganau M, Syrmos N, Martin AR, Jiang F, Fehlings MG. Intraoperative ultrasound in spine surgery: history, current applications, future developments. *Quant Imaging Med Surg.* 2018;8:261–267.

37. Kantelhardt SR, Bock CH, Larsen J, et al. Intraosseous ultrasound in the placement of pedicle screws in the lumbar spine. *Spine.* 2009;34:400–407.

38. Nojiri H, Miyagawa K, Yamaguchi H, et al. Intraoperative ultrasound visualization of paravertebral anatomy in the retroperitoneal space during lateral lumbar spine surgery. *J Neurosurg Spine.* 2019;31:334–337.

39. Haciyakupoglu E, Yuvruk E, Onen MR, Naderi S. The use of intraoperative ultrasonography in intradural spinal tumor surgery. *Turk Neurosurg.* 2019;29:237–241.

40. Zheng Y-P, Lee TT-Y, Lai KK-L, et al. A reliability and validity study for scolioscan: a radiation-free scoliosis assessment system using 3D ultrasound imaging. *Scoliosis Spinal Disord.* 2016;11:13.

41. Brink RC, Wijdicks SPJ, Tromp IN, et al. A reliability and validity study for different coronal angles using ultrasound imaging in adolescent idiopathic scoliosis. *Spine J.* 2018;18:979–985.

42. Stokes OM, O'Donovan EJ, Samartzis D, Bow CH, Luk KDK, Cheung KMC. Reducing radiation exposure in early-onset scoliosis surgery patients: novel use of ultrasonography to measure lengthening in magnetically-controlled growing rods. *Spine J.* 2014;14:2397–2404.

43. Yu E, Khan SN. Does less invasive spine surgery result in increased radiation exposure? A systematic review. *Clin Orthop Relat Res.* 2014;472:1738–1748.

44. Chin KR, Pencle FJR, Quijada KA, Mustafa MS, Mustafa LS, Seale JA. Decreasing radiation dose with fluoro-LESS standalone anterior cervical fusion. *J Spine Surg.* 2018;4:696–701.

45. Godzik J, Nayar G, Hunter WD, Tumialán LM. Decreasing radiation emission in minimally invasive spine surgery using ultra-low-radiation imaging with image enhancement: a prospective cohort study. *World Neurosurg.* 2019;122:e805–e811.

46. Wang TY, Harrison Farber S, Perkins SS, et al. Internally randomized control trial of radiation exposure using ultra-low radiation imaging versus traditional C-arm fluoroscopy for patients undergoing single-level minimally invasive transforaminal lumbar interbody fusion. *Spine.* 2017;42:217–223. https://doi.org/10.1097/brs.0000000000001720.

47. Huang Y-C, Urban JPG, Luk KDK. Intervertebral disc regeneration: do nutrients lead the way? *Nat Rev Rheumatol.* 2014;10:561–566.

48. Belykh E, Kalinin AA, Patel AA, et al. Apparent diffusion coefficient maps in the assessment of surgical patients with lumbar spine degeneration. *PLoS One.* 2017;12, e0183697.

49. Byvaltsev VA, Kolesnikov SI, Bardonova LA, et al. Assessment of lactate production and proteoglycans synthesis by the intact and degenerated intervertebral disc cells under the influence of activated macrophages: an in vitro study. *Bull Exp Biol Med.* 2018;166:170–173. https://doi.org/10.1007/s10517-018-4307-3.

50. Byvaltsev VA, Kolesnikov SI, Belykh EG, et al. Complex analysis of diffusion transport and microstructure of an intervertebral disk. *Bull Exp Biol Med.* 2017;164:223–228. https://doi.org/10.1007/s10517-017-3963-z.

51. Bibby SRS, Jones DA, Ripley RM, Urban JPG. Metabolism of the intervertebral disc: effects of low levels of oxygen, glucose, and pH on rates of energy metabolism of bovine nucleus pulposus cells. *Spine.* 2005;30:487–496.

52. Ishihara H, Urban JPG. Effects of low oxygen concentrations and metabolic inhibitors on proteoglycan and protein synthesis rates in the intervertebral disc. *J Orthop Res.* 1999;17:829–835. https://doi.org/10.1002/jor.1100170607.

53. Haughton V. Imaging intervertebral disc degeneration. *J Bone Joint Surg Am.* 2006;88:15. https://doi.org/10.2106/jbjs.f.00010.

54. Eguchi Y, Oikawa Y, Suzuki M, et al. Diffusion tensor imaging of radiculopathy in patients with lumbar disc herniation: preliminary results. *Bone Joint J.* 2016;98-B:387–394.

55. Raya JG. Techniques and applications of in vivo diffusion imaging of articular cartilage. *J Magn Reson Imaging.* 2015;41:1487–1504. https://doi.org/10.1002/jmri.24767.

56. Raya JG, Horng A, Dietrich O, et al. Articular cartilage: in vivo diffusion-tensor imaging. *Radiology.* 2012;262:550–559. https://doi.org/10.1148/radiol.11110821.

57. Novakofski KD, Pownder SL, Koff MF, Williams RM, Potter HG, Fortier LA. High-resolution methods for diagnosing cartilage damage in vivo. *Cartilage.* 2016;7:39–51. https://doi.org/10.1177/1947603515602307.

58. Gullbrand SE, Peterson J, Ahlborn J, et al. ISSLS prize winner: dynamic loading-induced convective transport enhances intervertebral disc nutrition. *Spine.* 2015;40:1158–1164.

59. Urban JPG, Holm S, Maroudas A, Nachemson A. Nutrition of the intervertebral disc. *Clin Orthop Relat Res.* 1982;296–302. https://doi.org/10.1097/00003086-198210000-00039.

60. Liu Q, Tawackoli W, Pelled G, et al. Detection of low back pain using pH level-dependent imaging of the intervertebral disc using the ratio of R1ρdispersion and −OH chemical exchange saturation transfer (RROC). *Magn Reson Med.* 2015;73:1196–1205. https://doi.org/10.1002/mrm.25186.

61. Paech D, Schuenke P, Koehler C, et al. T1ρ-weighted dynamic glucose-enhanced MR imaging in the human brain. *Radiology.* 2017;285:914–922. https://doi.org/10.1148/radiol.2017162351.

62. Peh S, Chatterjea A, Pfarr J, et al. Accuracy of augmented reality surgical navigation for minimally invasive pedicle screw insertion in the thoracic and lumbar spine with a new tracking device. *Spine J.* 2020;20:629–637. https://doi.org/10.1016/j.spinee.2019.12.009.

63. Longo DL, Bartoli A, Consolino L, et al. In vivo imaging of tumor metabolism and acidosis by combining PET and MRI-CEST pH imaging. *Cancer Res.* 2016;76:6463–6470. https://doi.org/10.1158/0008-5472.can-16-0825.

64. Keshari KR, Lotz JC, Link TM, Hu S, Majumdar S, Kurhanewicz J. Lactic acid and proteoglycans as metabolic markers for discogenic back pain. *Spine.* 2008;33:312–317. https://doi.org/10.1097/brs.0b013e31816201c3.

65. Galvez M, Asahi T, Baar A, et al. Use of three-dimensional printing in orthopaedic surgical planning. *JAAOS Glob Res Rev.* 2018;2:e071. https://doi.org/10.5435/jaaosglobal-d-17-00071.

66. Maki S, Furuya T, Horikoshi T, et al. A deep convolutional neural network with performance comparable to radiologists for differentiating between spinal schwannoma and meningioma. *Spine.* 2020;45:694–700.

67. Huang J, Shen H, Wu J, et al. Spine explorer: a deep learning based fully automated program for efficient and reliable quantifications of the vertebrae and discs on sagittal lumbar spine MR images. *Spine J.* 2020;20:590–599. https://doi.org/10.1016/j.spinee.2019.11.010.

68. Won D, Lee H-J, Lee S-J, Park SH. Spinal stenosis grading in magnetic resonance imaging using deep convolutional neural networks. *Spine.* 2020;45:804–812.

Index

Note: Page numbers followed by *f* indicate figures and *t* indicate tables.

CPI Antony Rowe
Eastbourne, UK
March 25, 2021